Experts' Perspectives on Medical Advances

This book series presents Chinese experts' perspectives on recent developments in clinical medicine. Written by leading Chinese experts in related fields, a wide variety of emerging and hot topics in internal medicine, surgery, oncology, neurosurgery, and ophthalmonology, etc., is covered by the series. Each title in this series covers a disease or a group of diseases, focusing on the basic knowledge, development and the latest research progress of clinical practice. This series is a practical and useful resource for researchers and practitioners in related subjects, as well as for general interest readers.

Jiangning Wang • Lei Gao
Editors

Refractory Wounds

Typical Cases and Analysis

Springer
科学技术文献出版社
SCIENTIFIC AND TECHNICAL DOCUMENTATION PRESS

Editors
Jiangning Wang
Department of Orthopedics
Beijing Shijitan Hospital
Capital Medical University
Beijing, China

Lei Gao
Department of Orthopedics
Beijing Shijitan Hospital
Capital Medical University
Beijing, China

ISSN 2948-1023 ISSN 2948-1031 (electronic)
Experts' Perspectives on Medical Advances
ISBN 978-981-96-2066-1 ISBN 978-981-96-2067-8 (eBook)
https://doi.org/10.1007/978-981-96-2067-8

The original submitted manuscript has been translated into English. The translation was done using artificial intelligence. A subsequent revision was performed by the author(s) to further refine the work and to ensure that the translation is appropriate concerning content and scientific correctness. It may, however, read stylistically different from a conventional translation.

Jointly published with Scientific and Technical Documentation Press

The print edition is not for sale in China (Mainland). Customers from China (Mainland) please order the print book from: Scientific and Technical Documentation Press.

This Springer imprint is published by the registered company Springer Nature Singapore Pte Ltd.
The registered company address is: 152 Beach Road, #21-01/04 Gateway East, Singapore 189721, Singapore

Preface

Characteristic Projects

The renowned expert team for comprehensive diagnosis and treatment of diabetic foot led by Professor Jiangning Wang was approved by the Beijing Municipal Hospital Administration Bureau on April 2, 2018, as the fourth batch of renowned expert teams in municipal hospitals (Beijing Medical Management Medical Care [2018] No. 10). Our team has created a comprehensive treatment model of multiple disciplinary team (MDT) collaboration centered on wound healing, which avoids the situation of traditional departments acting independently and fighting alone. We adopt a "joint operation" approach, conduct comprehensive examinations and meticulous diagnoses of patients, and formulate diagnostic and treatment plans suitable for specific conditions.

My team consists of orthopedic experts, orthopedic specialists, vascular surgery experts, plastic surgery specialists, diabetic foot experts, nutrition experts, blood purification experts, critical care medicine experts, pain management experts, prosthetic engineers, wound care therapists, and professional nurses, among others. We are a departmental team, not a hospital team. Our team primarily focuses on surgical comprehensive treatment, with internal medicine physicians assisting in management, nutritionists participating in dietary adjustments, rehabilitation technicians guiding functional exercises, foot disease shoe manufacturers producing functional supports, and foot disease therapists providing daily care. Currently, the MDT model within our department is recognized as the most ideal comprehensive treatment model for chronic diabetic foot wounds under existing medical conditions in China.

The MDT model of diagnosis and treatment within the department includes: ① Whole-body basic treatment (control of basic diseases, treatment of systemic complications, application of antibiotics, etc.); ② Critical illness management (respiratory and circulatory support, blood purification technology, etc.); ③ Reasonable diet, low-carb diet to control blood sugar; ④ Surgical comprehensive treatment (bone transplantation, pressure perfusion, vascular surgery intervention techniques, debridement, skin grafting and flap techniques, removal of dead bone, lumbar sympathetic ganglion block for pain treatment, application of negative pressure technology, etc.); ⑤ Other treatment methods (biological agents, micro-oxygen, ozone, etc.); ⑥ Lower limb load reduction and limb rehabilitation (supports, diabetic foot shoes, load-reducing insoles, limb exercise rehabilitation, appropriate traditional Chinese medicine massage to prevent joint flexion deformities, etc.); ⑦ Scientific and appropriate exercise; and ⑧ Traditional Chinese medicine.

Chronic non-healing wounds, commonly known as ulcers, are also referred to as chronic wounds. The International Wound Healing Society defines them as "wounds that cannot achieve anatomical and functional completeness through a normal, orderly, and timely repair process." Clinically, it often refers to wounds that have not healed or shown a tendency to heal after more than a month of treatment for various reasons. However, this one-month period is not absolute and depends on various factors such as wound size, cause, and individual general health status. Typically, if a wound cannot shrink by 10–15% per week or cannot shrink by 50% after a month, it is considered a chronic non-healing wound.

This book presents the main measures and experiences of my team in the clinical treatment of chronic non-healing wounds, summarizing and analyzing the problems encountered in the treatment of wounds such as diabetic foot ulcers, lower limb ischemic disease wounds, neuropathic wounds, pressure injury wounds, and tumor wounds through case analysis. It comprehensively introduces surgical techniques such as routine debridement, incision and drainage, dressing changes (dressing application), maggot bio-debridement therapy, skin grafting and flap techniques, negative pressure technology, skin stretching closure device technology, lower limb bone transfer technology, extracorporeal circulation pressurized perfusion technology, interventional treatment, three-dimensional reconstruction orthotic and footwear technology, comprehensive nutritional management and critical care management for diabetic patients (respiratory and circulatory support, blood purification technology), etc.

This book is a practical teaching book and also a guide that provides standards and guidance for wound treatment. It is hoped that readers engaged in the wound repair industry can expand their thinking on the treatment of non-healing wounds through reading this book, further enhance their wound repair diagnosis and treatment capabilities, and also hope that this book can improve the standardization level of this specialty.

Beijing, China — Jiangning Wang
Beijing, China — Lei Gao

Contents

About the Editors

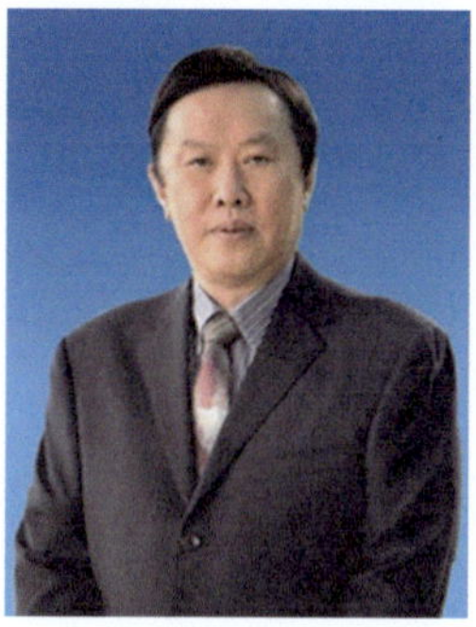

Jiangning Wang the leader of the orthopedic department at Beijing Shijitan Hospital affiliated with Capital Medical University, is a Chief Physician, Professor, and Doctoral Supervisor. He is an internationally renowned orthopedic expert and recipient of a special government allowance from the State Council. He is the Vice Chairman of the Association of International Medical Salvage of the Extremity, the Chairman of the Organ Infection and Injury Prevention Professional Committee of the Chinese Preventive Medicine Association, and the Chairman of the Beijing International Wound and Diabetic Foot Forum. He is an expert in the evaluation of the Ministry of Education's Science and Technology Progress Award and a peer reviewer for the National Natural Science Foundation. As the first author, he has published more than 30 papers in SCI-indexed journals. He has won one Science and Technology Progress Award from the Ministry of Education, three provincial and ministerial Science and Technology Progress Awards, two national invention patents, one US invention patent, and one Indian invention patent. He has undertaken three projects of the National Natural Science Foundation.

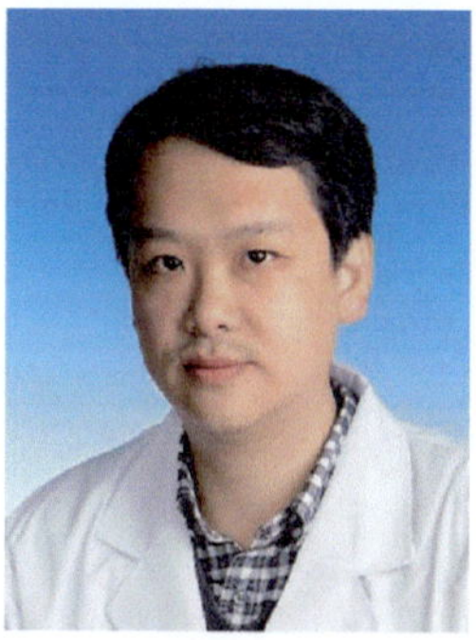

Lei Gao Deputy Chief Physician of the Orthopedic Department at Beijing Shijitan Hospital affiliated with Capital Medical University, is a member of the renowned team of diabetic foot experts. He mainly engages in reconstructive microsurgery and orthopedic work. He holds a doctorate from Capital Medical University and has studied at the Trauma Orthopedics Center of Ulm University in Germany. He was a visiting scholar at the Diabetic Foot Center of the General Hospital

Bad Cannstatt in Stuttgart, Germany, and he conducted research at the Schako Foot Research Center of the Mathias-Spital Hospital in Rheine, Germany. He has published many papers in SCI-indexed journals and domestic core journals. He is the second person in charge of two National Natural Science Foundation projects and three Capital Medical projects.

1 Application of Decellularized Allogeneic Dermis in the Repair of Diabetic Foot Wounds: Three Cases

Lei Gao and Jiangning Wang

1.1 Case Summary

1.1.1 Case 1

Patient, male, 49 years old. Admitted to the hospital due to redness, swelling, rupture, and pain in the right foot for 4 days.

[Present Illness History] The patient accidentally knocked his right foot 4 days ago. Without special treatment, the wound gradually increased in size. The patient experienced an increase in foot swelling and pain, and was treated at a top-tier hospital in Beijing on September 3, 2020. The diagnosis was diabetic foot infection. The patient was treated with Swotain for anti-infection, foot incision and drainage, and dressing changes. The foot swelling has now spread to the lower leg, with a large amount of purulent exudate from the wound. The patient sought further treatment in our hospital's emergency department and was admitted to our department with the diagnosis of "Type 2 Diabetic Necrotizing Fasciitis." Since the onset of the disease, the patient has not had a fever, has been in a general mental state, has been able to eat and defecate, and has recently lost 2 kg in weight.

L. Gao · J. Wang (✉)
Department of Orthopedics, Beijing Shijitan Hospital, Capital Medical University, Beijing, China
e-mail: gaolei3337@bjsjth.cn; wangjn@bjsjth.cn

[Past History] The patient has a three-year history of diabetes, has not regularly injected insulin, and has not regularly monitored blood sugar. The patient has a 14-year history of gout.

[Admission Examination] The right lower leg and foot are significantly swollen, with pitting edema and high skin temperature; the soft tissue of the skin on the lateral side of the foot is black and necrotic; there are four incisions on the front of the right ankle and the foot, the longest is about 6 cm, reaching the fascia; there are two incisions about 4 cm long on both sides of the ankle, and gray-black necrotic tissue can be seen in the incision (Fig. 1.1), a large amount of purulent exudate, foul smell, reduced foot toe sensation, limited right foot movement, and a weakened dorsalis pedis artery pulse.

[Admission Diagnosis] Type 2 diabetic necrotizing fasciitis, type 2 diabetic foot ulcer and peripheral vascular disease, type 2 diabetic foot ulcer and peripheral neuropathy, metabolic acidosis, hypoproteinemia, hyponatremia, renal function abnormality, hyperuricemia, mild anemia, coagulation function abnormality, lower limb edema, type 2 diabetes.

[Treatment and Outcome] After admission, the patient's basic condition was adjusted, and treatment was given for anti-infection, albumin supplementation, swelling and pain relief, blood transfusion, and wound dressing changes. The

J. Wang, L. Gao (eds.), *Refractory Wounds*, Experts' Perspectives on Medical Advances,
https://doi.org/10.1007/978-981-96-2067-8_1

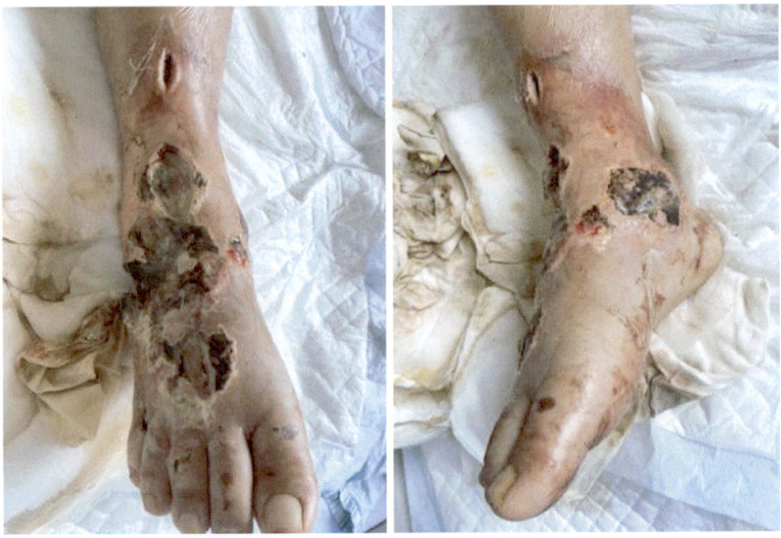

Fig. 1.1 Gray-black necrotic tissue can be seen in the incision

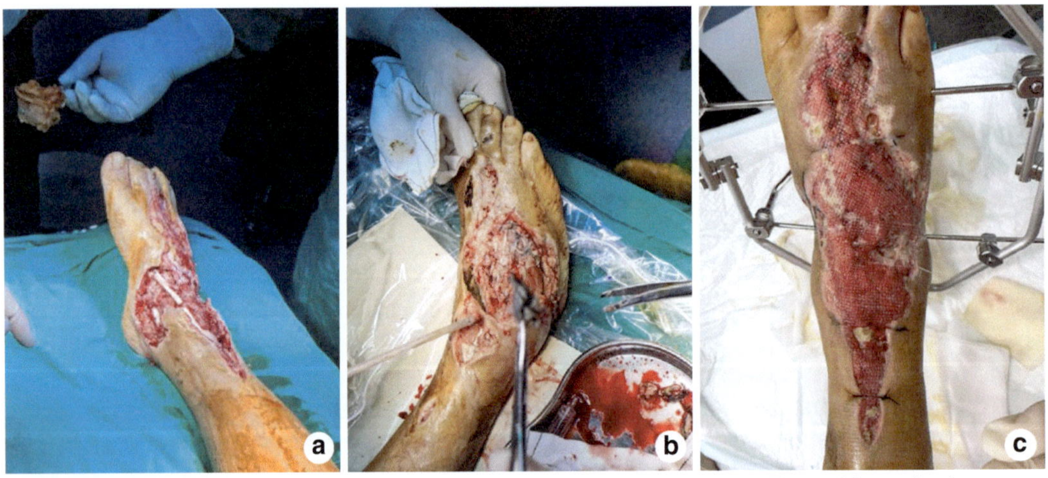

Debridement and exploration of the right foot were performed

The skin and subcutaneous tissue were dissected and drained

External fixator fixation

Fig. 1.2 Surgery under block anesthesia on September 11. (**a**) Debridement and exploration of the right foot were performed. (**b**) The skin and subcutaneous tissue were dissected and drained. (**c**) External fixator fixation

patient had surgical indications and no obvious surgical contraindications. On September 11, the patient underwent debridement and exploration of the right foot, incision and drainage of the skin and subcutaneous tissue, and external fixation (Fig. 1.2) under nerve block anesthesia. On September 27, the patient underwent debridement and exploration of the right foot and transplantation of decellularized allogeneic dermis (Fig. 1.3) under single lumbar anesthesia. After both surgeries, the patient was given anti-infection, neuroprotective treatment, albumin supplementation, swelling and pain relief, and blood transfusion treatment. On October 8, the patient underwent skin grafting and was discharged on October 18 with complete wound healing (Fig. 1.4).

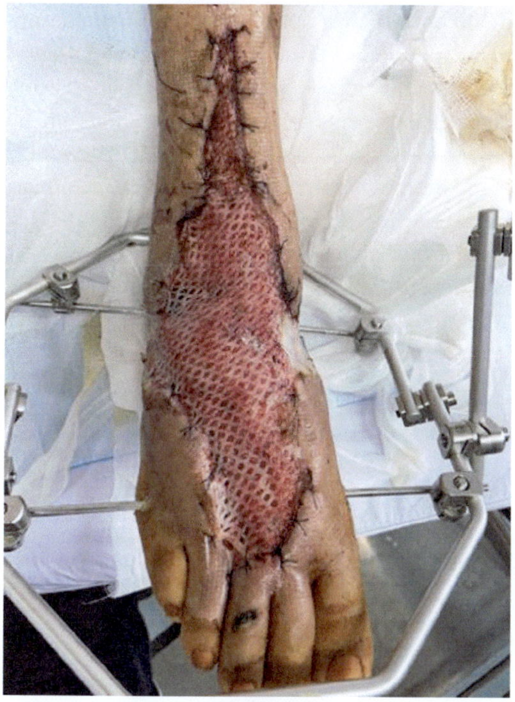

Fig. 1.3 Surgery on September 27

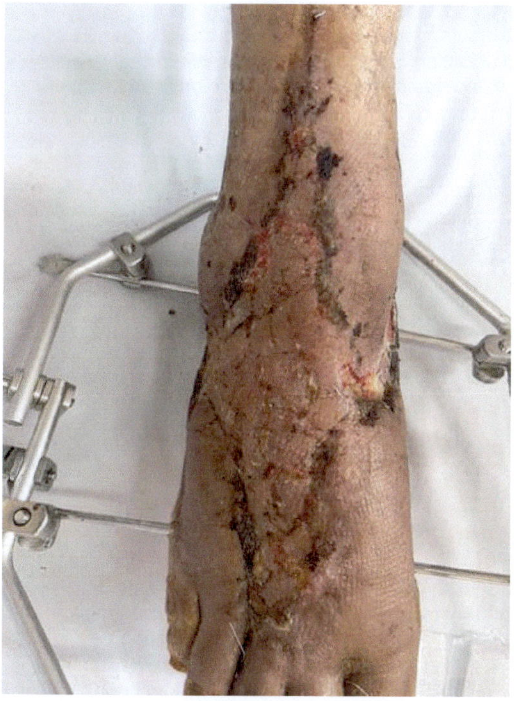

Fig. 1.4 Complete wound healing on October 18

1.1.2 Case 2

The patient, a 71-year-old man, was admitted to the hospital 5 days after gangrene of the metatarsal bone, 2 weeks after the amputation of the left big toe.

[Present Illness History] The patient underwent metatarsophalangeal joint amputation in an outside hospital due to gangrene of the left big toe 2 weeks ago. The infection of the big toe was not controlled after the operation, and the metatarsal bone developed secondary gangrene 5 days ago. The wound continued to deteriorate, accompanied by a large amount of purulent secretion. The patient came to our emergency department for further diagnosis and treatment and was admitted to our department with "diabetic foot gangrene." Since the onset of the disease, the patient has had no fever, general spirit, normal eating and defecation, and no recent weight loss.

[Past History] The patient had a 16-year history of diabetes, with poor blood sugar control.

[Admission Examination] Status after amputation of the left big toe (Fig. 1.5): the first metatarsal bone was exposed, the head of the metatarsal bone was black and necrotic, a large amount of purulent secretion could be seen in the

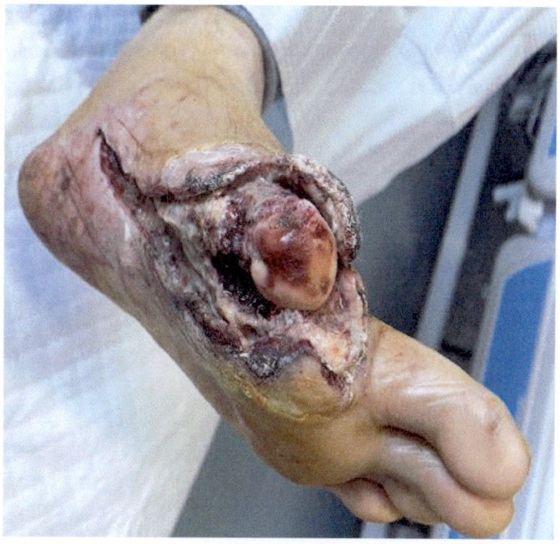

Fig. 1.5 Patient's foot at the time of admission situation (lateral position)

wound cavity, the sensation of the toes was reduced, the movement of the left foot was slightly limited, and the pulsation of the dorsalis pedis artery and the posterior tibial artery was weakened.

[Admission Diagnosis] Type 2 diabetic foot gangrene, metatarsal osteomyelitis, foot soft tissue infection, type 2 diabetes.

Diabetic foot ulcers and peripheral vascular disease, type 2 diabetic foot ulcers and peripheral neuropathy, hypoproteinemia, hyponatremia, renal dysfunction, mild anemia, coagulation dysfunction.

[Treatment and Outcome] After admission, the patient's basic condition was adjusted, and treatments such as anti-infection, albumin supplementation, swelling and pain relief, blood transfusion, and wound dressing change were given. The patient had surgical indications and no obvious surgical contraindications. After thoroughly removing the necrotic tissue, a decellularized allogeneic dermis and autologous blade-thick skin were transplanted together (Fig. 1.6). Postoperative anti-infection, nutritional nerve, albumin supplementation, swelling and pain relief, and blood transfusion treatment were given, and the wound eventually completely healed (Fig. 1.7).

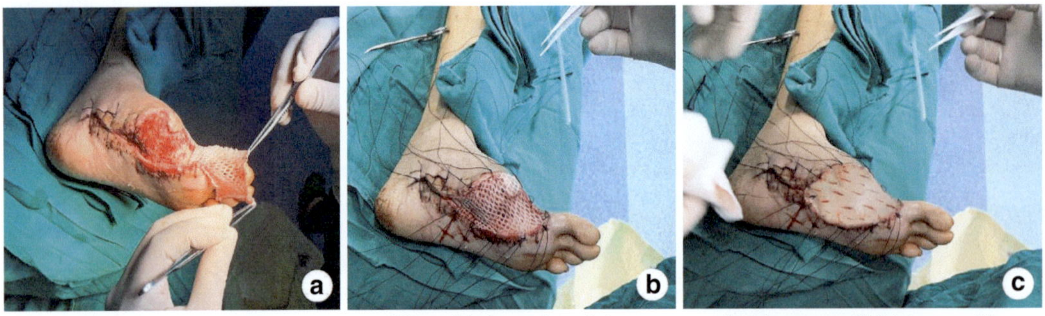

The wound area was 4.5 cm×5.0 cm after debridement and metatarsal stump dressing | The grid-shaped acellular allogeneic dermis was covered on the wound surface | Autologous split-thickness skin was overlaid on the surface of acellular allogeneic dermis

Fig. 1.6 During surgery. (**a**) The wound area was 4.5 cm × 5.0 cm after debridement and metatarsal stump dressing. (**b**) The grid-shaped acellular allogeneic dermis was covered on the wound surface. (**c**) Autologous split-thickness skin was overlaid on the surface of acellular allogeneic dermis

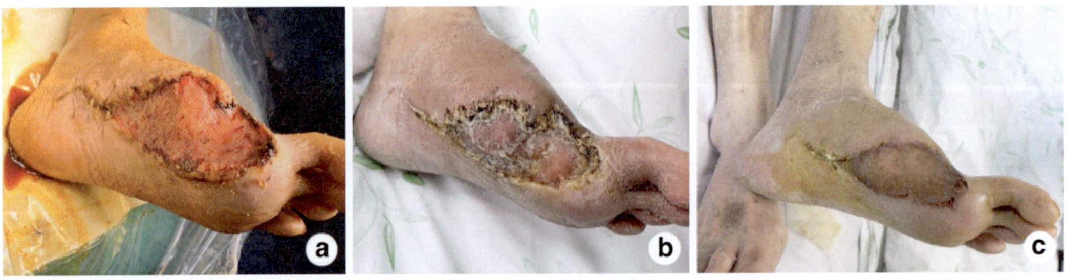

The autologous split-thickness skin survived 7 days after operation | Wound condition of 3 months after surgery | Wound condition of 10 months after surgery

Fig. 1.7 After surgery. After surgery. (**a**) The autologous split-thickness skin survived 7 days after operation. (**b**) Wound condition of 3 months after surgery. (**c**) Wound condition of 10 months after surgery

1.1.3 Case 3

Patient, female, 54 years old. Admitted to the hospital due to nonhealing ulcer on the right lower leg for over 20 days.

[Present Illness History] The patient developed a foot ulcer a year ago due to shoe friction, which healed after about a year of dressing changes. Twenty days ago, without any obvious cause, an ulcer appeared on the outside of the right lower leg, the skin turned black, initially about the size of a "fingernail cap," the wound gradually enlarged, now about the size of a "palm," with exudate and purulent secretion, local stabbing pain, no fever or discomfort, and the effect of dressing change was not good. Since the onset of the disease, the patient's spirit has been good, eating and bowel movements have been normal, and there has been no significant change in weight.

[Past History] History of hypertension for over 30 years, treated with oral aspirin enteric-coated tablets, nifedipine controlled-release tablets, and betaloc; history of hyperlipidemia, treated with oral atorvastatin calcium tablets; history of type 2 diabetes for 12 years, treated with oral acarbose and insulin injections.

[Admission Examination] General condition is okay, bilateral lung sounds are coarse, abdomen is soft, no tenderness, liver and spleen are not enlarged under the ribs, heart sounds are strong. Ulcer on the outside of the right lower leg, area about 15.0 cm × 7.0 cm, wound with black scab, necrotic tissue under the scab accompanied by purulent secretion and inflammatory exudate, local tenderness, pigmentation at the wound edge; scar at the Achilles tendon, fluctuation felt on both sides when pressed, no tenderness, ankle and toe movement possible, dorsal foot artery pulsation present, peripheral blood circulation is good (Fig. 1.8).

[Admission Diagnosis] Lower limb soft tissue infection, type 2 diabetic necrotizing fasciitis, type 2 diabetic peripheral vascular disease, type 2 diabetes, hypoproteinemia, mild anemia, hypertension, hyperlipidemia.

[Treatment and Outcome] After admission, complete the examination, exclude surgical contraindications, explain the condition to the patient and family, and sign the surgical treatment informed consent form. First, debride under the wound scab to promote wound repair and protect the wound (Fig. 1.9). After the wound is dry, remove the scab and apply negative pressure drainage to the wound to promote granulation tissue growth. At the same time, debride the Achilles tendon and remove the bilateral pouches. After the granulation tissue grows well, apply allogeneic dermis and autologous split-thickness skin graft to the wound (Fig. 1.10). Change the dressing of the wound, and the wound gradually heals (Fig. 1.11).

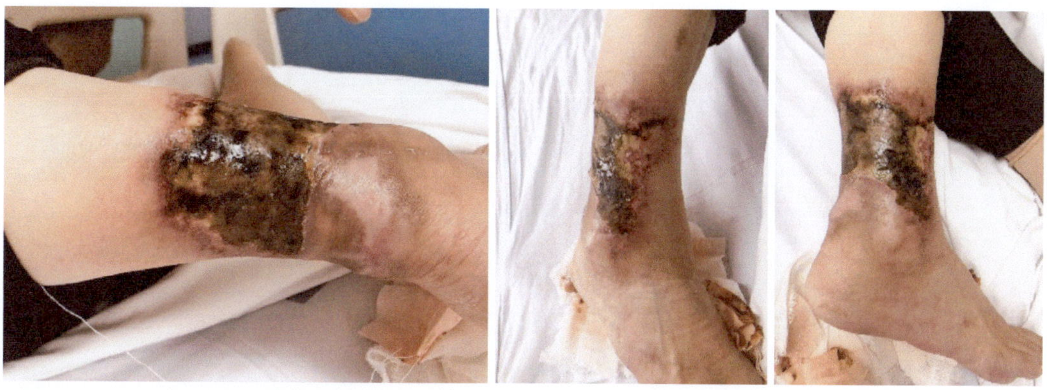

Fig. 1.8 Wound at the time of admission

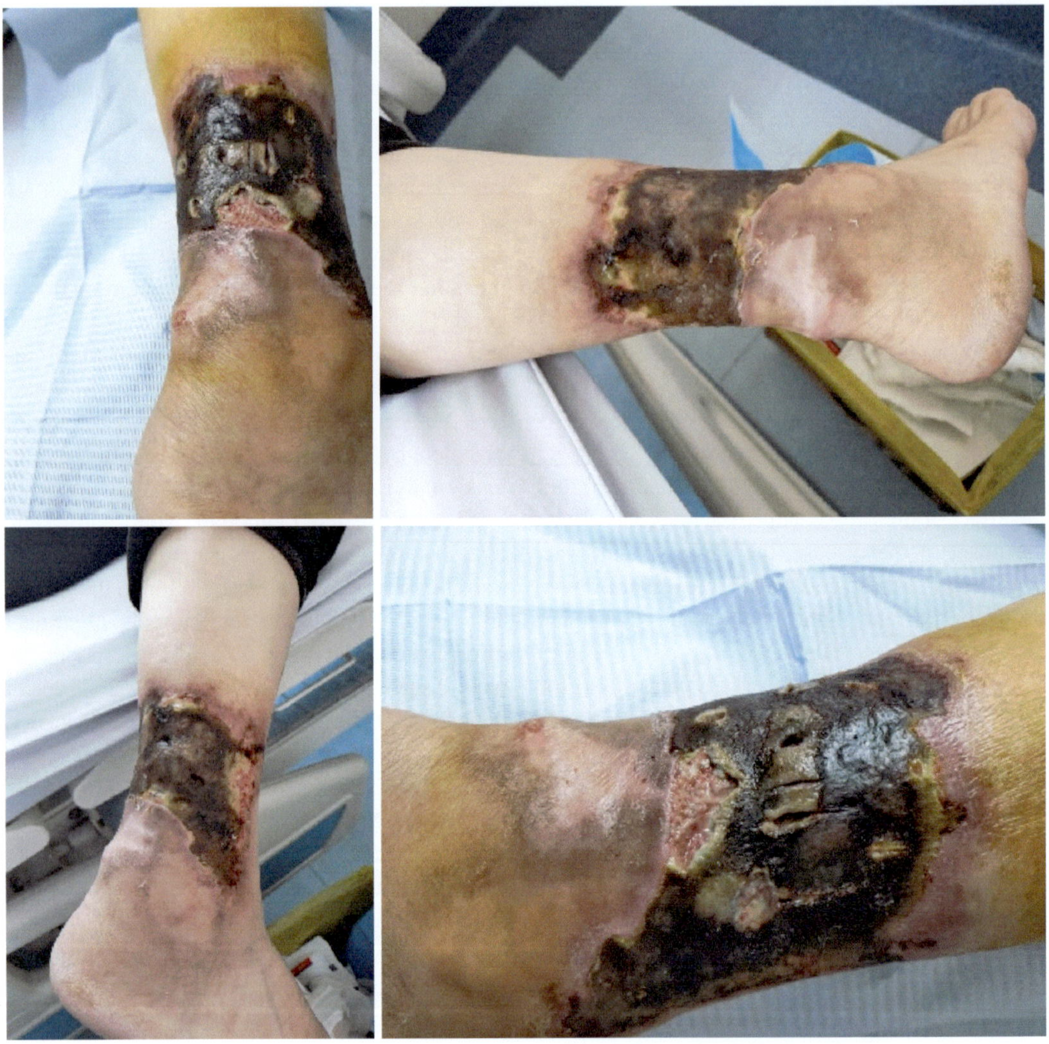

Fig. 1.9 Debridement under the wound scab, promoting wound repair and protecting the wound

Fig. 1.10 Applying allogeneic dermis and autologous split-thickness skin graft to the wound

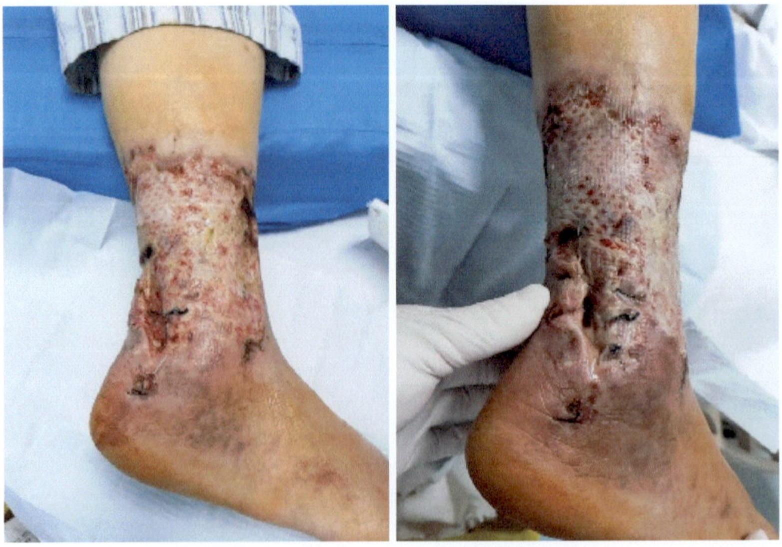

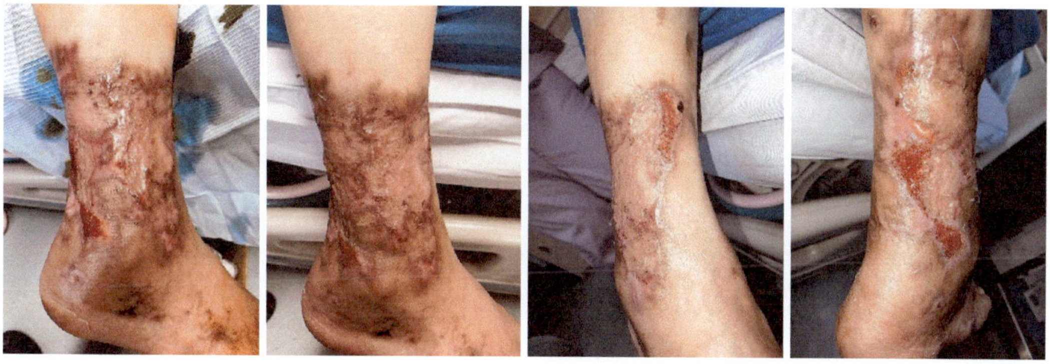

Fig. 1.11 Final healing of the wound

1.2 Case Analysis

1.2.1 Clinical Application of Decellularized Allogeneic Dermis

Decellularized allogeneic dermis (Beijing Jieya Leifu Biotechnology Co., Ltd. J-1 type) has significant value in plastic wound repair. The decellularized allogeneic dermis, being the main part of its structure, has the same structure and components as the extracellular matrix of dermal cells. During the production process, cellular components that trigger host immune rejection are removed, leaving an intact basement membrane, which can induce cell regeneration and expansion, is non-antigenic, and promotes the formation of new blood vessels and epithelial cells. For various wound depressions, different materials or tissues are needed for filling, and decellularized allogeneic dermis can serve as a patch, being one of the effective methods for filling and repairing wounds. It has the functions of scar contraction, plastic loosening, composite skin coverage, and wound repair, and can save autologous skin, with effects comparable to autologous full-thickness skin.

The application of decellularized allogeneic dermis and autologous blade-thick skin for composite transplantation to repair wounds, the matrix components of decellularized allogeneic dermis can effectively regulate fibroblast proliferation, enabling the retained basement membrane to effectively induce the growth and differentiation of new epithelial cells, thereby providing good conditions for the survival of autologous epidermis and its tight connection with the dermis layer, effectively promoting wound healing, and making the reconstructed skin have good elasticity and appearance. Moreover, the firm bond between the autologous epidermis and allogeneic dermis helps to maintain and improve the skin's abrasion and pressure resistance, and can effectively counteract the contraction phenomenon caused by the transplanted skin graft.

1.2.2 Methods of Composite Skin Transplantation

1. Preparation of decellularized allogeneic dermis. First, rinse repeatedly with physiological saline three times, cut off the floating fibrous tissue, and wrap it with wet saline gauze for standby. Be careful not to soak it in saline to prevent the skin graft from swelling.
2. Two methods of composite skin transplantation: one-step method and two-step method.

   ① One-step method: The decellularized allogeneic dermis and autologous blade-thick skin are transplanted to the wound at the same time, and the operation is completed in one time. Advantages: reduce patient pain, save time, save medical expenses, have more indications, and good postoperative effects.

   ② Two-step method: First, the decellularized allogeneic dermis or artificial dermis is transplanted into the wound. After establishing blood circulation (about 10–14 days postoperatively), the autologous blade-thick skin is transplanted, requiring two operations. It is suitable for artificial dermis or wounds with poor conditions.

1.2.3 Preparation and Requirements of the Skin Receiving Area

① Completely remove scars, various lesions, or necrotic tissues; retain vital tissues; the wound base should be flat; hemostasis should be thorough; and skin grafting should not be suitable on the fat layer. ② For infected wounds, prepare for surgery carefully, carry out dressing changes, local soaking or bathing, reduce wound secretions, control infection. During the operation, granulation tissue is scraped off, and if fibrous plaques are formed, they are also removed. Before and after scraping, rinse repeatedly three times with 1% hydrogen peroxide solution, physiological saline, metronidazole solution, to reduce the amount of bacteria in the wound, so as not to affect the survival of the skin graft.

1.2.4 Tissue Engineering Characteristics of Decellularized Allogeneic Dermis

Decellularized allogeneic dermal matrix is a tissue engineering material, which is a kind of non-vital tissue treated specially, only retaining the intact basement membrane and dermal extracellular matrix, which can provide good conditions for the migration and colonization of epithelial cells. Decellularized allogeneic dermis mainly removes highly antigenic epidermal cells and dermal fibroblasts through biochemical and cellular biological methods, effectively reducing antigenicity, alleviating inflammatory response, reducing immune rejection of the body, while preserving the three-dimensional framework structure and components of non-antigenic extracellular matrix effectively.

Bibliography

1. Zelen CM, Orgill DP, Serena T, et al. A prospective, randomised, controlled, multicentre clinical trial examining healing rates, safety and cost to closure of an acellular reticular allogenic human dermis versus standard of care in the treatment of chronic diabetic foot ulcers. Int Wound J. 2017;14(2):307–15.
2. Campitiello F, Mancone M, Della Corte A, et al. To evaluate the efficacy of an acellular flowable matrix in comparison with a wet dressing for the treatment of patients with diabetic foot ulcers: a randomized clinical trial. Updat Surg. 2017;69(4):523–9.
3. Widjaja W, Tan J, Maitz PKM. Efficacy of dermal substitute on deep dermal to full thickness burn injury: a systematic review. ANZ J Surg. 2017;87(6):446–52.
4. Pirayesh A, Hoeksema H, Richters C, et al. Glyaderm (®)dermal substitute: clinical application and long-term results in 55 patients. Burns. 2015;41(1):132–44.
5. Bohac M, Varga I, Polak S, et al. Delayed post mastectomy breast reconstructions with allogeneic acellular dermal matrix prepared by a new decellularization method. Cell Tissue Bank. 2018;19(1):61–8.
6. Specht M, Kelm S, Mirastschijski U. Suitability of biological acellular dermal matrices as a skin replacement. Handchir Mikrochir Plast Chir. 2020;52(6):533–44.
7. Goodarzi P, Falahzadeh K, Nematizadeh M, et al. Tissue engineered skin substitutes. Adv Exp Med Biol. 2018;1107:143–88.

A Case of Comprehensive Treatment for Diabetic Foot Necrotizing Fasciitis

2

Lei Gao and Jiangning Wang

2.1 Case Summary

The patient, a 55-year-old male, was admitted to the hospital due to redness, swelling, and rupture of the skin on the lateral side and dorsum of his left foot for 3 weeks, and increased purulent exudate for 3 days.

[Present Illness History] The patient had a skin rupture on the lateral side of the fifth metatarsophalangeal joint of his left foot with bloody exudate 3 weeks ago. He was treated with dressing changes at a local community hospital. During this period, the patient self-administered traditional Chinese medicine at home, but the effect was not good. One day ago, he underwent a debridement surgery at a local tertiary hospital outpatient clinic. The wound did not improve after the surgery. He came to our hospital for further treatment and was admitted to our department with "diabetic foot necrotizing fasciitis."

[Past Medical History] The patient's general health condition was average, with a history of diabetes for over 21 years. He irregularly took metformin orally, and his blood sugar control was not good. He denied a history of coronary heart disease and cerebral infarction, denied a history of hepatitis B and tuberculosis and close contact history, denied a history of trauma, denied a history of blood product transfusion, denied a history of drug and food allergies, and his vaccinations were up to date.

[Admission Examination]

1. Specialized physical examination. There was a skin rupture wound about 3.0 cm × 4.0 cm in size on the dorsum of the left foot. The wound edge was irregular, reaching the tendon, with grayish-white purulent exudate; the exudate had an odor, and the skin around the wound was slightly red and swollen; on the lateral side of the fifth metatarsophalangeal joint of the left foot, there was a wound about 1.5 cm. There is a skin ulcer of 1.2 cm × 1.2 cm in size, reaching the fascia layer, accompanied by bloody secretions. Exudation, red and swollen skin on the outer side of the left foot, with three drainage wounds of about 0.5 cm × 0.5 cm in size, slight tenderness around the skin, slightly low skin temperature, slightly limited flexion and extension of the toes of the left foot, reduced peripheral blood circulation and sensation (Fig. 2.1).
2. Laboratory examination. ① Biochemical profile: alanine aminotransferase 8 U/L, aspartate aminotransferase 9 U/L, total bilirubin 8.5 μmol/L, direct bilirubin 3.3 μmol/L,

L. Gao · J. Wang (✉)
Department of Orthopedics, Beijing Shijitan Hospital, Capital Medical University, Beijing, China
e-mail: gaolei3337@bjsjth.cn; wangjn@bjsjth.cn

J. Wang, L. Gao (eds.), *Refractory Wounds*, Experts' Perspectives on Medical Advances,
https://doi.org/10.1007/978-981-96-2067-8_2

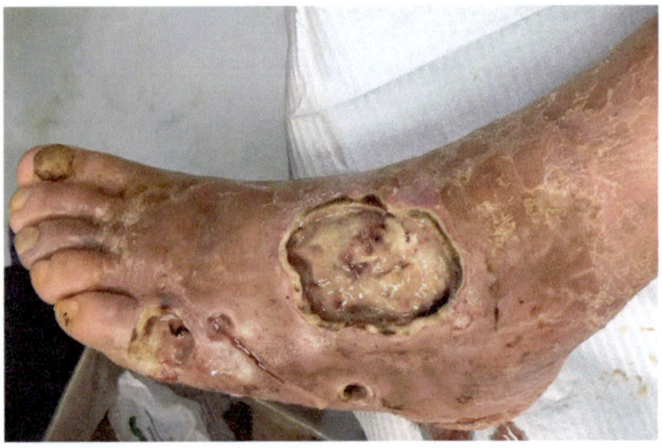

Fig. 2.1 Condition of the left foot wound upon admission

indirect bilirubin 5.1 μmol/L, total protein 63.8 g/L, sodium 138 mmol/L, chloride 103 mmol/L, calcium 2.26 mmol/L, phosphorus 1.1 mmol/L, serum iron 8.8 μmol/L, serum magnesium 0.87 mmol/L, potassium 3.73 mmol/L, creatinine 52 μmol/L, uric acid 154 μmol/L, serum glucose 12.8 mmol/L, creatine kinase 29 U/L, lactate dehydrogenase 141 U/L, globulin 31.1 g/L, albumin 32.7 g/L, alkaline phosphatase 129 U/L, blood urea nitrogen 3.98 mmol/L. ② Blood routine (venous blood): White blood cells (WBC) 12.73×10^9/L, neutrophil percentage 82.4%, platelets (PLT) 410×10^9/L, hemoglobin (HGB) 144 g/L. ③ C-reactive protein (CRP) 60.14 mg/L. ④ Procalcitonin (PCT) 0.03 ng/mL.

3. Imaging examination. ① Left foot X-ray: The joints of the left foot are in good alignment, there is marginal osteophyte formation in some phalanges, and some spaces are narrowed. The bone quality of the distal phalanges of the second to fourth toes of the left foot is not good, and the bone density at the distal end is slightly high (Fig. 2.2).

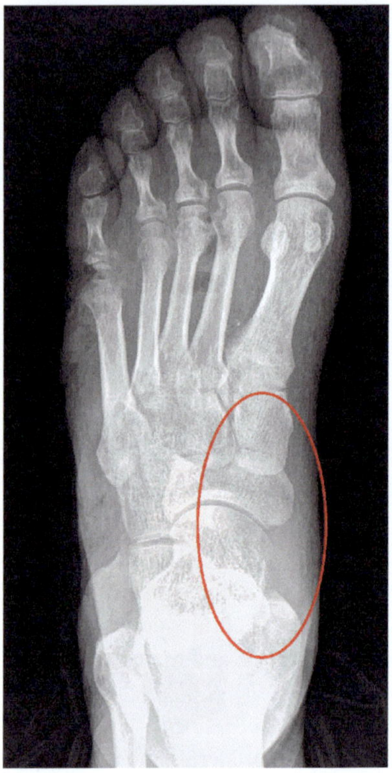

Fig. 2.2 Left foot X-ray

Diagnosis: Changes in some distal phalanges of the left foot, consistent with diabetic foot changes; degenerative changes in the left foot. ② Foot computed tomography (CT): Both feet's joints are in position, some bones show osteogenesis, joint surfaces are smooth, the cortical bone of the third metatarsal bone of the left foot is slightly rough. Gas shadows can be seen within the soft tissue from the dorsum of the left foot to the toes (Fig. 2.3). Diagnosis: The left foot shows signs of diabetic foot; both feet show signs of degeneration. ③ CT angiography (CTA) of both lower limbs: Bilateral iliac arteries, femoral arteries, popliteal arteries, anterior and posterior tibial arteries, and peroneal arteries show multiple punctate calcifications on the wall, and multiple mild to moderate stenoses in the lumen. Swelling of the soft tissue of the left lower limb and both feet (Fig. 2.4). Diagnosis: Arteriosclerosis of the lower limbs; swelling of the soft tissue of the left lower limb and both feet. ④ Lower limb venous ultrasound: Good compressibility of the femoral, popliteal, and intermuscular veins of both legs, no obvious abnormal echo in the lumen. ⑤ Color Doppler flow imaging (CDFI) shows blood flow filling in the above vessels; pulsed wave Doppler imaging shows normal blood flow spectrum; no obvious abnormalities in the vessels within the examination range. ⑥ Lower limb arterial ultrasound: Thickening of the intima in the femoral and popliteal arteries of

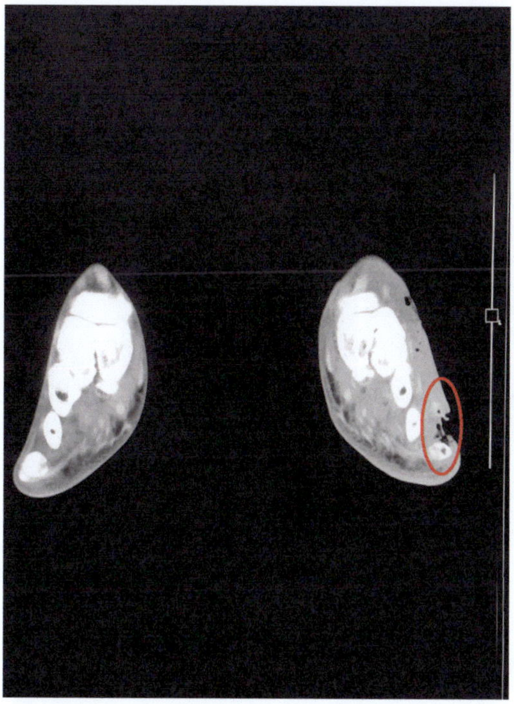

Fig. 2.3 Foot CT

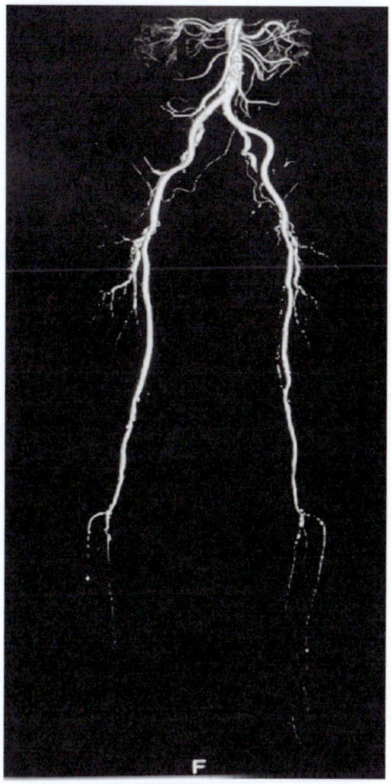

Fig. 2.4 Lower limb CTA

both legs, not smooth, multiple low echo and strong echo plaques can be seen on the wall, causing mild stenosis of the lumen of the opening of the left superficial femoral artery and the lower segment of the left popliteal artery, occlusion of the lumen of the middle and upper segment of the left superficial femoral artery. Diagnosis: Widespread arteriosclerosis of both lower limbs and segmental stenosis, occlusion of the middle and upper segment of the left superficial femoral artery. ⑦ Cardiac ultrasound: Normal cardiac chamber size, aorta, and pulmonary artery are not wide; no obvious abnormalities in valve structure and motion; normal left ventricular wall thickness, no obvious abnormal motion. ⑧ Foot magnetic resonance imaging (MRI): Significant swelling of the soft tissue of the left foot, local defect of the subcutaneous soft tissue around the fifth toe bone of the dorsum of the foot, slightly long T1 abnormal signal in the bone of the fifth metatarsophalangeal joint, high signal in the short time inversion recovery sequence (STIR), multiple small patchy and linear slightly high signals seen in the remaining second to fourth toe bones, metatarsal bones, multiple tarsal bones, and calcaneocuboid bones. Liquid abnormal signal seen in the left ankle joint cavity (Fig. 2.5). Diagnosis: Left foot matches MRI changes of diabetic foot; local soft tissue defect with significant bone marrow edema in the fifth metatarsal joint (high possibility of osteomyelitis); multiple bone signal abnormalities in the left foot, suggesting bone marrow edema; effusion in the left ankle joint.

[Diagnosis] Type 2 diabetic foot gangrene, necrotizing fasciitis, type 2 diabetes, type 2 diabetic foot ulcer and peripheral neuropathy, type 2 diabetic foot ulcer and peripheral vascular disease, soft tissue infection of the foot (left).

[Treatment and Outcome] After admission, the patient was given wound dressing changes, symptomatic treatment such as anti-infection, swelling reduction, circulation improvement, neurotrophic and anticoagulant drugs. Wound dressing changes were performed using alginate cavity drainage, and silver ion hydrogel dressing

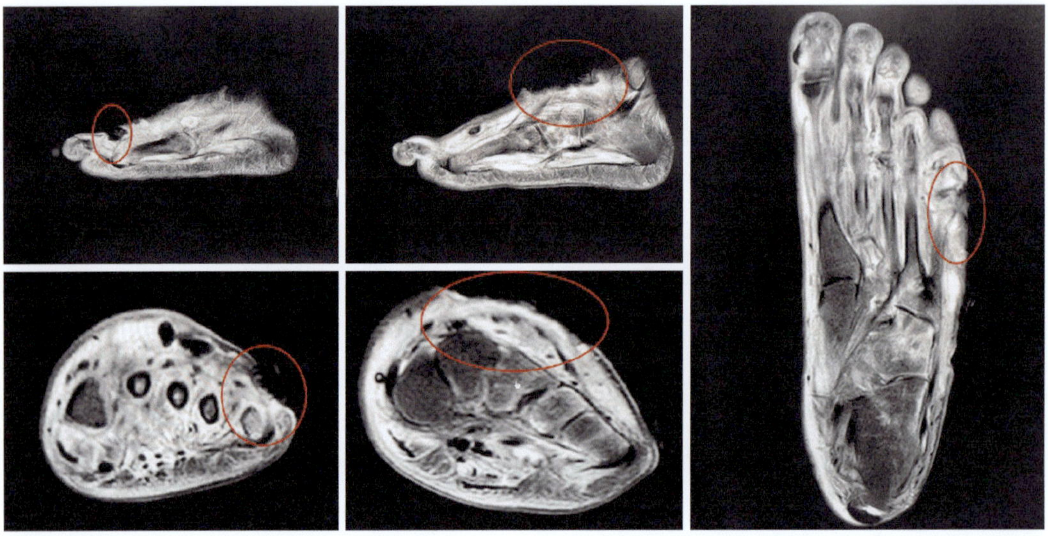

Fig. 2.5 Foot MRI

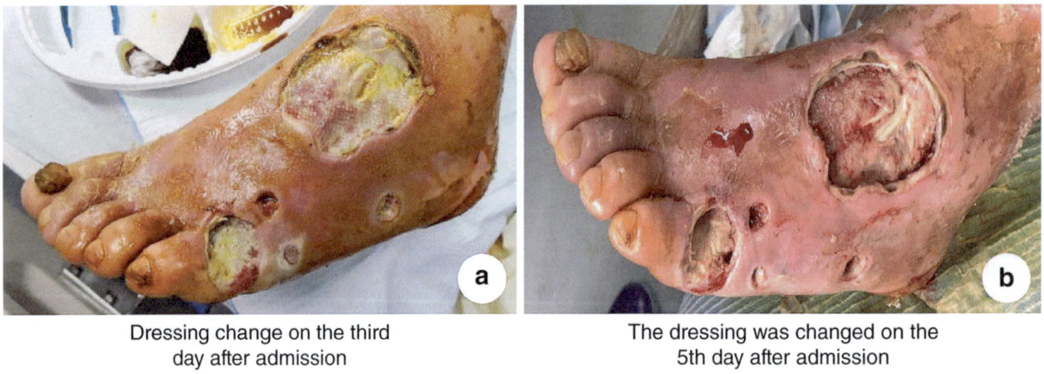

Fig. 2.6 Wound. (**a**) Dressing change on the third day after admission. (**b**) The dressing was changed on the fifth day after admission

was applied to the dorsal foot wound (Fig. 2.6). Antibacterial drugs covering staphylococci and streptococci were used.

One week after admission, debridement of necrotic tissue in the left foot was performed under nerve block anesthesia, along with vascular nerve tendon exploration, incision, and drainage. After the operation, symptomatic treatments such as anti-infection, swelling reduction, circulation improvement, and neurotrophic and anticoagulant drugs were continued under the premise of insulin control of blood sugar, and silver ion gel dressing was applied to the postoperative wound, with alginate dressing used for cavity drainage (Fig. 2.7).

On the first day after surgery, a routine blood test and related infection indicators were reviewed. ① Full biochemical profile: alanine aminotransferase 16 U/L, aspartate aminotransferase 21 U/L, total bilirubin 11.3 μmol/L, direct bilirubin 3.9 μmol/L, indirect bilirubin 7.4 μmol/L, total protein 67.6 g/L, sodium 139 mmol/L, chloride 99 mmol/L, calcium 2.12 mmol/L, phosphorus 1.04 mmol/L, serum iron 7.5 μmol/L, serum magnesium 0.96 mmol/L, potassium 3.85 mmol/L, creatinine 46 μmol/L, uric acid 130 μmol/L, serum glucose 11.05 mmol/L, creatine kinase 36 U/L, lactate dehydrogenase 164 U/L, globulin 31.6 g/L, albumin 32 g/L, alkaline phosphatase 102 U/L, urea nitrogen 3.14 mmol/L. ② Routine blood test (venous blood): WBC 7.29 × 10^9/L, neutrophil percentage 75.4%, PLT 361 × 10^9/L, HGB 107 g/L. ③ CRP 5.13 mg/L. ④ PCT 0.03 ng/mL. To promote wound healing, on the fourth day after the first surgery, the patient underwent left foot vascular nerve tendon exploration, necrotic tissue debridement, skin grafting, and vacuum sealing drainage (VSD) surgery. One week after the surgery, the patient underwent left foot necrotic tissue debridement and VSD device removal surgery. After routine dressing changes, anti-infection, and diuretic symptomatic treatment, the skin graft area healed well, and inflam-

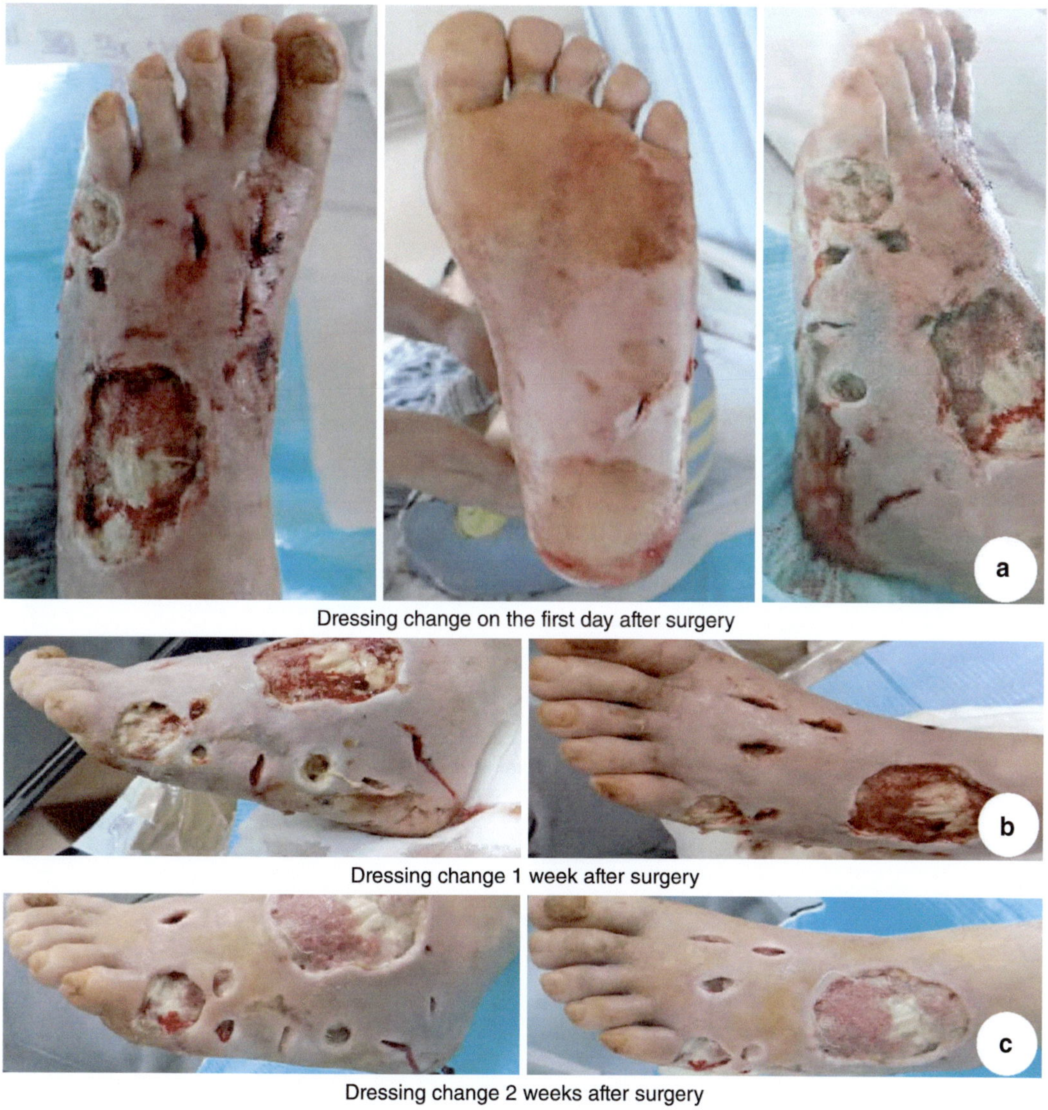

Fig. 2.7 Postoperative wound condition after the first surgery in hospital. (**a**) Dressing change on the first day after surgery. (**b**) Dressing change 1 week after surgery. (**c**) Dressing change 2 weeks after surgery. (**d**) Dressing change 4 weeks after surgery.

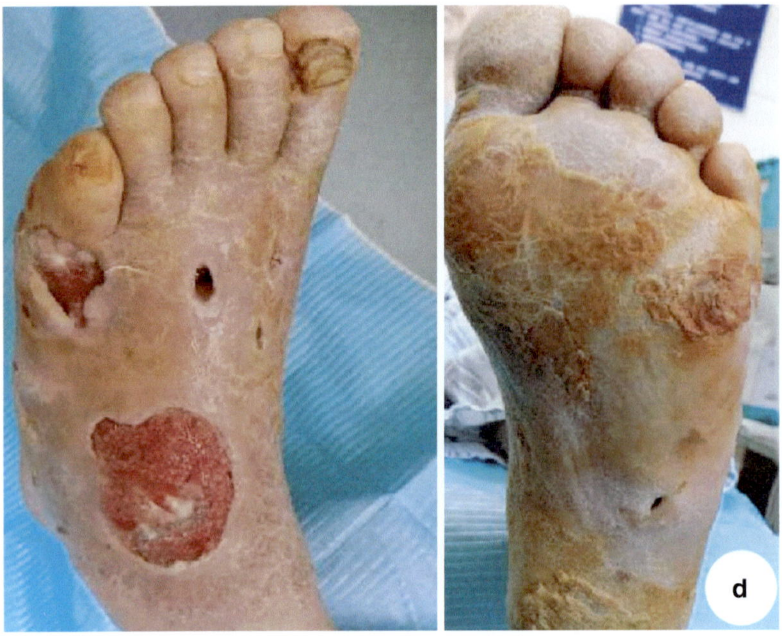

Dressing change 4 weeks after surgery

Fig. 2.7 (continued)

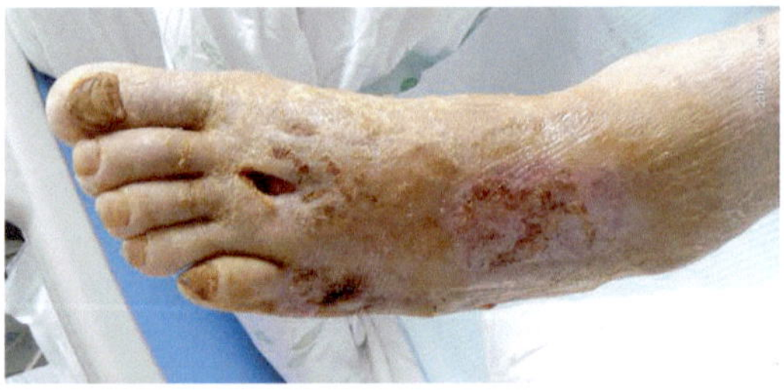

Fig. 2.8 Post-grafting wound recovery

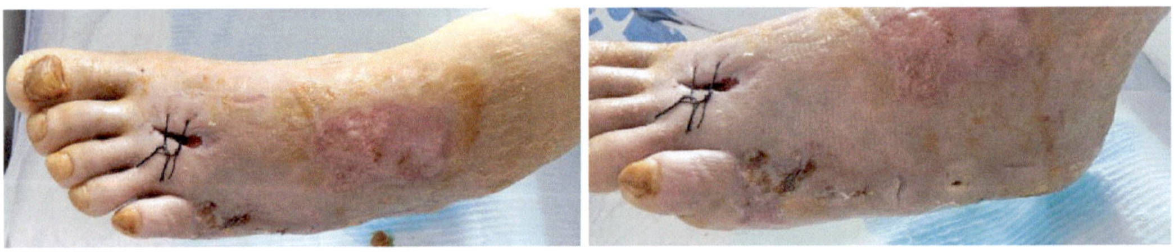

Fig. 2.9 Post-fat grafting wound

matory granulation tissue was visible at the distal end of the dorsal foot wound (Fig. 2.8). Three days after the vacuum removal, the patient underwent left foot vascular nerve tendon exploration, necrotic tissue debridement, and fat grafting surgery (Fig. 2.9). After the surgery, the wound was dressed, and the wound healed 2 weeks later (Fig. 2.10).

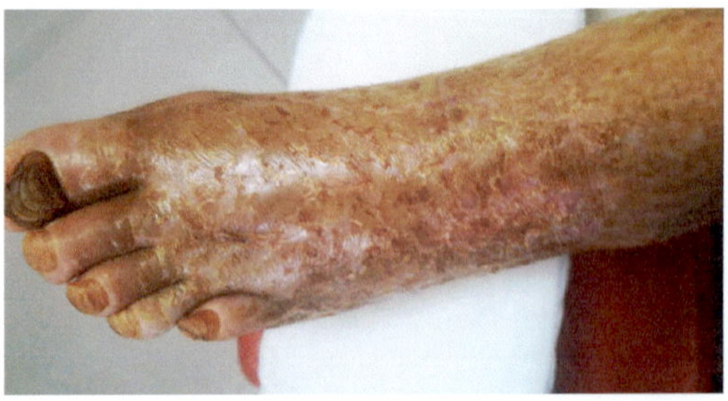

Fig. 2.10 Wound 2 weeks after fat grafting

2.2 Case Analysis

2.2.1 Surgical Treatment of Acute Infection of Necrotizing Fasciitis in Diabetic Foot

The patient in this case was diagnosed with gangrene of the diabetic foot combined with necrotizing fasciitis. For wounds in the acute infection stage, the necrotic tissue should be thoroughly debrided first, and incision and drainage should be performed for skin tissues with high tension to make the wound relatively clean. During the operation, the principle was to remove as much necrotic tissue from the wound as possible, and the necrotic fascia tissue should be removed to the greatest extent. For many patients with severe foot infections, the risk of local infection spreading to the whole body was high, so the thorough debridement in the first stage was particularly important.

2.2.2 Use of Antimicrobial Drugs After Debridement of Necrotizing Fasciitis in Diabetic Foot

After the first stage of debridement, antimicrobial drugs should be used for anti-infection treatment. Narrow-spectrum antimicrobial drugs should be chosen for mild or moderate infections; initial treatment should be chosen based on the most common pathogens and known local antimicrobial drug sensitivity data; empirical medication (broad-spectrum) should be adjusted based on culture results and clinical response to the initial treatment plan. It should be noted that bacterial culture of the infected wound can identify the pathogenic bacteria, and the specimens after debridement should be cultured aerobically and anaerobically. Reliable culture specimens should be the scrapings from the base of the ulcer after debridement, aspirated purulent secretions, tissue fragments obtained surgically, etc. The culture results of swab (swab) specimens obtained from the surface of the ulcer before debridement are unreliable.

Almost all cases should cover positive cocci and negative bacilli. Combined with bacterial culture results, drugs proven to be effective in treating skin and soft tissue infections can be selected, including semi-synthetic penicillins, cephalosporins, β-lactamase inhibitors, clindamycin, fluoroquinolones, carbapenems, and thiazolone. Ertapenem, linezolid, and piperacillin/tazobactam have significant effects in treating secondary skin and tissue infections (including diabetic foot infections).

2.2.3 Experience in Taking Bacterial Culture Specimens from Infected Wounds

① Samples should be obtained from all infected wounds. ② Samples should be taken after debridement. ③ Samples should be taken with a sterile scalpel or skin scraper. ④ Pus and aspirates need to be taken with a sterile puncture needle and syringe. ⑤ Samples should be quickly sent for examination, using sterile containers and appropriate culture media, for aerobic and anaerobic culture, and Gram staining should be performed as much as possible. It is not appropriate to: ① culture uninfected wounds; ② obtain samples without first debriding; ③ obtain specimens by wiping the wound or draining the wound.

2.2.4 Closure of the Wound in Diabetic Foot Necrotizing Fasciitis

Autologous skin grafting is a commonly used method in the clinical treatment of soft tissue defects in diabetic foot, divided into thin skin grafts, medium-thickness skin grafts, and full-thickness skin grafts. Because full-thickness skin grafts have higher requirements for the condition of the wound and the donor skin area is limited, they cannot be used for large-area wound coverage, and are currently not commonly used for wound repair in diabetic foot. Thin skin grafts and medium-thickness skin grafts are more commonly used in clinical practice, both of which have a high survival rate. Among them, thin skin grafts are more likely to survive than medium-thickness skin grafts, because the donor skin area still contains part of the dermis and can heal on its own, so the donor skin area is relatively unrestricted.

2.2.5 Application of Negative Pressure Technology in Wound Repair

This case used a negative pressure dressing made of cotton material, which was soft, nonirritating, low allergenic, and had good compliance, making it easy to fill according to the shape of the wound. At the same time, Prof. Wang Jiangning's team improved the suction cup and suction tube device of negative pressure, combining the suction cup drainage with the tube drainage, to keep the wound and wound cavity as clean as possible, and promote the growth of granulation tissue under the condition of smooth drainage of secretions.

2.2.6 Conclusion

Diabetic foot is one of the serious complications in diabetic patients. For the treatment of acute infectious wounds of diabetic foot necrotizing fasciitis, on the basis of internal medicine control of blood sugar, applying anti-infectives, lowering lipid levels, improving microcirculation, nutritional nerves, and surgical methods should be adopted first; necrotic tissue debridement combined with negative pressure treatment is followed; skin grafting repair after the wound is fresh; and finally the wound is healed to avoid amputation.

Bibliography

1. Kooiman TJM, De Groot M, Hoogenberg K, et al. Self-tracking of physical activity in people with type 2 diabetes: a randomized controlled trial. Comput Inform Nurs. 2018;36(7):340–9.
2. Keukenkamp R, Merkx MJ, Busch Westbroek TE, et al. An explorative study on the efficacy and feasibility of the use of motivational interviewing to improve footwear adherence in persons with diabetes at high risk for foot ulceration. J Am Podiatr Med Assoc. 2018;108(2):90–9.
3. Jeffcoate WJ, Vileikyte L, Boyko EJ, et al. Current challenges and opportunities in the prevention and management of diabetic foot ulcers. Diabetes Care. 2018;41(4):645–52.
4. Lazzarini PA, Pacella RE, Armstrong DG, et al. Diabetes-related lower-extremity complications are a leading cause of the global burden of disability. Diabet Med. 2018;35:1297–9.
5. Jiangning W, Lei G, Tiangui C, et al. Professor Wang Jiangning's team's comprehensive diagnosis and treatment of diabetic foot cases. Beijing: Science and Technology Literature Publishing House; 2018.

3 A Case of Repairing Diabetic Foot Ulcer with Injectable Platelet-Rich Fibrin

Lei Gao and Jiangning Wang

3.1 Case Summary

The patient, a 50-year-old male, was admitted to the hospital due to an unhealed rupture of the right foot for more than 8 months.

[Present Illness History] The patient developed a rupture in the skin of the right foot due to unreasonable weight-bearing 8 months ago, accompanied by secretion exudation. After self-medication, there was no improvement. During this period, he continued to bear weight and walk, and the area of the foot rupture gradually increased. He came to our hospital for further diagnosis and treatment, and was admitted to our department with the diagnosis of "diabetic foot ulcer." Since the onset of the disease, the patient's spirit, diet, and sleep had been normal, and there had been no weight loss.

[Past History] The patient was generally healthy. He denied having hypertension, hyperlipidemia, coronary heart disease, and stroke history; denied having hepatitis, tuberculosis history, and close contact history; denied having a history of trauma; denied having a history of blood product transfusion; denied having a history of drug and food allergies. Vaccination was carried out as planned. He had a history of diabetes for more than 21 years, and he usually controlled his blood sugar by injecting insulin subcutaneously (Gansulin 30 R injection, 20 IU in the morning and 20 IU in the evening), but the effect was not good. Three years ago, due to Charcot's foot, he underwent necrotic bone removal surgery on his right foot in our hospital + External fixation surgery, a year ago due to a foot ulcer on the right foot; debridement was performed in our hospital.

[Admission Examination]

1. Specialized physical examination. The right lower leg and foot were significantly swollen; a 5.0 cm × 4.0 cm wound could be seen on the sole of the right foot, with inflammatory granulation tissue visible inside and secretions seeping out; the wound was concave, about 1.0 cm deep. The flexion and extension of the right ankle and toes were slightly limited, the pulse of the foot arteries was weakened, and the peripheral blood circulation and sensation were reduced (Fig. 3.1).
2. Laboratory examination. ① Biochemical profile: alanine aminotransferase 9 U/L, aspartate aminotransferase 12 U/L, total bilirubin 24.7 μmol/L, sodium 142 mmol/L, chloride 99 mmol/L, calcium 2.17 mmol/L, phosphorus 1.03 mmol/L, serum iron 9.2 μmol/L, serum magnesium 0.8 mmol/L, potassium

L. Gao · J. Wang (✉)
Department of Orthopedics, Beijing Shijitan Hospital, Capital Medical University, Beijing, China
e-mail: gaolei3337@bjsjth.cn; wangjn@bjsjth.cn

J. Wang, L. Gao (eds.), *Refractory Wounds*, Experts' Perspectives on Medical Advances,
https://doi.org/10.1007/978-981-96-2067-8_3

3.37 mmol/L, creatinine 57 μmol/L, uric acid 257 μmol/L, serum glucose 14.32 mmol/L, albumin 36.2 g/L, total cholesterol 5.74 mmol/L, triglycerides 1.78 mmol/L, urea nitrogen 6.21 mmol/L. ② Blood routine

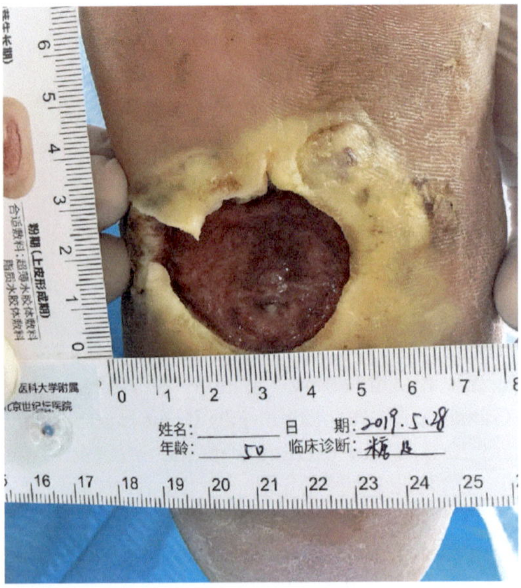

Fig. 3.1 Right foot wound at admission

(venous blood): WBC 5.77 × 109/L, neutrophil percentage 85.4%, PLT 238 × 10^9/L, HGB 179 g/L. ③ CRP 37.2 mg/L, erythrocyte sedimentation rate (ESR) 39 mm/h, PCT 0.09 ng/mL, D-dimer 278 ng/mL, glycated hemoglobin (HBA1c) 8.4%.

3. Imaging examination. ① Foot anteroposterior and lateral X-ray (right): Multiple tarsal bone destruction in the right foot, with corresponding joints involved; distal phalangeal bone destruction of the first toe; peripheral soft tissue swelling, incomplete skin on the lateral base of the fifth metatarsal, a large amount of gas density shadow can be seen. Diagnosis: Right foot surface. The current condition is consistent with changes in diabetic foot (Fig. 3.2).

   ② Foot CT: Multiple round low-density cystic changes in the distal tibia, talus, calcaneus, several tarsal bones, and distal first toe bone on the right side. The density inside the bone marrow cavity is unevenly increased, the bone edge is rough and not smooth, and some bone destruction is obvious. Subcutaneous gas shadows can be seen on the sole of the right

Fig. 3.2 Right foot anteroposterior and lateral X-ray film

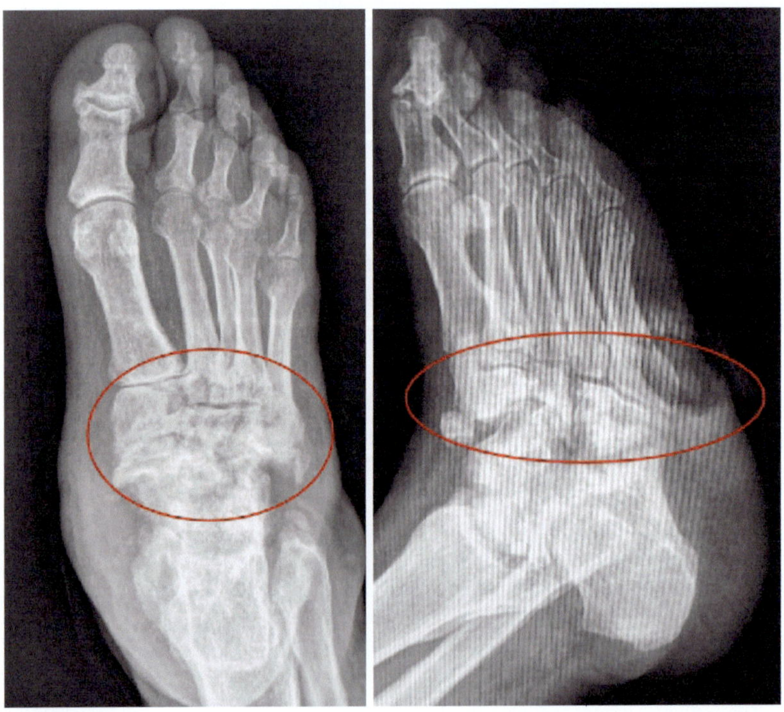

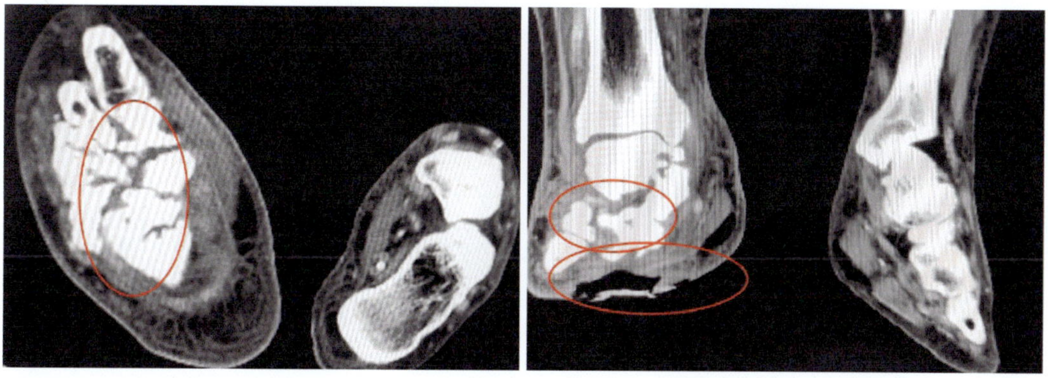

Fig. 3.3 CT of the right foot showing bone dissolution

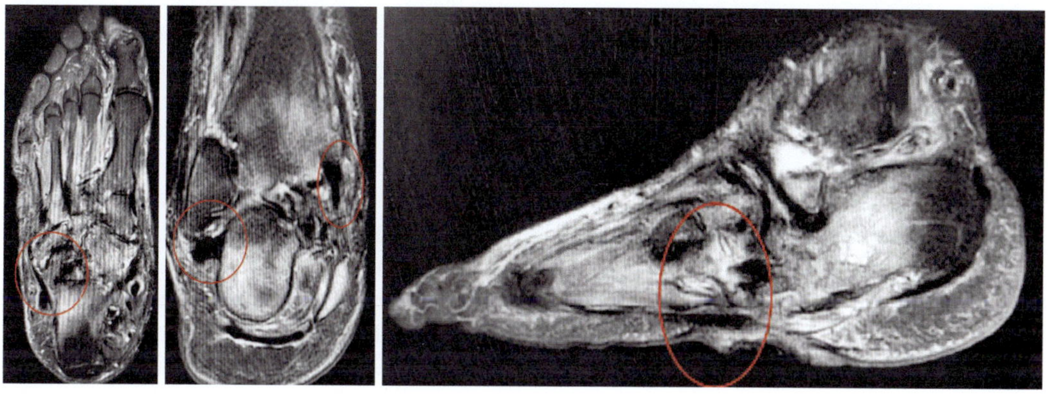

Fig. 3.4 MRI of the right foot

foot, and the skin is locally discontinuous. The bone morphology of the left foot is still acceptable, and no obvious bone destruction changes are seen. Diagnosis: Multiple bone abnormalities in the right foot, considered consistent with changes in diabetic foot bones, progressed compared to before, and there is a possibility of subcutaneous soft tissue infection and rupture on the sole of the right foot (Fig. 3.3). ③ Right foot MRI: Swelling of the soft tissues of the right foot, the skin edge of the mid-foot bottom shows a serrated change, the alignment of the bones in the mid-foot is disordered, the gap disappears, and many bones are deformed. Short time of inversion recovery (STIR) sequence shows slightly high signal in a flocculent pattern. The cortical bone of the talus, calcaneus, and lower end of the tibia is rough, and a small patchy slightly long T1 abnormal signal is seen inside; STIR shows a high signal, and a small round higher signal is seen inside. The base of the fourth and fifth metatarsal bones shows a small patchy slightly long T1 abnormal signal in the marrow cavity, and STIR shows a slightly high signal. The course of the Achilles tendon is continuous, and a linear slightly high signal is seen inside. Abnormal fluid signal is seen in the right ankle joint. Diagnosis: The right foot is consistent with the MRI manifestation of diabetic foot, Charcot joint formation, multiple abnormal signals in the marrow cavity of multiple bones in the mid-foot, hindfoot, and lower end of the tibia; abnormal signal in the right Achilles tendon, Achilles tendonitis; right ankle joint effusion (Fig. 3.4).

4. Vascular examination. ① Lower limb arterial ultrasound: Arteriosclerosis of both lower limbs. ② Lower limb venous ultrasound: No obstruction was seen in the deep and superficial

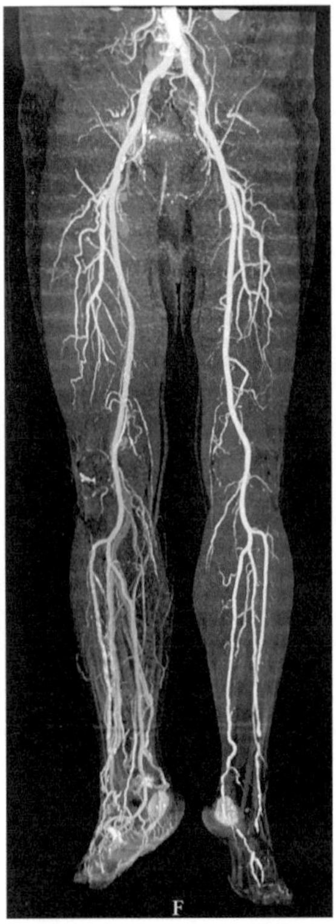

Fig. 3.5 Lower limb arteriography

veins of both lower limbs. ③ computed tomography angiography (CTA) of both lower limbs: Lower segment of the abdominal aorta, multiple eccentric atherosclerotic plaques and calcified plaques were seen on the walls of the bilateral common iliac arteries, internal and external iliac arteries, femoral arteries, popliteal arteries, anterior and posterior tibial arteries, and peroneal arteries. There was varying degrees of narrowing in the local lumen, especially in the deep arteries of the bilateral lower legs. During the arterial scan, multiple deep and superficial veins in the right lower limb were prematurely enhanced. The soft tissue density in the right lower leg was lower than that on the opposite side. The deep and superficial veins in the right ankle and foot were thickened, tortuous, and disordered (Fig. 3.5).

[Preliminary Diagnosis] Type 2 diabetic foot ulcer and peripheral neuropathy, type 2 diabetic foot ulcer and peripheral vascular disease, type 2 diabetic Charcot's joint disease, foot soft tissue infection (right), type 2 diabetic foot, type 2 diabetes, hyperlipidemia.

[Treatment and Outcome] After admission, the patient's insulin was adjusted to control blood sugar within a reasonable range. At the same time, symptomatic treatment was given for anti-infection, swelling reduction, circulation improvement, and neurotrophic drugs. After completing preoperative preparations, debridement of necrotic tissue on the right foot + platelet-rich fibrin (PRF) injection repair surgery were performed under local anesthesia. The patient was placed in the supine position. After satisfactory anesthesia, the surgical area was routinely disinfected, sterile drapes were laid, and a 5.0 cm × 4.0 cm wound was found on the right foot. The wound was concave with a large amount of inflammatory granulation tissue formation, and necrotic tissue formation was seen around the wound. The inflammatory granulation tissue in the wound was removed with a curette, and after the necrotic tissue around the wound was excised, fresh bloody fluid was seen seeping out from the wound. After the wound was rinsed three times with hydrogen peroxide, sterile saline, and dilute iodine, the bleeding was completely stopped with absorbable hemostatic gauze. About 6 mL of liquid PRF prepared by a centrifuge was drawn with a 1-mL syringe and evenly injected into the central part of the wound and the 1, 3, 5, 7, 9, 11 points of the wound edge. The wound was dressed with oil gauze and fixed with sterile gauze (Figs. 3.6 and 3.7).

Postoperative treatment continues under the premise of insulin control of blood sugar, including anti-infection, swelling reduction, circulation improvement, and symptomatic treatment with nutritional nerve drugs. The wound is treated with alginate dressing for drainage and silver ion gel dressing for dressing change (Fig. 3.8).

To accelerate wound healing, debridement + PRF injection repair surgery was performed again on the necrotic tissue of the right foot bottom under local anesthesia on the 14th day after surgery (Figs. 3.9 and 3.10).

Postoperative treatment continues under the premise of insulin control of blood sugar, includ-

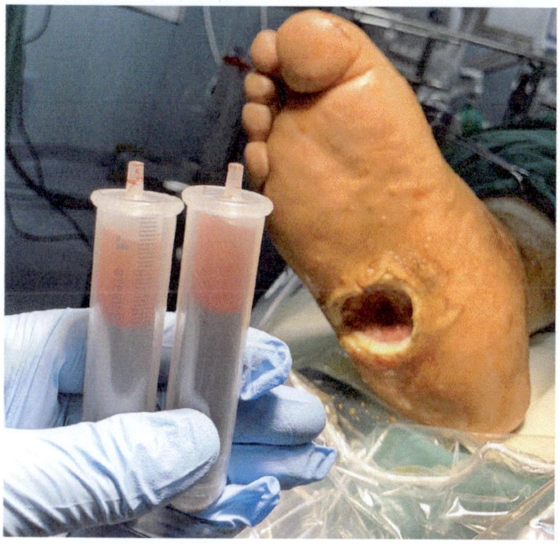

Fig. 3.6 Necrotic tissue of the right foot bottom debridement + PRF injection repair surgery

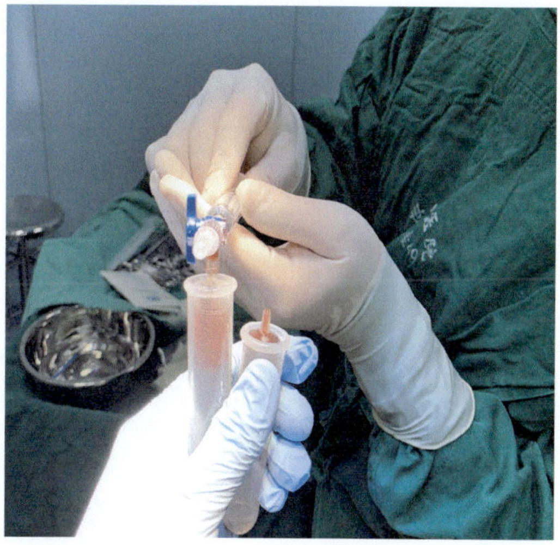

Fig. 3.7 Extraction of prepared liquid PRF

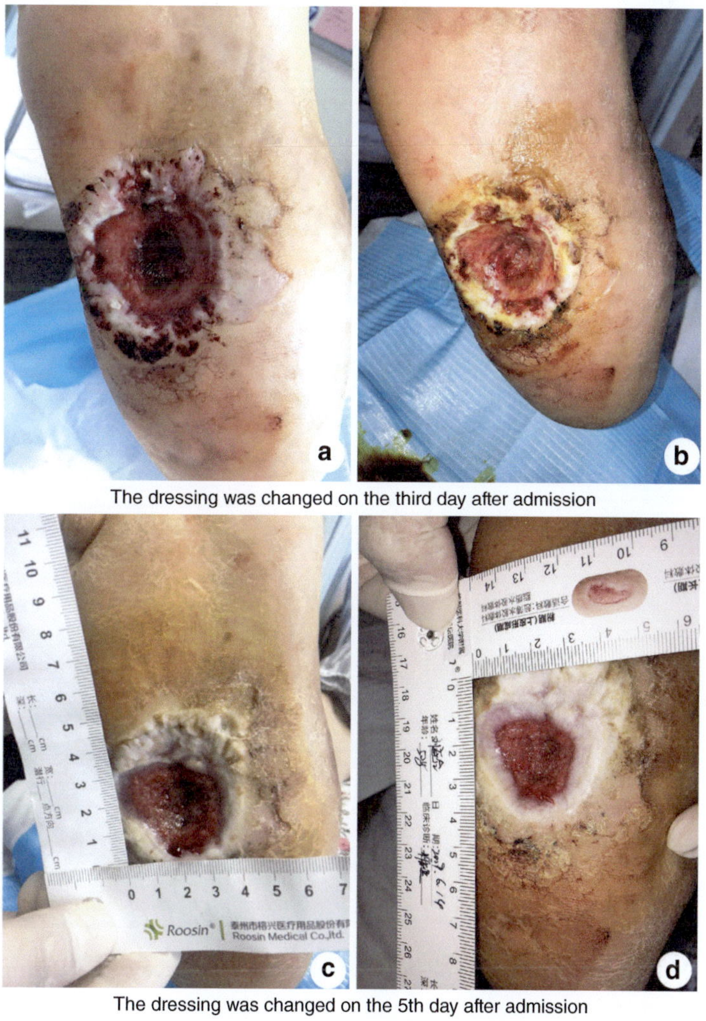

Fig. 3.8 Postoperative wound. (**a**) The dressing was changed on the third day after admission. (**b**) The dressing was changed on the fifth day after admission

ing anti-infection, swelling reduction, circulation improvement, and symptomatic treatment with nutritional nerve drugs. The wound is treated with alginate dressing for drainage and silver ion gel dressing for dressing change (Fig. 3.11).

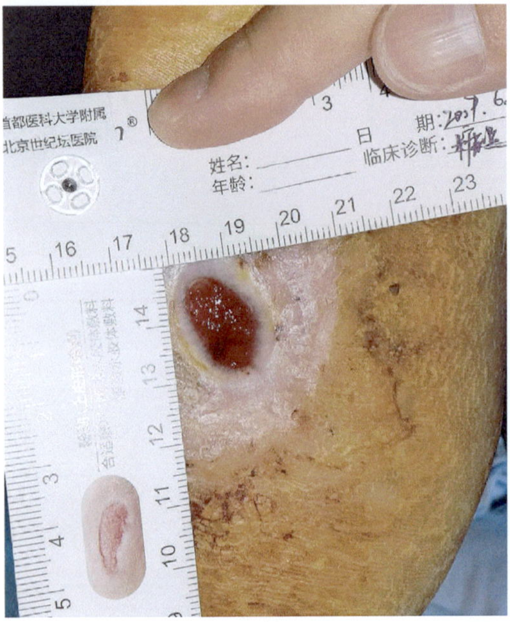

Fig. 3.9 The wound reduced to 2.0 cm × 1.5 cm on the 14th day after surgery

The patient's wound healed 27 days after admission, as shown in Fig. 3.12, which depicts the appearance of the patient's foot. Due to the presence of Charcot's foot, a second phase of biomechanical three-dimensional reconstruction was required, along with the production of pressure-relieving orthotic insoles and footwear, to ensure walking function while preventing the recurrence of foot ulcers.

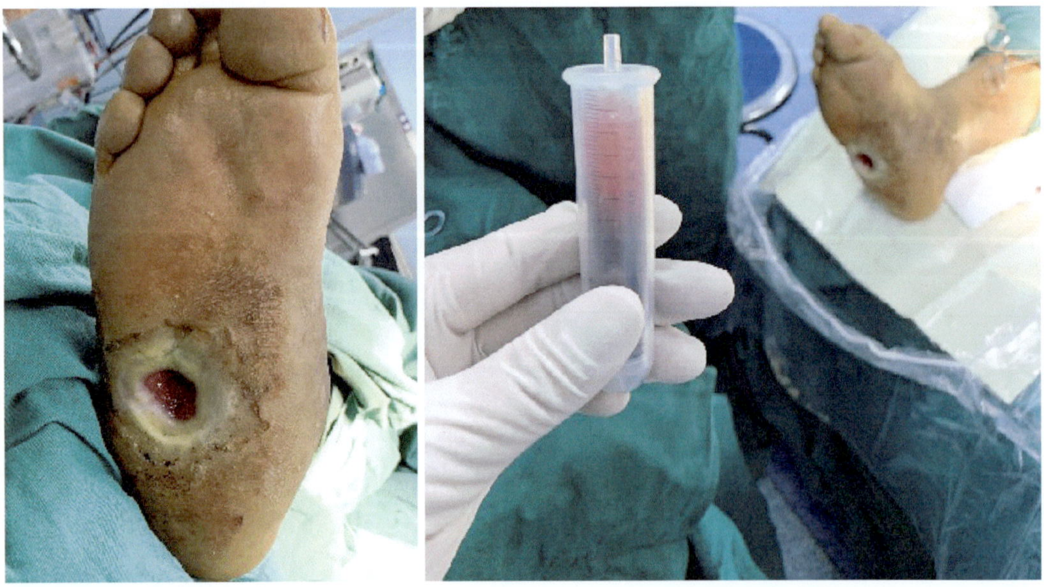

Fig. 3.10 Debridement + PRF injection repair surgery on necrotic tissue of right foot bottom

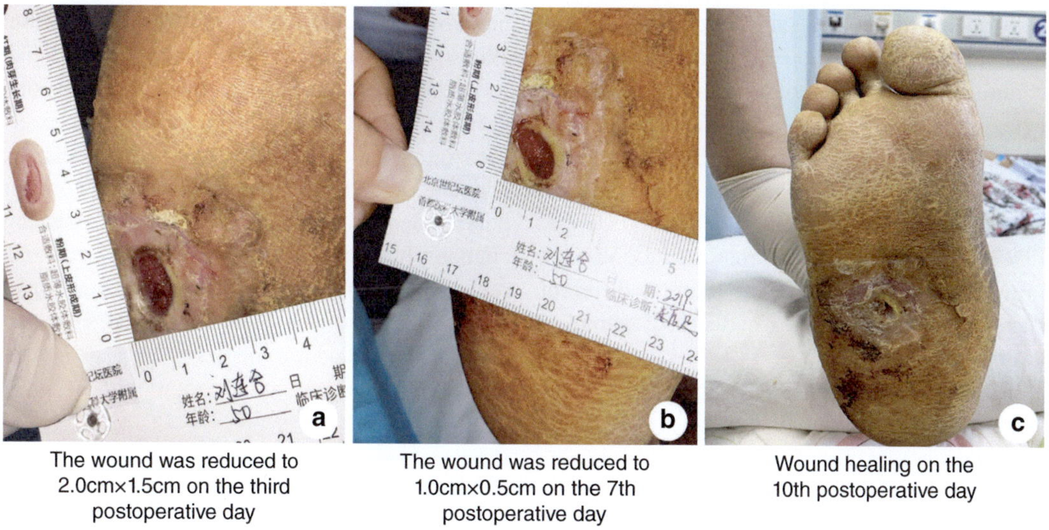

Fig. 3.11 Wound after the second surgery. (**a**) The wound was reduced to 2.0 cm × 1.5 cm on the third postoperative day. (**b**) The wound was reduced to 1.0 cm × 0.5 cm on the seventh postoperative day. (**c**) Wound healing on the tenth postoperative day

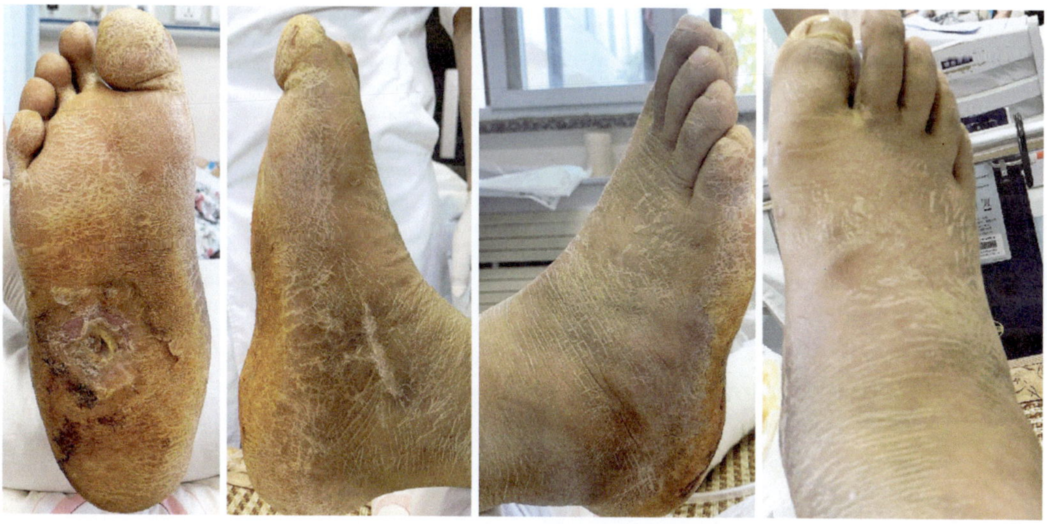

Fig. 3.12 Appearance of the right foot sole, medial side, lateral side, and dorsum

3.2 Case Analysis

3.2.1 The Mechanism of Action of Injectable PRF in Wound Repair

The standard preparation process for PRF involves placing venous blood in a dry centrifuge tube without anticoagulant. Under the strong centrifugal force of the centrifuge, substances with different sedimentation rates in the blood are separated, achieving blood stratification: the upper layer is the pale yellow platelet plasma layer, the bottom layer is the red cell fragment layer, and between them is the fibrin gel layer rich in platelets. By changing the centrifugation program, an injectable form of PRF (i-PRF) can be formed without using any anticoagulants. The latter appears similar to PRP in appearance, but contains the highest concentrations of leukocytes, platelets, growth factors, and fibrinogen. Thus, the new generation of PRF possesses both solid and liquid forms.

PRF is rich in VEGF, bFGF, TGF-β1, PDGF-AB, IGFs, matrix proteins, etc. Various growth factors play different roles at different stages, forming a complex network of signaling molecule regulation.

PDGF is a key growth factor in the early stages of tissue healing, promoting the proliferation and chemotaxis of stem cells, fibroblasts, and chondrocytes; TGF-β can enhance the proliferation of fibroblasts, promote the secretion of the matrix and the deposition of bone matrix; TGF-β can inhibit the formation of osteoclasts and bone resorption; VEGF can promote endothelial cell migration and mitosis, and is a powerful angiogenic factor. A unique feature of PRF is the role of fibrin, which slowly forms a three-dimensional, loose, and elastic fibrin clot through equilateral connections, facilitating the integration of cell factors, providing a place for cell adhesion, migration, and differentiation, and its three-dimensional structure allows it to slowly release growth factors and cell factors during the wound healing process, thereby prolonging the action time of factors in the wound.

3.2.2 Offloading Treatment of Charcot's Foot Wound

The patient in this case has Charcot's foot, and 3 years ago, due to foot ulcers, he underwent necrotic bone removal and external fixation. When asked about the patient's postoperative recovery, he reported that he did not take any load reduction measures after the removal of the external fixator, walked normally with weight-bearing, and a foot ulcer reappeared a year ago. After debridement, the wound healed with dressing changes, but he still did not take any formal load reduction measures after the operation, leading to the recurrence of the ulcer. It can be seen that regular load reduction measures are a guarantee to prevent the recurrence of foot ulcers.

Bibliography

1. Chiaravalloti AJ, Zubkov B, Zubkov A. Treatment of a chronic cutaneous surgical wound with platelet-rich fibrin. Dermatologic Surg. 2018;44(3):449–52.
2. Yang L, Jiangning W. Progress in the application of platelet-rich blood products in tissue wound healing. Chin J Med Aesthetics Beauty. 2018;24(3):159–61.
3. Miron RJ, Fujioka-Kobayashi M, Hernandez M, et al. Injectable platelet rich fibrin (i-PRF):opportunities in regenerative dentistry? Clin Oral Investig. 2017;21(8):2619–27.
4. Balse N, Baliga S. Evaluation of wound healing and bone regeneration using autologous platelet-rich plasma and platelet-rich fibrin postextractions: a comparative study. Indian J Heal Sci Bio Res (KLEU). 2017;10(2):167–72.
5. Jiangning W, Lei G, Tiangui C, et al. Professor Wang Jiangning's team's in-depth analysis of diabetic foot comprehensive diagnosis and treatment cases. Beijing: Science and Technology Literature Publishing House; 2018.

4 Two Cases of Lower Extremity Diabetic Necrotizing Fasciitis Wounds

Xinyuan Qin, Tiangui Chen, and Jiangning Wang

4.1 Case Summary

4.1.1 Case 1

Patient, male, 45 years old. The main reason for hospitalization was swelling in the distal right lower leg for 10 days, worsening with pain for 2 days.

[Present Illness] The patient experienced swelling in the distal right calf without any obvious cause 10 days ago. After receiving puncture treatment at a local hospital, the swelling slightly subsided. However, the swelling worsened again 2 days ago, accompanied by pain. The patient came to our hospital for further treatment. The outpatient department admitted the patient with "Type 2 Diabetic Necrotizing Fasciitis." The patient's general health condition is average, and his diet, sleep, and bowel movements have been normal since the onset of the disease, with occasional low fever.

[Past History] The patient denies a history of hypertension. He has a two-year history of diabetes and has been treated with insulin injections (16 IU of Humalog before breakfast, lunch, and dinner, and 10 IU of Lantus before bedtime). He has a history of cirrhosis and has been treated with hepatoprotective drugs orally. He has a history of surgery (spleen removal in a Beijing hospital in 2016), blood product transfusion, and drug allergy (sulfa drugs).

[Admission Examination]

1. Specialist examination. The distal right calf to the dorsum of the right foot is significantly swollen, soft, with poor mobility, adhered to the skin, with a sense of fluctuation, obvious tenderness, and limited ankle joint movement (Fig. 4.1).
2. Laboratory examination. White Blood Cell (WBC) $14.71 \times 10^9/L$, neutrophil percentage 85.2%, Hemoglobin (HGB) 48 g/L, albumin 26.3 g/L, C-Reactive Protein (CRP) 159.82 mg/L.
3. Imaging examination. CT of the calf +3D reconstruction: Swelling of the soft tissue under the skin of the right calf, right ankle, and right foot, with strip-like slightly high-density shadows; the muscles are more swollen than the opposite side, showing multiple patchy slightly low-density shadows, CT value about 23 HU, especially in the posterior muscles (gastrocnemius, soleus), with unclear boundaries (Fig. 4.2).

[Treatment and Outcome] After admission, the patient completed preoperative examinations and urgently underwent necrotizing fasciotomy +

X. Qin · T. Chen · J. Wang (✉)
Department of Orthopedics, Beijing Shijitan Hospital, Capital Medical University, Beijing, China
e-mail: doctorqin1987@163.com; csy800808@163.com; wangjn@bjsjth.cn

J. Wang, L. Gao (eds.), *Refractory Wounds*, Experts' Perspectives on Medical Advances,
https://doi.org/10.1007/978-981-96-2067-8_4

necrotic tissue debridement + vascular nerve tendon exploration surgery on the right calf (Fig. 4.3). Postoperative wound drainage and dressing changes were performed, along with symptomatic treatments such as anti-infection, improving circulation, correcting hypoalbuminemia, correcting anemia, and nutritional support. After the patient's condition stabilized, debridement, fat grafting, and VSD negative pressure suction surgeries were performed successively (Fig. 4.4).

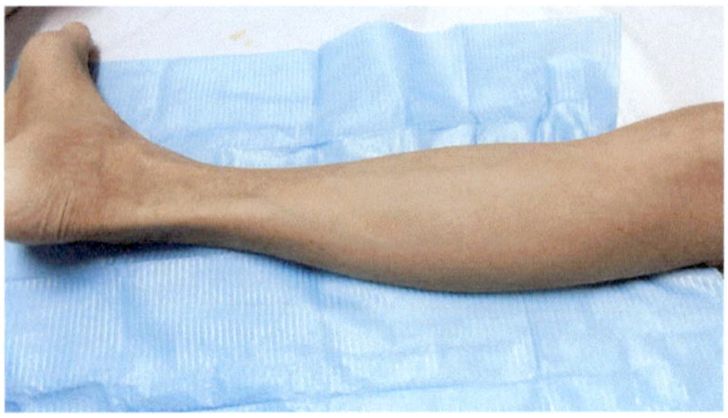

Fig. 4.1 Patient's right calf

After multiple incisions for drainage, multiple surgical debridements, and culture of necrotic tissue from the deep wound and antibiotic use guided by drug sensitivity, the patient's sepsis turned negative, the infection gradually subsided, and suturing was given after the wound granulation was fresh. One week after the suturing, the wound healed well, and the patient was discharged smoothly.

4.1.2 Case 2

Patient, male, 43 years old. The main reason for admission was nonhealing ulcers in the sacrococcygeal area, right hip, and right thigh for more than 3 months.

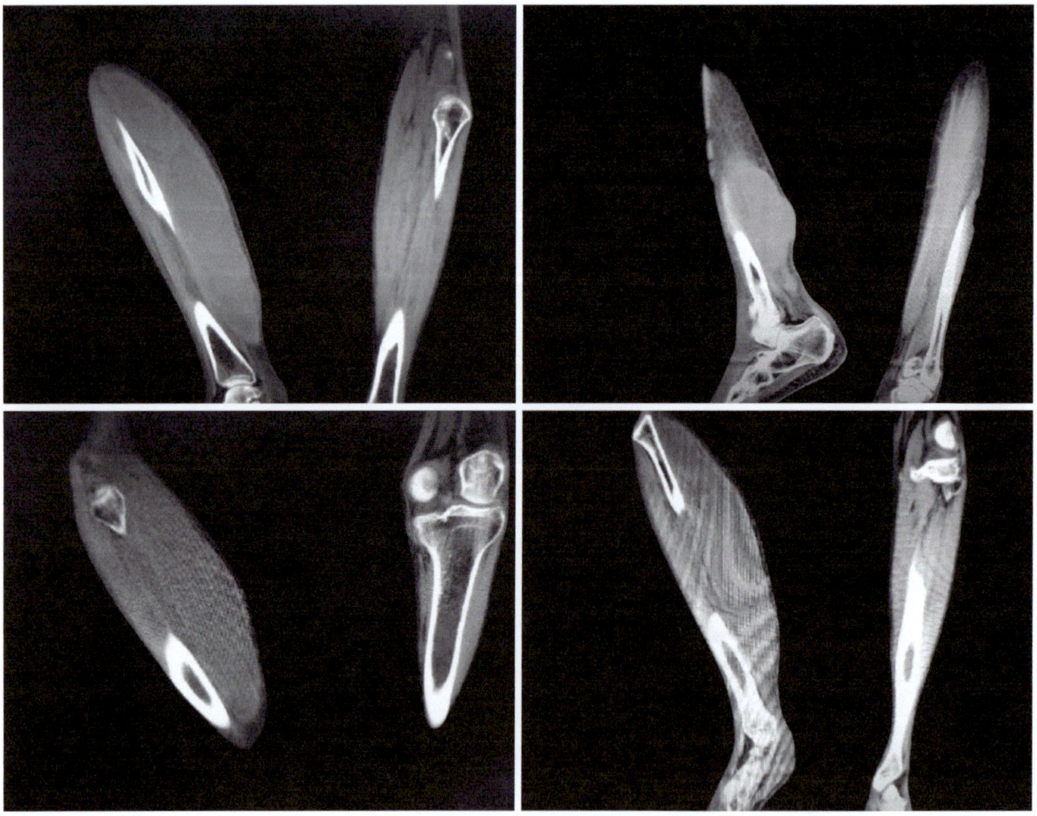

Fig. 4.2 Imaging examination

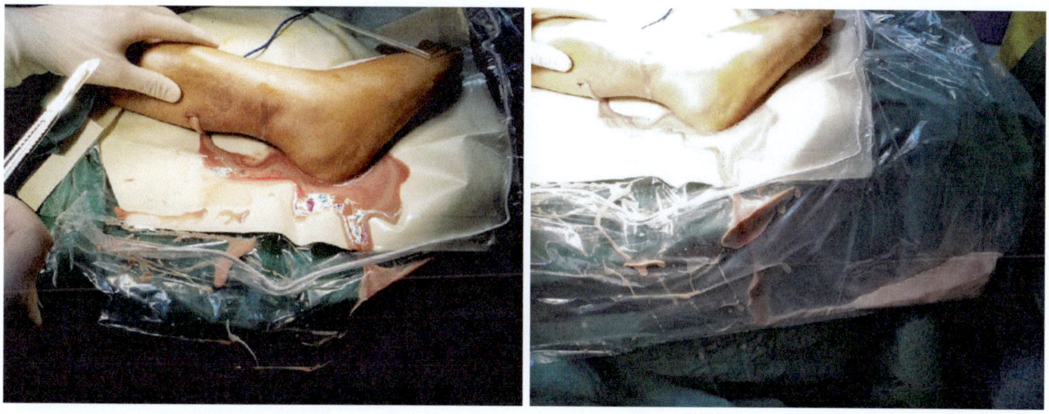

Fig. 4.3 Emergency surgery on the right lower leg

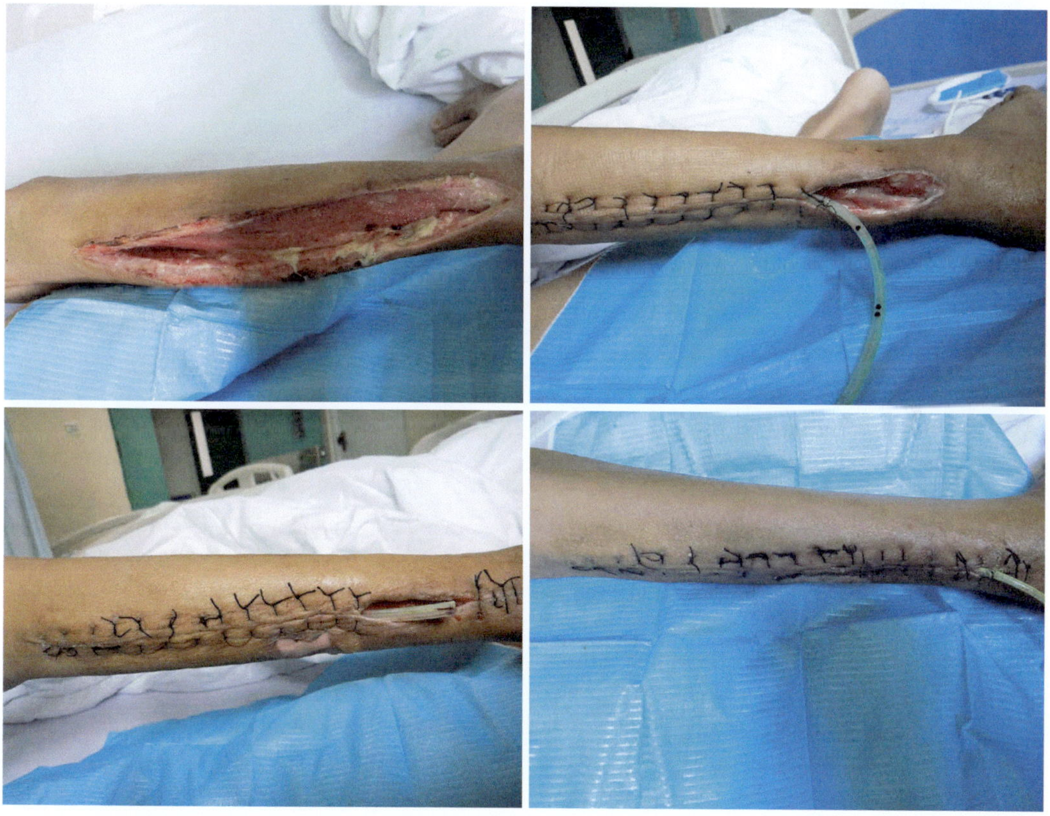

Fig. 4.4 Continued surgical treatment after the patient's condition stabilizes

[Present Illness History] The patient had been bedridden for a long time, and 3 months ago, ulcers appeared in the sacrococcygeal area, right hip, and right thigh. He changed the dressing at home, but the wound never healed, with yellow pus oozing out, accompanied by an odor. He did not pay much attention to it. One day ago, he had a fever, reaching a maximum of 39.0 °C, and was given anti-infection (specific drugs unknown), fever reduction, and dressing change treatment at a local hospital. The symptoms did not significantly alleviate, so he came to our hospital's emergency department for further diagnosis and treatment, and was admitted to the hospital with "soft tissue infection."

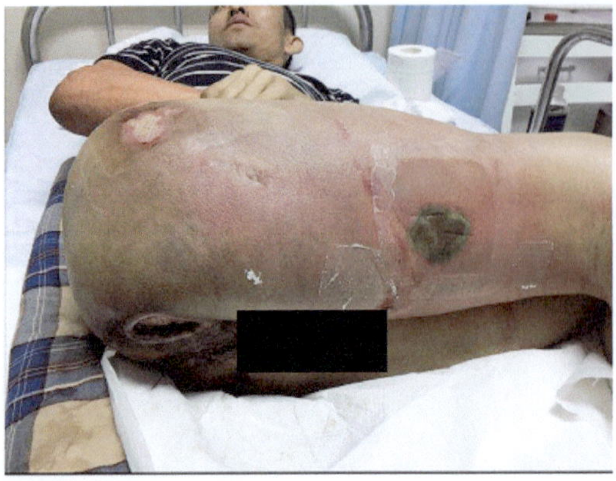

Fig. 4.5 Thigh wound

[Past Medical History] The patient was paralyzed in the lower limbs due to tuberculous meningitis 20 years ago. He has a history of type 2 diabetes, but it is not specifically controlled; he has a history of syringomyelia. He denies a history of hypertension, hyperlipidemia, coronary heart disease, denies a history of hepatitis and close contact, denies a history of surgery, trauma, blood product transfusion, denies a history of drug and food allergies. Vaccinations were carried out as planned.

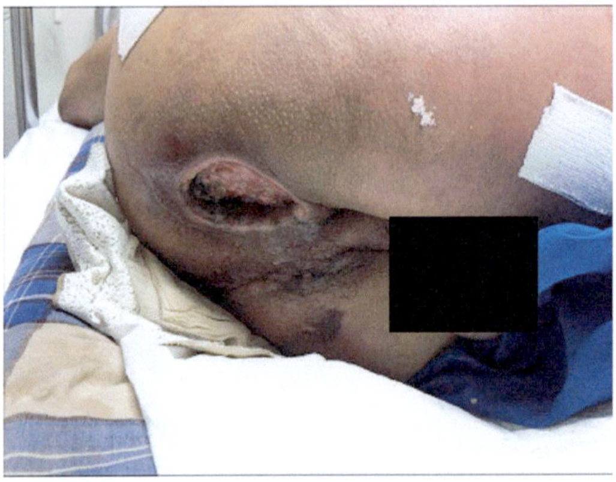

Fig. 4.6 Sacrococcygeal wound

[Admission Examination]

1. Specialist examination. Normal development, malnutrition, clear consciousness, semi-recumbent position, expression in pain; the patient was wheeled into the ward, cooperative during the examination. A wound approximately 10.0 cm × 5.0 cm in size can be seen in the sacrococcygeal area, the wound is dirty, with a large amount of necrotic secretion visible, reaching the bone tissue, with a severe odor; a wound approximately 7.0 cm × 5.0 cm in size can be seen on the back of the right thigh, the wound is dirty and dark, with a large amount of necrotic secretion visible, the depth is unmeasurable, with a severe odor; two wounds approximately 4.0 cm × 4.0 cm in size can be seen on the right hip, the wound is not clean, with a small amount of secretion visible, no odor, the wound edge is neat, proliferative scar tissue can be seen around it. The skin of the right thigh and right buttock is obviously red and swollen, with obvious tenderness (Figs. 4.5 and 4.6).
2. Laboratory examination. ① Blood routine: WBC 15.03 × 10^9/L, neutrophil percentage 92.8%, HGB 91 g/L. ② Blood biochemistry: albumin 19.8 g/L. ③ CRP 88.75 mg/L. ④ Dynamic ESR 39 mm/h. ⑤ PCT 1.42 ng/mL. ⑥ The results of deep wound bacterial culture are *Staphylococcus aureus, Escherichia coli*, and *Streptococcus dysgalactiae*.
3. Imaging examination. Pelvis + right thigh CT + three-dimensional reconstruction: gas density shadow in the right buttock, pelvis, and right thigh soft tissue, considering infection (Fig. 4.7).

[Treatment and Outcome] After admission, the patient was given symptomatic treatment such as

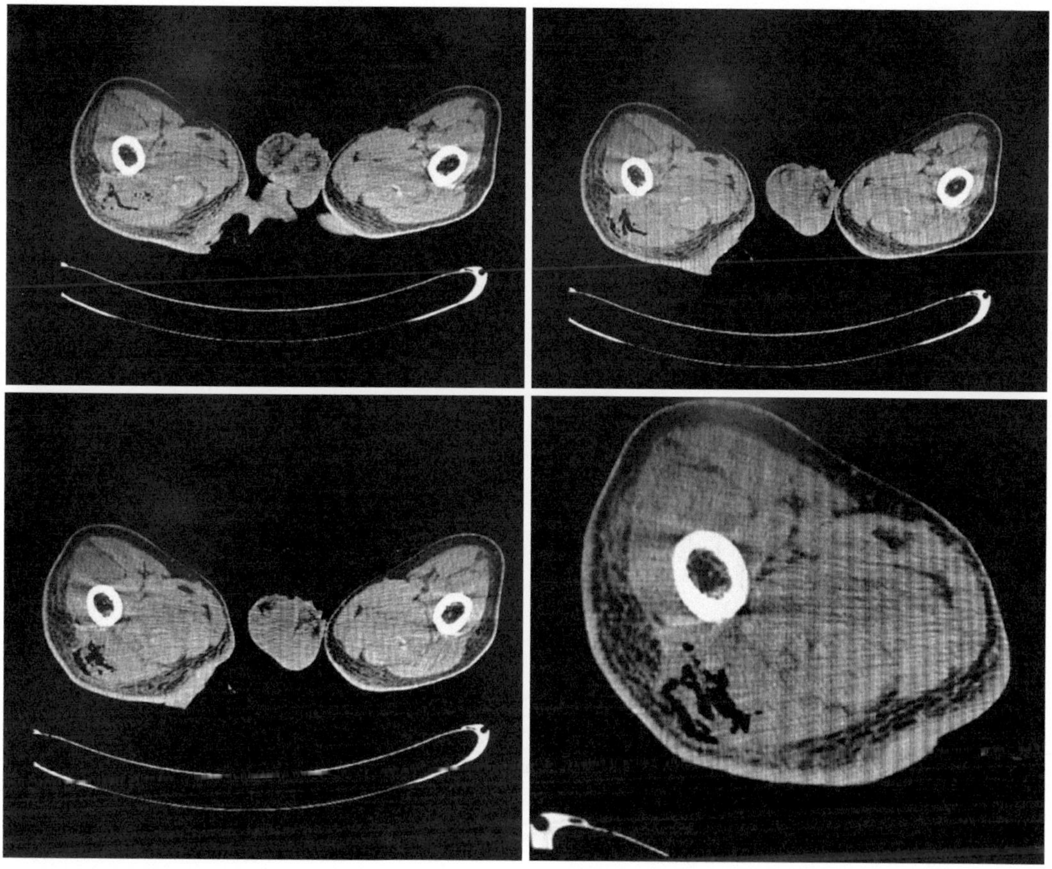

Fig. 4.7 Imaging examination

anti-infection, improving circulation, correcting hypoalbuminemia, nutritional support, and so on. After excluding surgical contraindications, necrotic fascia incision and drainage of the right buttock and right thigh + necrotic tissue debridement + vascular nerve tendon exploration surgery were performed under anesthesia, and the wound was drained and dressed after surgery (Fig. 4.8).

After multiple incision drainage, multiple surgical debridement treatments, deep necrotic tissue culture of the wound guided by drug sensitivity, and the use of antimicrobial drugs, the patient's sepsis turned negative, the infection gradually reduced, and after the wound granulation was fresh, suturing was given. Two weeks after the suturing, the wound healed, the sutures were removed, all inflammation indicators dropped to normal, and the patient was successfully discharged (Fig. 4.9).

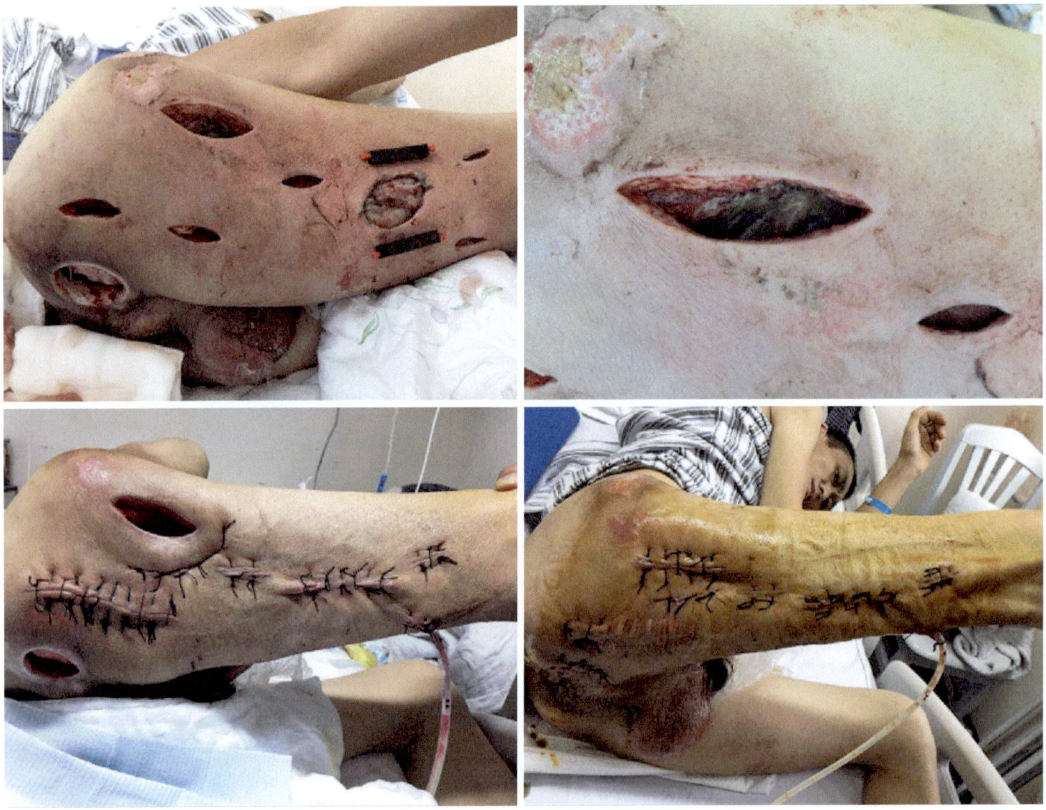

Fig. 4.8 Treatment situation

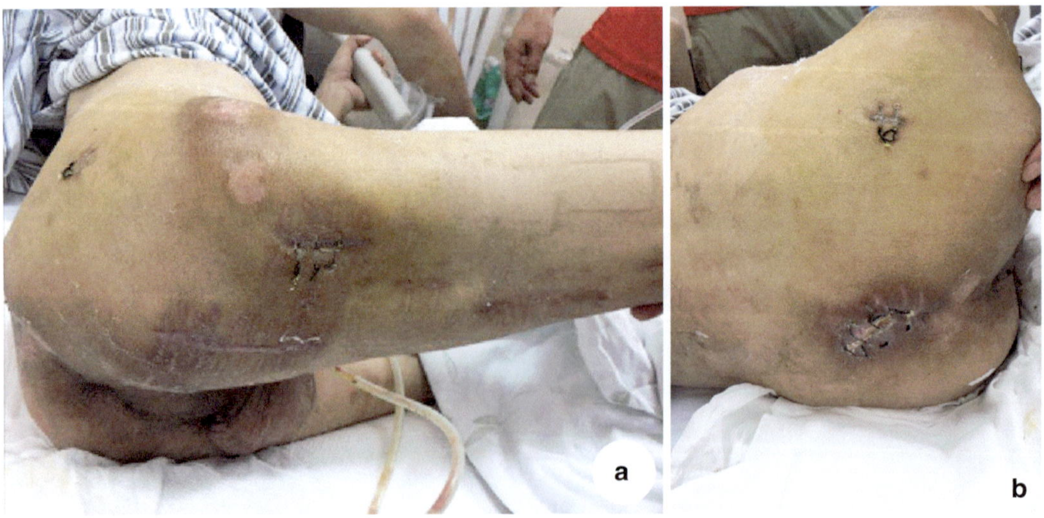

Fig. 4.9 Wound healing. (**a**) Buttock wound. (**b**) Sacrococcygeal wound

4.2 Case Analysis

4.2.1 Type 2 Diabetic Necrotizing Fasciitis

Necrotizing fasciitis (NF) is a rapidly progressing infectious disease, with the infection spreading along the deep and superficial fascia, not involving the muscle layer tissue, forming thrombi in the involved vessels, causing necrosis of the skin, subcutaneous tissue, and fascia in the corresponding area. The infection is often accompanied by sepsis, septicemia, and multiple organ failure, etc. The lesions often occur in the abdomen, perineum, and limbs, with the limbs being the most common, and there are also reports of the disease in the head and neck. NF involving the perineum, vulva, and perianal area is also known as Fournier's gangrene. The presentation of NF is similar to cellulitis, but progresses more rapidly. Because it is relatively rare clinically, it is very difficult to distinguish, so it is easy to misdiagnose. In Canada, four out of every 100,000 people have NF; in Florida, USA, only 1.3 cases per 100,000 people are diagnosed. Although the incidence of NF is not high, the mortality rate is as high as about 20%, and the hospital stay is long, the condition is dangerous, and the cost is huge. Spanish scholars have found that the average hospital stay for NF survivors is 27.54 days, with an average cost of 25,108.67 euros, and 32.4% of patients need to be admitted to the intensive care unit. Arifi and others reported that the average hospital stay for NF patients is 43 days.

At present, the medical community has not yet formed a consensus on how to effectively manage NF. Diabetes is the most common cause of NF, accounting for 18–60%. As the incidence of diabetes in our country continues to rise, the number of patients with NF combined with diabetes is gradually increasing. If not diagnosed in time or improperly treated, it can lead to severe sepsis, amputation, and even life-threatening conditions. Therefore, how to reduce the mortality rate of patients with NF combined with diabetes and preserve limb function to the greatest extent has gradually attracted the attention of clinical doctors. Early diagnosis, the use of sufficient and effective antibiotics, and active and thorough drainage are the keys to treatment. At present, wound repair mainly involves surgical debridement and amputation. However, the wounds of patients with NF combined with diabetes are different from general surgical wounds, not only the onset is urgent, the progress is fast, the disease is severe, the condition is dangerous, the prognosis is poor, but also the course of the disease is long, the treatment is difficult, the effect is slow, the cost is high, the recurrence rate is high, the disability and mortality rate is high, and the difficulty of repair is relatively large.

4.2.2 Differential Diagnosis of NF Combined with Diabetes

NF combined with diabetes should be differentiated from the following diseases. ① Erysipelas. Local patchy erythema, high skin temperature, no edema, clear boundaries, accompanied by lymphangitis and lymph node lesions, soft tissue swelling or skin necrosis is relatively light, systemic symptoms are lighter. ② Cellulitis. It only involves the subcutaneous tissue, the fascia is normal, often accompanied by lymphatic invasion, imaging shows subcutaneous tissue thickening, fat tissue density increased, accompanied by strip-like irregular enhancement, with or without subcutaneous and superficial fascial effusion, deep structures are normal. Effective treatment with sensitive antibiotics. ③ Streptococcal necrosis. Mainly caused by beta-hemolytic streptococcus infection. Skin necrosis occurs, not involving the fascia. Early local skin redness and swelling, with blisters, containing bloody serum and bacteria. After the epidermis necrosis, it dries and scabs, similar to burn scabs. ④ *Clostridium perfringens* gas gangrene. It is common in deep contaminated wounds, characterized by rapid muscle necrosis, severe local pain, often accompanied by systemic poisoning and central nervous system changes. ⑤ Aerobic streptococcal myositis. Mainly involves the muscles, often accompanied by rapidly developing gangrene and severe local pain. ⑥ Other diseases, such as fasciitislipomembranous syndrome, diabetic gangrene, gangrenous pyoderma, etc.

4.2.3 Treatment of NF Combined with Diabetes

Early diagnosis and treatment are the keys to improving the survival rate of patients with NF combined with diabetes. Current clinical treatment mainly includes internal medicine treatment and surgical debridement.

4.2.3.1 Internal Treatment

① Infection control for NF. In the treatment of infections combined with diabetes, broad-spectrum antibiotics should be actively used. The principle is to adopt a "step-down therapy." Before the results of bacterial culture and sensitivity tests are clear, antibiotics should be used in combination. The antibacterial spectrum should include antibiotics that are sensitive and effective against both Gram-positive and Gram-negative bacteria, taking into account anaerobic bacteria, to quickly control the infection and reduce the loss of subcutaneous tissue. Subsequently, the antibiotic treatment plan can be further adjusted according to the results of the sensitivity test and the patient's clinical effect. The antibacterial spectrum of penicillin and aminoglycoside antibiotics can cover almost all pathogens. ② Blood sugar control. Use insulin to lower blood sugar to near normal. General experience suggests that controlling blood sugar within 10.0 mmol/L is beneficial for controlling wound infection and promoting granulation growth. ③ Supportive treatment. This includes nutritional support and correction of water and electrolyte disorders. Adequate nutritional support can help reduce morbidity and mortality. For patients with anemia and hypoproteinemia, fresh blood or blood products (albumin or plasma, etc.) can be transfused. Nasal feeding or intravenous high nutrition, elemental diet, etc. can be used to ensure sufficient calorie intake. If necessary, total parenteral nutrition should be given, and the nutritional calories should be at least twice the basic metabolism.

4.2.3.2 Surgical Debridement for Necrotizing Fasciitis (NF)

Once diagnosed, aggressive surgical intervention and debridement are crucial. However, NF in patients with diabetes is very complex. Aggressive surgical debridement can not only exacerbate local tissue ischemia and edema, progressive tissue necrosis, and gradually enlarge the necrotic area, but it may also lead to severe complications such as heart, brain, and kidney. Therefore, surgical debridement is more suitable for NF patients with diabetes. This debridement method is divided into three stages of treatment. The first stage is the basic treatment stage: this stage requires active drainage, and there is no rush to perform large-scale thorough debridement. Only by fully opening, draining, and exposing the wound tissue can the further development of NF be effectively controlled and prepared for the next stage of treatment. When necessary, multiple extensive incisions should be made, and the width of the incision should be larger than the edge of the wound. The second stage is the necrotic removal stage: after infection control, microcirculation improvement, and complication correction, the debridement is mostly done by surgical debridement, focusing on necrotic removal, increasing drainage, and gradually removing necrotic tissue. The fascial space between the separated incisions and the subcutaneous tissue and fascia should be fully freed and removed, and thorough debridement should be performed until fresh tissue bleeding. The third stage is the muscle regeneration stage: various muscle regeneration methods are used to promote granulation tissue regeneration and achieve wound healing. In addition, VSD technology is very effective in treating complex wounds. Hyperbaric oxygen therapy is commonly used in clinical practice as an auxiliary treatment, which can promote the growth of granulation tissue, promote repair, and accelerate healing.

Bibliography

1. Malghem J, Lecouvet FE, Omoumi P, et al. Necrotizing fasciitis: contribution and limitations of diagnostic imaging. Joint Bone Spine. 2013;80(2):146–54.

2. Kani R, Mcgeer A, Low DE, et al. Population-based surveillance for group a streptococcal necrotizing fasciitis: clinical features, prognostic indicators, and microbiologic analysis of seventy-seven cases. Ontario Group a Streptococcal study. Am J Med. 1997;103(1):18–24.
3. Mulla ZD, Gibbs SG, Amnoff DM. Correlates of length of stay, cost of care, and mortality among patients hospitalized for necrotizing fasciitis. Epidemiol Infect. 2007;135(5):868–76.
4. Khamnuan P, Chongruksut W, Jearwattanakanok K, et al. Necrotizing fasciitis: risk factors of mortality. Risk Manag Healthc Policy. 2015;8:1–7.
5. Jiménez-Pacheco A, Arrabal-Polo M, Arias-Santiago S, et al. Fournier gangrene: description of 37 cases and analysis of associated health care costs. Actas Dermosifiliogr. 2012;103(1):29–35.
6. Arifi HM, Duci SB, Zatriqi VK, et al. A retrospective study of 22 patients with necrotising fasciitis treated at the University Clinical Center of Kosovo (2005—2010). Int Wound J. 2013;10(4):461–5.
7. Hung CC, Chang SC, Lin SF, et al. Clinical manifestations, microbiology and prognosis of 42 patients with necrotizing fasciitis. J Formos Med Assoc. 1996;95(12):917–22.
8. Dufel S, Martino M. Simple cellulitis or a more serious infection? J Fam Pract. 2006;55(5):396–400.
9. Ayestaray B, Dudrap E, Chartaux E, et al. Necrotizing pyoderma gangrenosum: an unusual differential diagnosis of necrotizing fasciitis. J Plast Reconstr Aesthet Surg. 2010;63(8):655–8.
10. Barr KL, Chhatwal HK, Wesson SK, et al. Pyoderma gangrenosum masquerading as necrotizing fasciitis. Am J Otolaryngol. 2009;30(4):273–6.
11. Bucca K, Spencer R, Orford N, et al. Early diagnosis and treatment of necrotizing fasciitis can improve survival: an observational intensive care unit cohort study. ANZ J Surg. 2013;83(5):365–70.
12. Sroczyński M, Sebastian M, Rudnicki J, et al. A complex approach to the treatment of Fournier's gangrene. Adv Clin Exp Med. 2013;22(1):131–5.
13. Childers BJ, Potyondy LD, Nachreiner R, et al. Necrotizing fasciitis: a fourteen-year retrospective study of 163 consecutive patients. Am Surg. 2002;68(2):109–16.
14. Leiblein M, Marzi I, Sander AL, et al. Necrotizing fasciitis: treatment concepts and clinical results. Eur J Trauma Emerg Surg. 2018;44(2):279–90.
15. Pastore AL, Palleschi G, Ripoli A, et al. A multistep approach to manage Fournier's gangrene in a patient with unknown type II diabetes: surgery, hyperbaric oxygen, and vacuum-assisted closure therapy: a case report. J Med Case Rep. 2013;7:1.
16. Devaney B, Frawley G, Frawley L, et al. Necrotising soft tissue infections: the effect of hyperbaric oxygen on mortality. Anaesth Intensive Care. 2015;43(6):685–92.

Case of Necrotizing Fasciitis of the Neck in a Patient with Diabetes

5

Shuo Wang, Jiangning Wang, and Lei Gao

5.1 Case Summary

Patient, male, 56 years old. Admitted to the hospital due to elevated blood sugar for over 4 years and skin infection in the neck for over half a month.

[Medical History] The patient was found to have elevated blood sugar during a physical examination 4 years ago, with random blood sugar levels of 11–12 mmol/L; no symptoms of polyphagia, polydipsia, polyuria, or weight loss. He self-administered metformin hydrochloride 0.25 g (before meals), supplemented with exercise to lower blood sugar, irregular blood sugar monitoring, random blood sugar fluctuated between 7 and 12 mmol/L, no symptoms of blurred vision or numbness in the limbs. Half a month ago, a carbuncle appeared on the skin of the back of the neck, gradually enlarged into an abscess, and treated with anti-infection and dressing changes at a community hospital; specific medication unknown and no improvement. A week ago, he visited our outpatient clinic for incision and regular dressing changes, added acarbose 100 mg (before meals) and glimepiride 120 mg (before breakfast) to lower blood sugar, the wound became more red and swollen, and has not healed to date. He was admitted to the hospital for further diagnosis and treatment with the diagnosis of "diabetic necrotizing fasciitis."

[Past History] Hypertension for over 20 years, highest systolic pressure 160 mmHg, currently taking amlodipine 5 mg (before breakfast) for blood pressure control, and aspirin enteric-coated tablets 100 mg (before breakfast) for antiplatelet therapy. No history of hepatitis B, tuberculosis, or contact history; no other chronic cardiovascular and cerebrovascular disease history; no history of surgery, trauma, or blood transfusion; no food or drug allergy history.

[Family History] His brother and sister have diabetes and are treated with oral hypoglycemic drugs.

[Admission Examination]
The patient underwent various examinations after being transferred to our department from the endocrinology department.

1. Specialist examination: A 2.0 cm × 4.0 cm oblique incision can be seen on the neck, with a large amount of yellow purulent fluid flowing out, and local skin redness and swelling (Fig. 5.1).
2. Laboratory examination. CRP 225.37 mg/L, PCT 0.87 ng/mL, albumin 25.8 g/L, WBC

S. Wang · J. Wang (✉) · L. Gao
Department of Orthopedics, Beijing Shijitan Hospital, Capital Medical University, Beijing, China
e-mail: shenkemao@qq.com; wangjn@bjsjth.cn; gaolei3337@bjsjth.cn

J. Wang, L. Gao (eds.), *Refractory Wounds*, Experts' Perspectives on Medical Advances,
https://doi.org/10.1007/978-981-96-2067-8_5

17.05 × 10^9/L, neutrophils 15.3 × 10^9/L.L, ketone bodies have turned negative.

3. Radiological examination. Neck MRI: Occipital and posterior neck unevenly swollen, subcutaneous local fat largely missing, muscle and interstitial signals diffusely increased (Fig. 5.2).

[Preliminary Diagnosis] Type 2 diabetic necrotizing fasciitis, type 2 diabetic peripheral vascular disease, type 2 diabetic peripheral neuropathy, type 2 diabetic ketoacidosis; sepsis; hypertension level 3, extremely high risk; hypokalemia; hypochloremia; hyponatremia; hypocalcemia; hypoproteinemia; constipation; coagulation dysfunction; elevated tumor markers; abnormal lung imaging diagnosis.

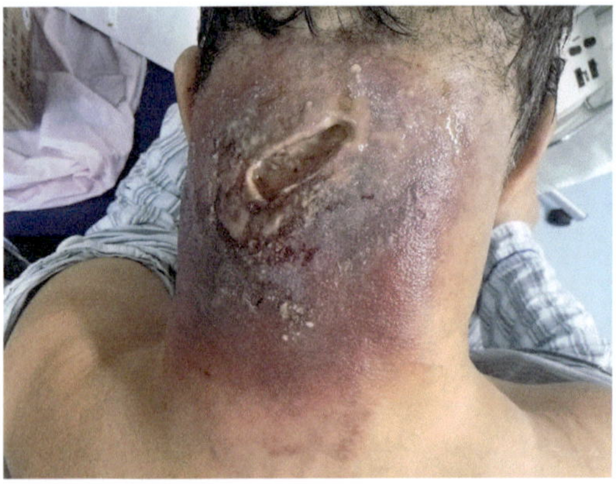

Fig. 5.1 The patient's neck when transferred to our department

[Treatment and Outcome] After admission, the patient was given anti-infection, swelling reduction, and symptomatic treatment to improve circulation. Multiple debridement and VSD surgical treatment were performed in our department. After the operation, the skin tension on the right side of the neck wound was small, and it healed after local suturing; the wound on the left side of the neck was larger, and the skin was stretched with a closure device, followed by a skin grafting operation, and the wound gradually healed (Figs. 5.3, 5.4, 5.5, 5.6, 5.7, 5.8, 5.9 and 5.10).

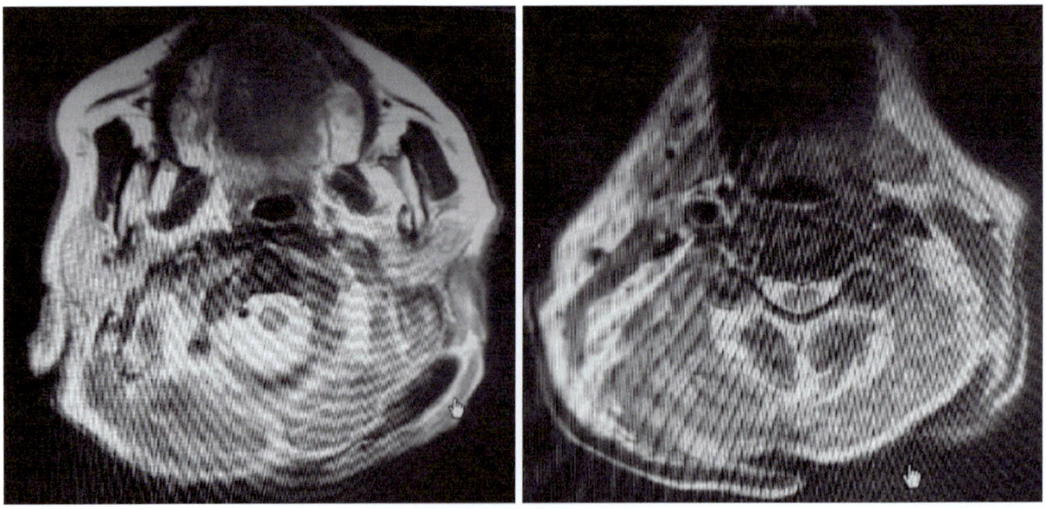

Fig. 5.2 Neck MRI shows large area of loss in the occipital and posterior neck

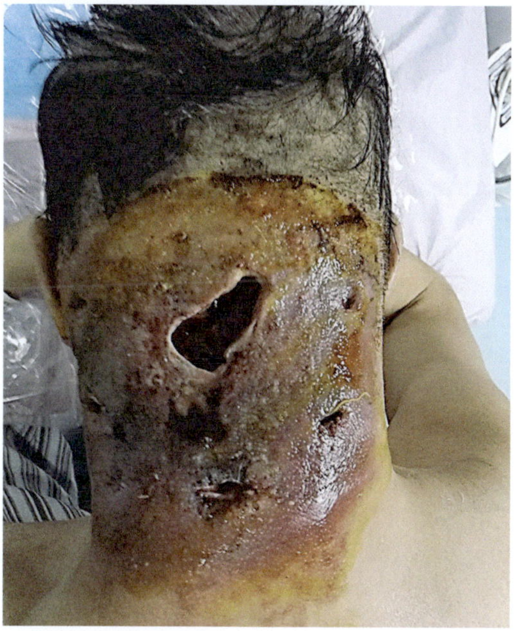

Fig. 5.3 Drainage of pus cavity in the wound, discharge of pus in the wound

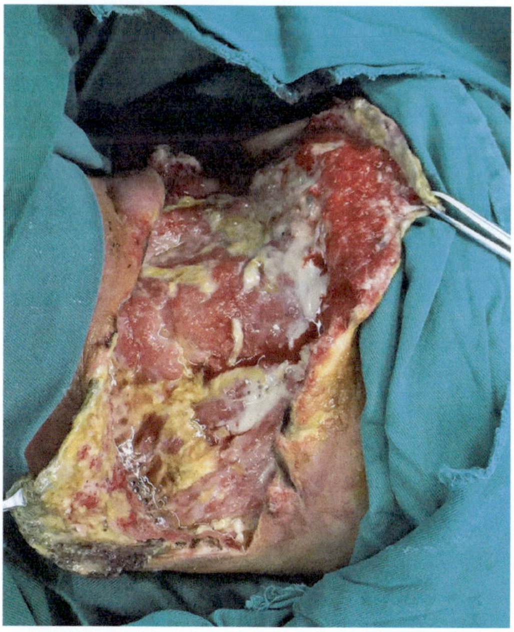

Fig. 5.4 Multiple necrotic tissues removed after surgery

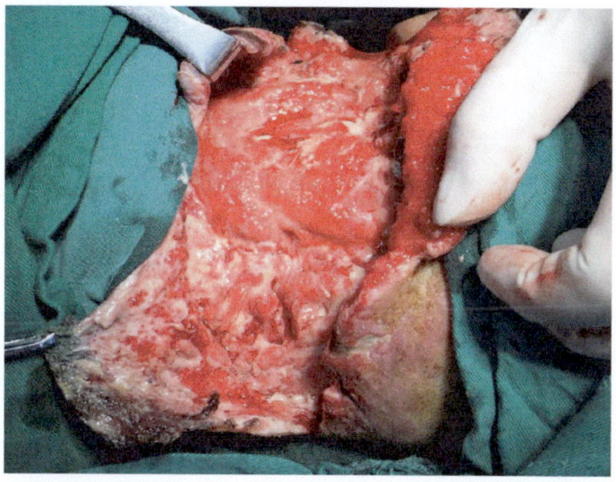

Fig. 5.5 After surgery to remove necrotic tissue

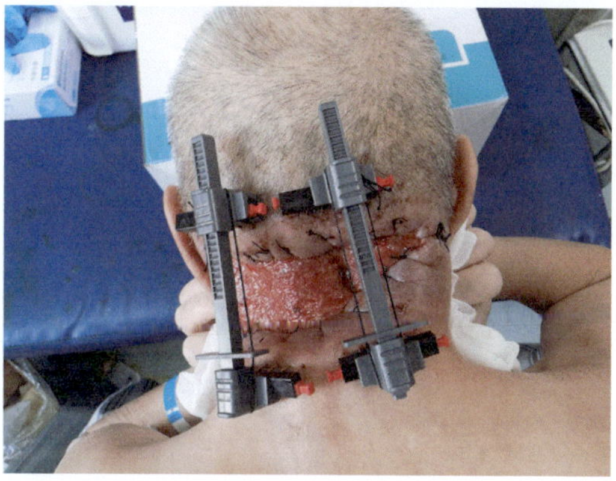

Fig. 5.6 Skin stretched with closure device

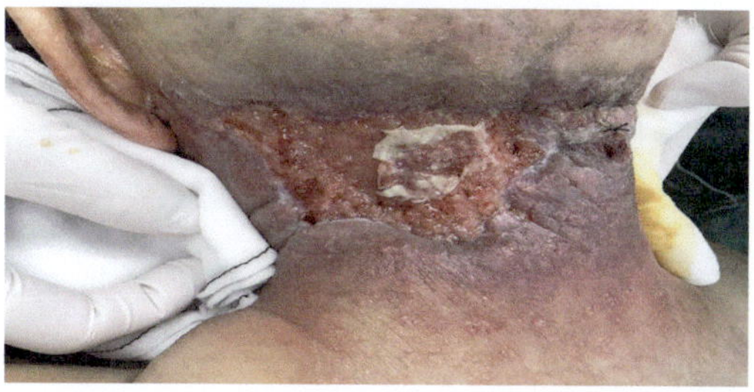

Fig. 5.7 Local skin grafting, survival of the graft after grafting

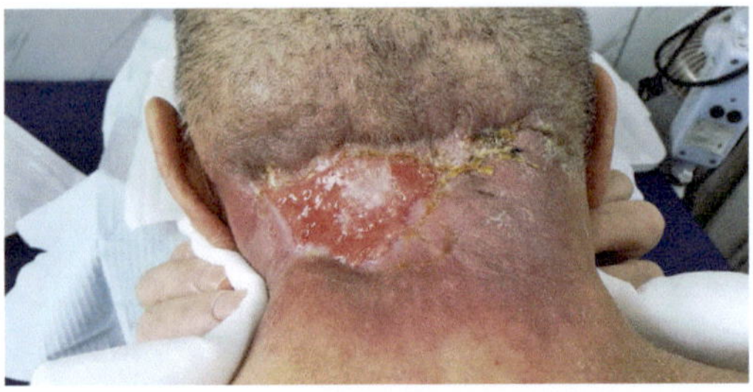

Fig. 5.8 14 days after skin grafting, discharged, regular dressing changes after discharge

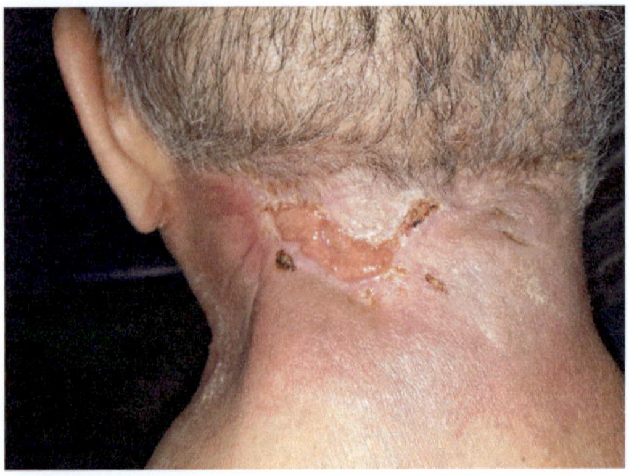

Fig. 5.9 One week after discharge, the wound area has significantly reduced

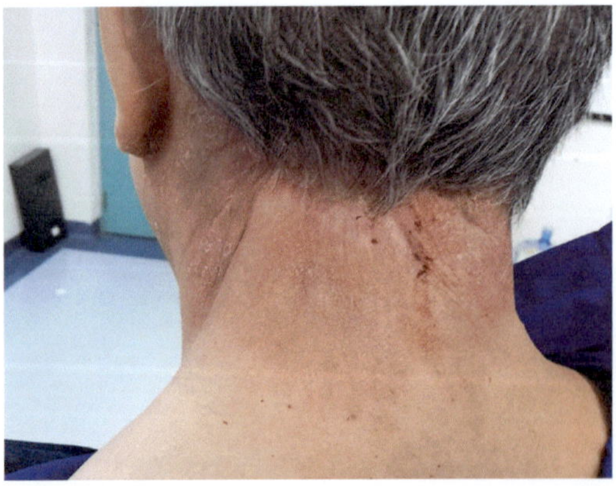

Fig. 5.10 Five weeks after discharge, the wound is completely healed

5.2 Case Analysis

Necrotizing fasciitis is a necrotizing soft tissue infection that mainly involves the superficial fascia and subcutaneous tissue. It is a serious infection in surgery, and it is more serious when combined with diabetes. Low anti-infection ability is an important basis for the occurrence of this disease. Another important reason for the high mortality rate of this disease is that it is treated as a common infection, leading to delays in diagnosis and treatment. Our department has encountered cases of necrotizing fasciitis patients showing signs of shock and several cardiac arrests. It can be said that the time from the appearance of the symptoms of this disease to the adoption of surgical treatment is the most important factor determining the prognosis. The patient, in this case, had poor basic blood sugar control, did not pay attention to the neck ulcer, and the anti-infection drugs and local expansion time were delayed. The superficial fascia and fat tissue were basically infected, the local muscles were involved, the area was wide, and the infection was heavy, which was the main reason for the multiple surgeries and long recovery time in the later stage.

The diagnosis of diabetic necrotizing fasciitis is more significant than treatment, early and thorough debridement and anti-infection can greatly reduce treatment time and cost. In addition, due to the large wound surface, it is necessary to supplement nutrition and control blood sugar, which is the basis for promoting wound healing.

Bibliography

1. Yi L, Xianying Z, Cheng Z, et al. Diagnosis and treatment of necrotizing fasciitis. Chin J Comprehen Clin. 2002;18(8):728–9.
2. Delong X, Shipeng Z, Tao Y, et al. Diagnosis and treatment of necrotizing fasciitis. Chin J Gen Surg. 2000;9(3):264–5.
3. Nia L, Lihui Z. Research progress on necrotizing fasciitis combined with diabetes. Med Rev. 2017;23(24):4921–5.
4. Chengliang D, Zairong W, Xueqin Z, et al. VSD technology treatment of diabetes combined with acute necrotizing fasciitis and infectious shock 1 case. Chin Emerg Med. 2016;36(7):667–8.
5. Yuzhi S, Chaohui Z, Jinghua M, et al. Furan regeneration method combined with small incision drainage treatment of diabetic foot acute necrotizing fasciitis. Chine J Integr Trad West Med Surg. 2014;6:578–80.

6. Jiali S, Ying W, Zheng Z, et al. Retrospective analysis of the diagnosis and treatment of neck necrotizing fasciitis. Chin J Otorhinolaryngol Skull Base Surg. 2019;5(1):78–83.
7. Yan F, Zibing W, Bing Z, et al. Clinical efficacy observation of modified negative pressure closed drainage in the treatment of perianal necrotizing fasciitis. Chin J Colorectal Dis Electr J. 2019;8(1):54–7.
8. Han Zhijie. Research progress on the diagnosis and treatment of necrotizing fasciitis [Master's thesis]. Hebei Medical University; 2018.

One Case of Skin Flap Repair of Diabetic Necrotizing Fasciitis Wound in the Buttocks

6

Tianbo Li, Jiangning Wang, and Lei Gao

6.1 Case Summary

Patient, male, 66 years old. The main reason for admission was redness, swelling, and rupture of the left buttock with blackened skin for 7 days.

[Present Illness] The patient developed redness, swelling, and rupture in the left buttock area without any obvious cause 7 days ago. After seeking treatment at a local hospital and receiving simple wound dressing changes, there was no significant relief. The red and swollen area gradually enlarged, and the surface skin turned black. The patient came to our hospital for further treatment. During the course of the disease, the patient's body temperature rose to 38.9 °C and the patient's spirit and appetite were not good.

[Past History] The patient has a five-year history of diabetes, has not been treated regularly, and has not checked blood sugar on time.

[Admission Examination]

1. Specialist examination. The skin of the left buttock is about 16.0 cm × 16.0 cm red and swollen, the skin temperature is increased, and there is about 10.0 cm × 10.0 cm black and red skin rupture and hard scab in the middle, with obvious tenderness, and there is a sense of fluctuation when touched (Fig. 6.1).
2. Laboratory examination. ① Blood routine: WBC 16.05 × 10^9/L, neutrophil percentage 91.3%, HGB 115 g/L. ② Blood biochemistry: albumin 24.9 g/L, serum glucose (fasting) 16.9 mmol/L, glycated hemoglobin 9.5%. ③ CRP 101.1 mg/L; ESR 60 mm/h. ④ PCT 1.1 μg/L. ⑤ The result of bacterial culture of wound secretions is *Staphylococcus aureus*.
3. Imaging examination. CT and B-ultrasound both suggest that there is a liquid echo under the red and swollen area.

[Treatment and Outcome] After admission, the patient was prepared for emergency surgery and underwent necrotic tissue debridement and abscess drainage under spinal anesthesia. During the operation, a large amount of pus was seen under the skin, accompanied by fascial necrosis (Fig. 6.2). After the operation, anti-infection, hypoglycemic, nutritional support, and other treatments were given, and the wound was changed daily (Fig. 6.3). After 1 month of treatment, ① Blood routine: WBC 8.05 × 10^9/L, neutrophil percentage 71.3%, HGB 108 g/L.

② Blood biochemistry: albumin 34.9 g/L, serum glucose (fasting) 7.9 mmol/L, glycated hemoglobin 6.5%. ③ CRP 13.2 mg/L. ④ ESR 21.0 mm/h. ⑤ PCT 0.05 μg/L. After the

T. Li · J. Wang (✉) · L. Gao
Department of Orthopedics, Beijing Shijitan Hospital, Capital Medical University, Beijing, China
e-mail: ltb32167@126.com; wangjn@bjsjth.cn; gaolei3337@bjsjth.cn

J. Wang, L. Gao (eds.), *Refractory Wounds*, Experts' Perspectives on Medical Advances,
https://doi.org/10.1007/978-981-96-2067-8_6

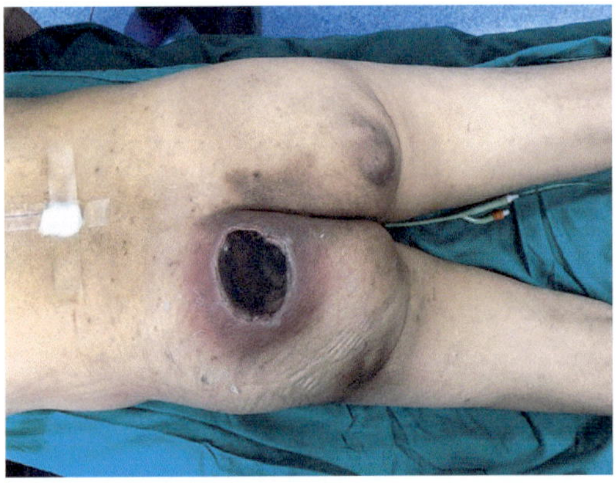

Fig. 6.1 Pre-admission situation

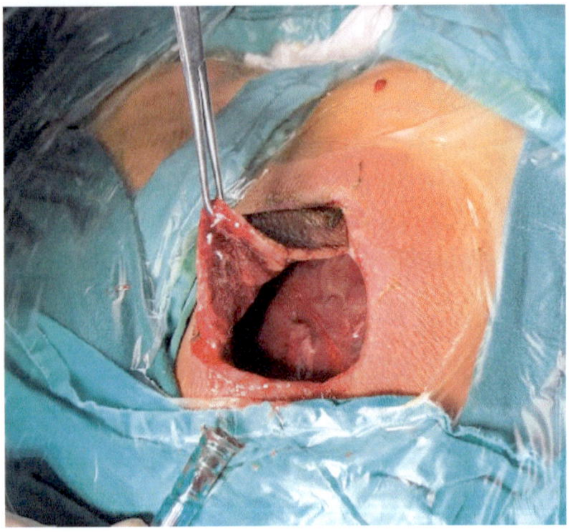

Fig. 6.2 During the surgery, a large amount of pus and necrotic fascia can be seen subcutaneously

patient's overall condition was good, a local flap transplantation was performed under spinal anesthesia in the left buttock (Fig. 6.4). The skin at the edge of the incision turned black post-surgery (Fig. 6.5), daily dressing changes were administered (Fig. 6.6), up to 1 month post-surgery.

One month after the second surgery, the laboratory results showed as follows: ① Blood routine: WBC 4.05 × 10^9/L, neutrophil percentage

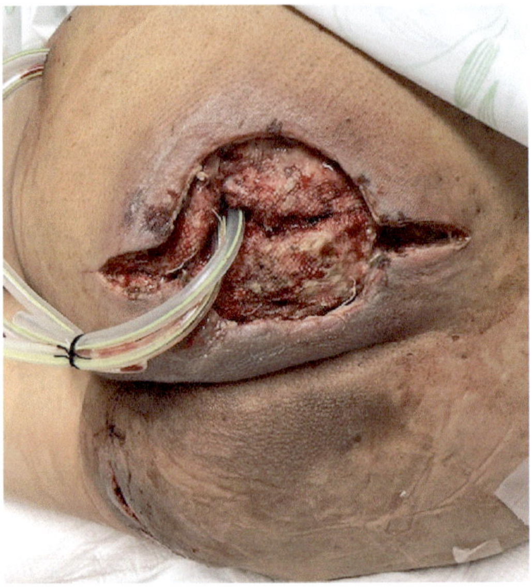

Fig. 6.3 Dressing change 1-week post-surgery

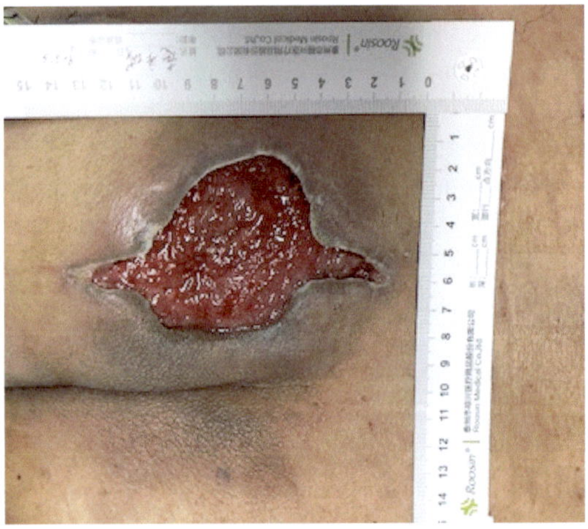

Fig. 6.4 Dressing change 1-month post-surgery

53.3%, HGB 120 g/L. ② Blood biochemistry: albumin 38.9 g/L, fasting blood glucose 6.9 mmol/L, glycated hemoglobin 6.1%. ③ CRP 12.1 mg/L. ④ ESR 14.0 mm/h. ⑤ PCT 0.03 μg/L. Specialist examination: The wound on the left buttock has basically completely healed (Fig. 6.7).

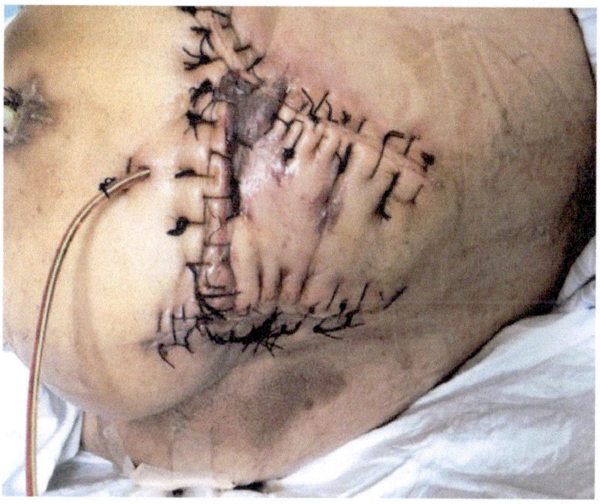

Fig. 6.5 After the skin flap transfer surgery, the skin at the edge of the incision turned black, but the skin flap survived basically

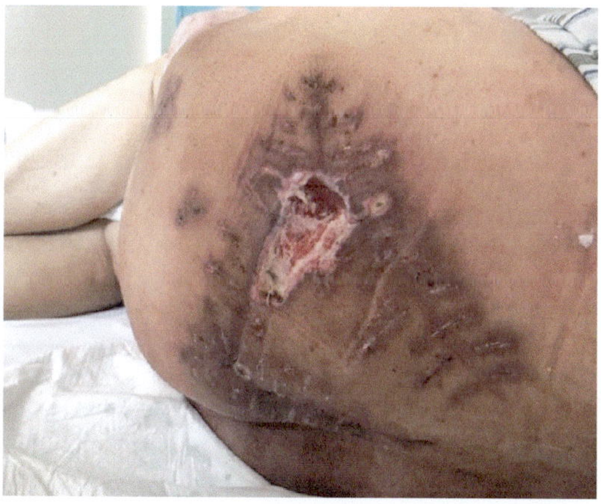

Fig. 6.6 Dressing change 3 weeks after the skin flap transfer surgery

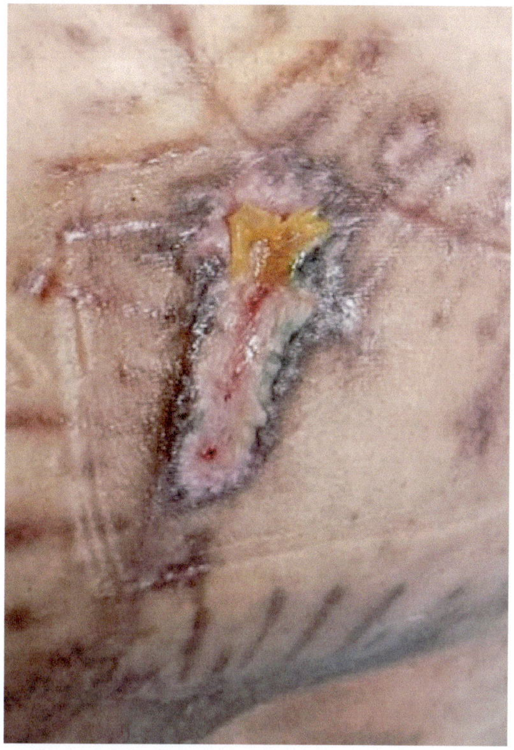

Fig. 6.7 Photo at the time of dressing change 5 weeks after skin flap transplantation, the wound has basically healed

6.2 Case Analysis

Necrotizing fasciitis is a rare acute infectious disease in clinical practice, characterized by necrotic soft tissue infection that invades subcutaneous tissues and fascia, with rapid onset, wide range of impact, and high mortality rate. Diabetes combined with necrotizing fasciitis is complex and progresses quickly, often accompanied by systemic symptoms such as high fever and chills. If not treated in time, it can lead to patient death due to sepsis or pyemia. Early diagnosis, active drainage, and the use of effective antibiotics are key to treatment. A skin flap is a tissue with blood supply, which has a high survival rate, strong anti-infection ability, certain elasticity, good filling effect. Treating diabetic foot ulcers with skin flap repair not only can repair the patient's wound, restore it to normal tissue structure and morphology, but also increase the wear resistance of local tissues, effectively protecting important tissues such as tendons and bones.

Bibliography

1. Kulasegaran S, Cribb B, Vandal AC, et al. Necrotizing fasciitis:11-year retrospective case review in South Auckland. ANZ J Surg. 2016;86(10):826–30.
2. Goh T, Goh LG, Ang CH, et al. Early diagnosis of necrotizing fasciitis. Br J Surg. 2014;101(1):e119–25.
3. Wang JM, Lim HK. Necrotizing fasciitis: eight-year experience and literature review. Braz J Infect Dis. 2014;18(2):137–43.
4. Xin W, Zhiqiang M, Jianchun Y, et al. Diagnosis and treatment of necrotizing fasciitis. Chin J Basic Clin Gen Surg. 2014;21(10):1289–91.

7 A Case of Diabetic Foot Complicated with Osteomyelitis and Refractory Wound

Zeyang Yu, Jiangning Wang, and Lei Gao

7.1 Case Summary

The patient, a 72-year-old male, was admitted to the hospital 3 days after incision and drainage due to a nonhealing wound on the lateral side of his right first toe, which had been ulcerated and necrotic for over 2 months.

[Medical History] The patient suffered a wound on the lateral side of his right first toe due to an external injury 2 months ago. He did not pay much attention to it at the time and treated it at home with disinfectants and dressings, without any specific symptomatic treatment. The wound did not heal, and 1 month ago, the wound further enlarged and was accompanied by a fever, reaching a maximum of 39 °C. The wound was about 3.0 cm × 2.0 cm in size, with pus and a foul smell. He took oral anti-infection medication at home and mistakenly used 95% alcohol for disinfection, which caused a burn on the wound, but he still did not seek medical treatment. Three days ago, the patient had a fever, the pain in the wound intensified, and the redness and swelling worsened. He was admitted to a tertiary hospital in an emergency, diagnosed with type 2 diabetic foot infection, and underwent incision and drainage of the wound. The wound still had a large amount of purulent exudate and a foul smell. The patient came to our hospital for further diagnosis and treatment, and was admitted to our department with the diagnosis of "type 2 diabetic foot with infection."

[Past History] The patient has had type 2 diabetes for 19 years, with the highest blood sugar level reaching 28 mmol/L. He usually takes metformin and pioglitazone for treatment, but his blood sugar control is poor. In 2015, he lost sight in his right eye due to retinal hemorrhage. A year ago, a physical examination at a tertiary hospital showed atherosclerosis in both lower limb arteries. He has no history of food or drug allergies, has had foot debridement surgery, no history of blood transfusion, and denies other medical history. He has been smoking for 30 years, up to 60 cigarettes/day.

[Admission Examination]

1. Specialist examination. The right foot was significantly swollen, the skin of the first toe was purplish, and an S-shaped drainage incision about 16 cm long was visible from the bottom of the toe to the middle of the foot. The first metatarsal bone was exposed, a large amount of soft tissue was gray-black and necrotic, and there was a large amount of purulent and serous exudate with a foul smell

Z. Yu · J. Wang (✉) · L. Gao
Department of Orthopedics, Beijing Shijitan Hospital, Capital Medical University, Beijing, China
e-mail: xiaobo723810@126.com; wangjn@bjsjth.cn; gaolei3337@bjsjth.cn

J. Wang, L. Gao (eds.), *Refractory Wounds*, Experts' Perspectives on Medical Advances,
https://doi.org/10.1007/978-981-96-2067-8_7

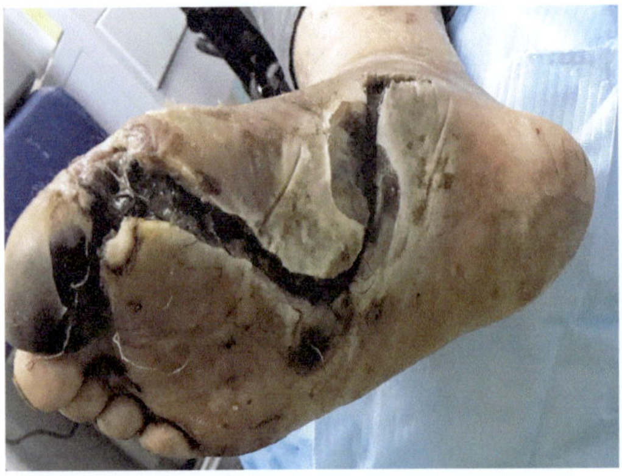

Fig. 7.1 Wound condition at the time of admission

(Fig. 7.1). The local touch pain was obvious, the active movement of the first and second toes was limited, the passive movement pain was intensified, the remaining three toes could move slightly, the skin sensation of the dorsum of the foot was reduced, the dorsal artery pulse was weak, and the posterior tibial artery pulse was acceptable.

2. General examination. Blood pressure 90/60 mmHg, body temperature 38.6 °C.
3. Laboratory examination. ① Blood routine: WBC 8.93 × 10^9/L, neutrophil percentage 7.4 × 10^9/L, HGB 82 g/L. ② Blood biochemistry: albumin 21.7 g/L. ③ CRP 262.4 mg/L. ④ BNP 993 pg/mL. ⑤ Myoglobin 66.6 ng/mL, Troponin <0.01 ng/mL. ⑥ Deep wound bacterial culture: *Staphylococcus aureus*, *Enterococcus faecalis*.
4. Imaging examination. Foot CT shows fracture and destruction of the distal first metatarsal and thumb of the right foot, with gas density shadow visible inside, and swelling of the soft tissue around the right foot and ankle joint, with patchy gas density shadow inside.

[Preliminary Diagnosis] Type 2 diabetic foot (right) with soft tissue infection, type 2 diabetic necrotizing fasciitis, chronic osteomyelitis of the first metatarsal of the right foot, type 2 diabetic peripheral neuropathy, septic shock, type 2 diabetes, lower extremity atherosclerotic occlusion, right eye blindness, post-debridement and drainage, hypoalbuminemia.

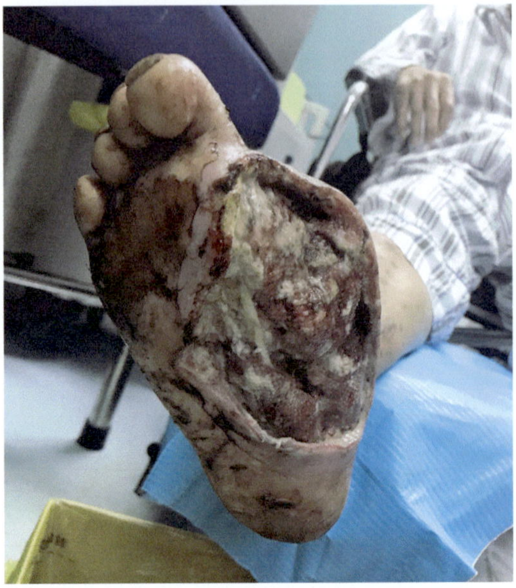

Fig. 7.2 After the first debridement surgery

[Treatment and Outcome] After admission, the patient was given symptomatic treatment for anti-infection, swelling reduction, circulation improvement, and neurotrophic and anticoagulant drugs. On the second day of admission, the first toe amputation + necrotic tissue debridement, and exploration surgery were performed under spinal anesthesia. After the surgery, the body temperature returned to normal, and the necrotic exudation of the wound was significantly reduced compared to before. Daily dressing changes were performed after the surgery, and the second debridement surgery was performed 1 week later, with regular dressing changes after the surgery. On the 14th and 20th days after the second surgery, the third and fourth debridement surgeries + Vacuum Sealing Drainage (VSD) treatment were performed. After 6 days of negative pressure drainage, the negative pressure was removed, and fresh granulation was visible. Symptomatic dressing changes were performed for 5 days, followed by skin grafting on the wound, and the wound healed well (Figs. 7.2, 7.3, 7.4, 7.5, 7.6 and 7.7).

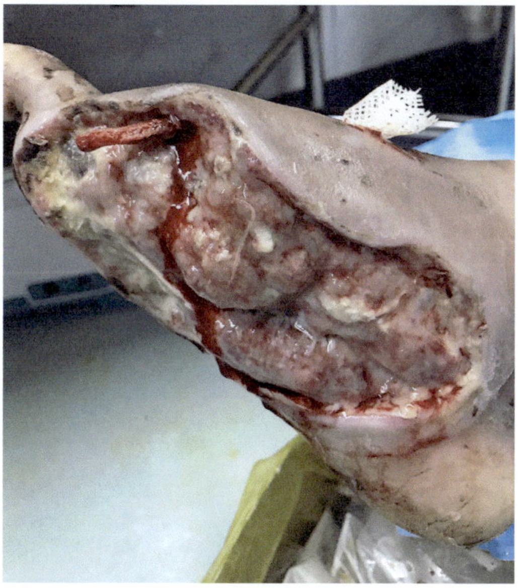

Fig. 7.3 After the second debridement surgery

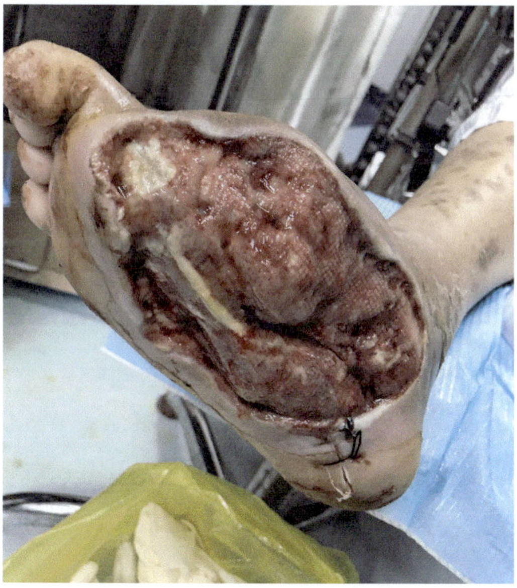

Fig. 7.4 After the third debridement + VSD surgery

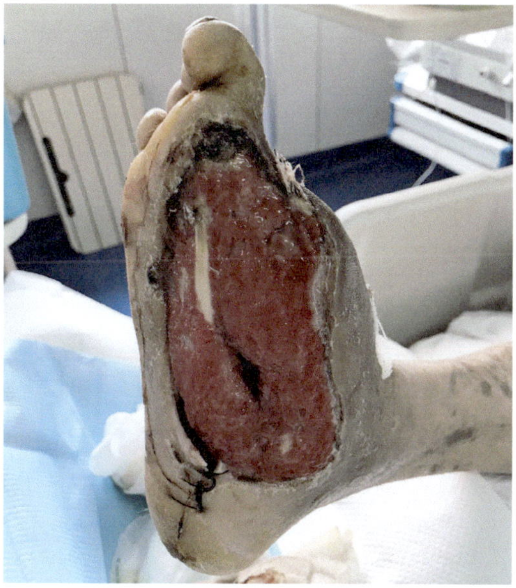

Fig. 7.5 After the fourth debridement + VSD surgery

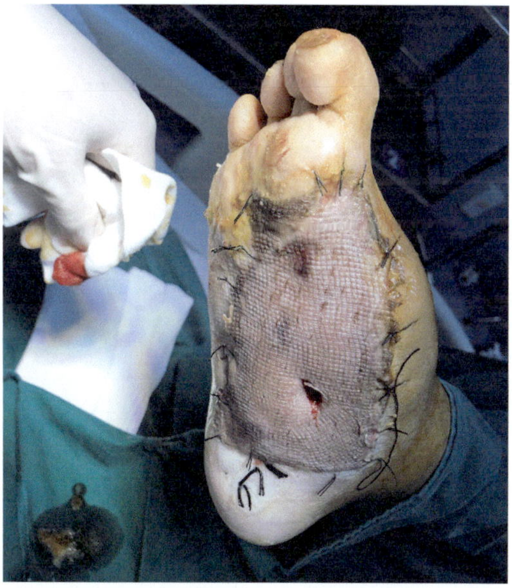

Fig. 7.6 After debridement and skin grafting

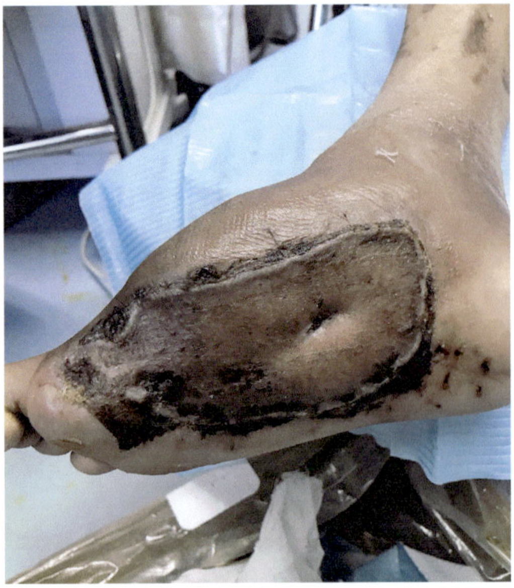

Fig. 7.7 Wound healing

7.2 Case Analysis

Diabetic foot osteomyelitis is a common complication in diabetic patients, with about 20% of diabetic foot infection patients having osteomyelitis. Clinically, osteomyelitis is often overlooked, and if diagnosis and treatment are not timely, it can often lead to serious complications such as amputation. Reports suggest that the risk of amputation due to osteomyelitis in patients with diabetic foot infection is four times that of simple soft tissue infection. Infections in patients with diabetic foot osteomyelitis are common in weight-bearing parts of the foot, such as the head of the first metatarsal, the head of the fifth metatarsal, and the heel. In addition, the base of the fifth metatarsal and heel of the foot can also be affected. About 90% of osteomyelitis occurs in the forefoot, with 5% each in the midfoot and hindfoot. Early diagnosis and rational treatment of diabetic foot osteomyelitis can effectively reduce the incidence of the disease and delay its progression. Diagnosis includes clinical physical examination, laboratory tests, and imaging studies. In addition to the use of sensitive antibiotics, thorough debridement surgery is crucial, which cannot be replaced by any antibiotics. Small-scale amputation can enable almost all patients to regain independent walking, and the functional evaluation is much higher than below-knee amputation, with a five-year survival rate after surgery of up to 43%.

For the treatment of diabetic infectious foot, timely debridement and toe amputation are particularly important in cases of severe infection, which can promptly improve symptoms of infectious shock. Through surgical debridement, toe amputation, symptomatic anti-infection treatment, the probability of wound healing greatly increases when the infection is under control.

Bibliography

1. Lavery LA, Peters EJ, Armstrong DG, et al. Risk factors for developing osteomyelitis in patients with diabetic foot wounds. Diabetes Res Clin Pract. 2009;83(3):347–52.
2. Mutluoglu M, Sivrioglu AK, Eroglu M, et al. The implications of the presence of osteomyelitis on outcomes of infected diabetic foot wounds. Scand J Infect Dis. 2013;45(7):497–503.
3. Acharya S, Soliman M, Egun A, et al. Conservative management of diabetic foot osteomyelitis. Diabetes Res Clin Pract. 2013;101(3):18–20.
4. Van Damme H, Rorive M, Martens DE, Noorthout BM, et al. Amputations in diabetic patients: a plea for foot-sparing surgery. Acta Chir Belg. 2001;101(3):123–9.

8 A Case of Limb Preservation in Type 2 Diabetic Foot Gangrene

Yefeng Yin, Jiangning Wang, and Lei Gao

8.1 Case Summary

The patient was admitted to the hospital due to gangrene of the right foot for more than 3 months.

[Medical History] The patient developed a rupture between the fourth and fifth toes of the right foot without any obvious cause in February 2019. The patient self-treated with saline washes, but saw no significant improvement. The ulcer area gradually expanded to the dorsum of the foot. The patient received wound dressing changes at an external hospital, but the wound area continued to expand. The patient continued to receive dressing changes in our hospital's department of plastic surgery in April. The right foot gradually turned black with pus seeping out. The patient sought further treatment in our department and was admitted to the hospital with "type 2 diabetic foot gangrene." Since the onset of the disease, the patient's spirit has been poor, with poor eating and sleeping habits, normal bowel movements, and no significant weight loss recently.

[Past History] In May 1979, the patient underwent surgery for a gastric perforation at a local hospital in Sichuan. In October 2016, the patient underwent surgery for lumbar tuberculosis at a tertiary hospital in Beijing, with a history of blood transfusion, but no transfusion reaction. The patient has a 28-year history of diabetes, treated with Glucobay, 1 tablet/time, 3 times/day, fasting blood glucose around 10 mmol/L. The patient has a history of hypertension for over 20 years, previously treated with oral medication (details unknown), stopped medication in 2017, blood pressure controlled at 110–120/50–60 mmHg. The patient has varicose veins in both lower limbs, which have not been treated.

[Admission Examination]

1. Specialist examination. Both lower limbs have dark red skin, reduced sensation, and muscle strength of level 3. Necrosis and gangrene of soft tissues from the distal end of the second to fifth toes to the ankle of the right foot, a soybean-sized necrosis on the skin near the ankle joint of the right tibia, purulent secretion around the necrotic tissue with a foul smell; a broad bean-sized necrosis of soft tissue on the skin near the ankle joint of the left lower limb, hard texture, no obvious exudation, poor blood circulation in both lower limbs, anterior tibial and posterior tibial arteries and dorsalis pedis artery not palpable, limited active movement of the right foot (Figs. 8.1 and 8.2).

Y. Yin · J. Wang (✉) · L. Gao
Department of Orthopedics, Beijing Shijitan Hospital, Capital Medical University, Beijing, China
e-mail: yefeng541009@163.com; wangjn@bjsjth.cn; gaolei3337@bjsjth.cn

J. Wang, L. Gao (eds.), *Refractory Wounds*, Experts' Perspectives on Medical Advances,
https://doi.org/10.1007/978-981-96-2067-8_8

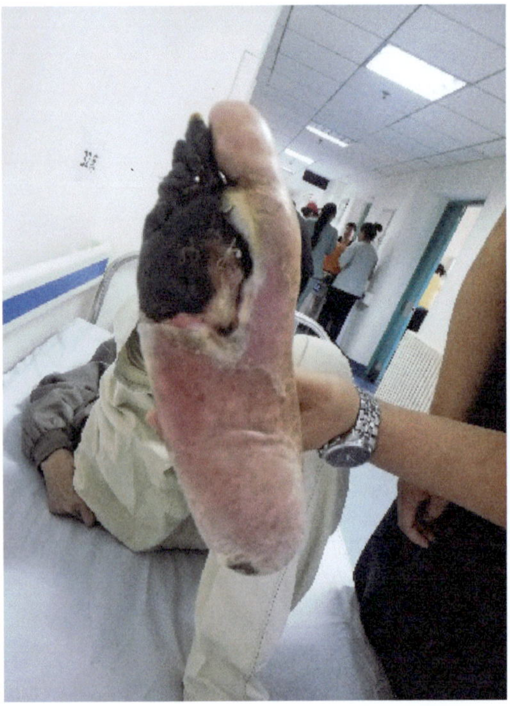

Fig. 8.1 Plantar side of the affected foot

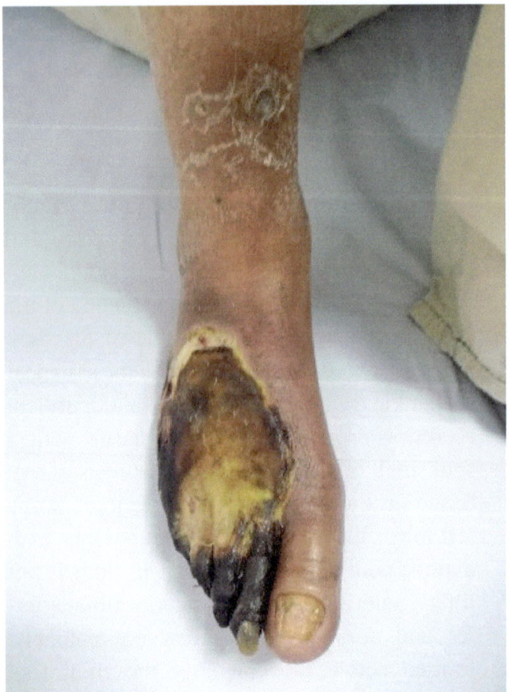

Fig. 8.2 Dorsal side of the affected foot

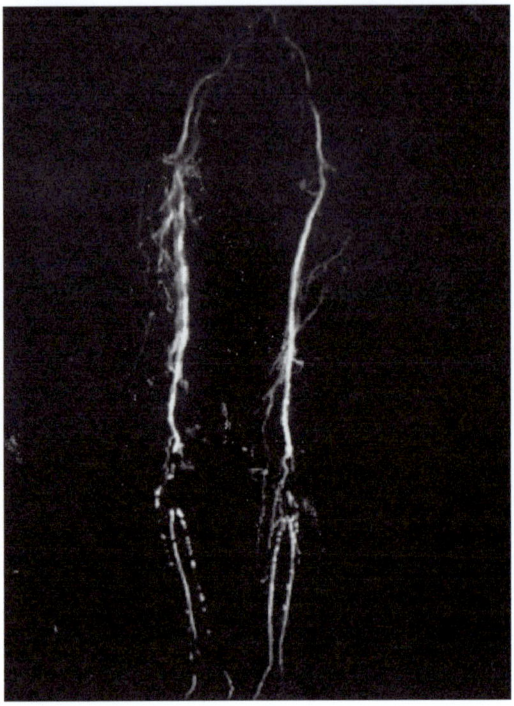

Fig. 8.3 Lower limb arterial CTA

2. Laboratory examination. Wound culture: *Pseudomonas aeruginosa*; serum glucose 35.52 mmol/L, albumin 28.3 g/L, WBC 11.82×10^9/L, neutrophil percentage 88.7%, neutrophils 10.5×10^9/L, CRP 119.31 mg/L.
3. Imaging examination. ① Lower limb arterial CTA: Multiple atherosclerosis in both lower limb CTA, local lumen multiple stenosis, bilateral arteries, anterior and posterior tibial arteries and peroneal arteries multiple moderate to severe stenosis, some lumen discontinuous enhancement (Fig. 8.3). ② Foot MRI: Abnormal signals in the skin and subcutaneous tissues, second to fifth metatarsal bones, multiple muscle groups and interstices of the right foot, considering it is related to diabetic foot, and ankle joint effusion (Fig. 8.4).

[Preliminary Diagnosis] Type 2 diabetic peripheral vascular disease and gangrene, type 2 diabetic foot ulcer and peripheral neuropathy, necrotizing fasciitis, lower limb soft tissue infection, lower limb varicose veins, type 2 dia-

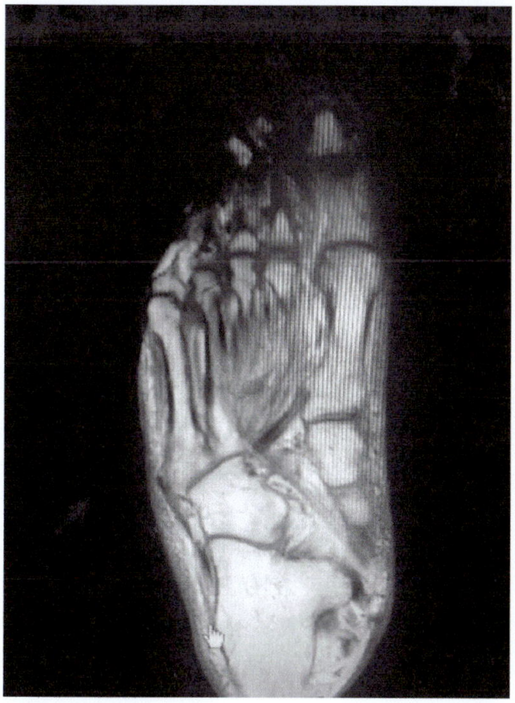

Fig. 8.4 MRI of the affected foot

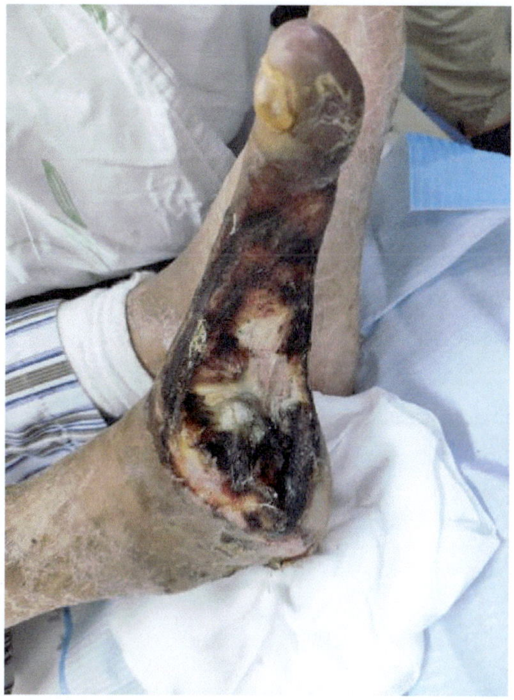

Fig. 8.5 Post-debridement wound blood circulation

betes, arterial stenosis (right), atherosclerosis, lacunar infarction.

[Treatment and Outcome] After the patient was admitted to the hospital, relevant examinations were completed, and treatments for infection, nutritional nerves, and circulation improvement were administered. Under general anesthesia, the patient underwent surgery for tendon, blood vessel, and nerve exploration, as well as necrotic skin and subcutaneous tissue debridement. Postoperative treatment included infection control, routine dressing changes, and other symptomatic treatments. The postoperative wound had poor blood circulation and slight exudation (Fig. 8.5). Due to postoperative anemia, two units of suspended red blood cells were transfused without any adverse reactions. Once the patient's condition stabilized, balloon angioplasty and arterial stent implantation were performed under local anesthesia (Figs. 8.6, 8.7 and 8.8).

Postoperative treatment included anticoagulation, infection control, routine dressing changes, and other symptomatic treatments. Once the lower limb circulation improved, another debridement and local flap repair surgery were performed under general anesthesia. Postoperative treatment included infection control, circulation improvement, nerve damage improvement, blood sugar control, routine dressing changes, and other treatments. The patient's vital signs were stable, and the flap had good blood circulation (Fig. 8.9). Laboratory tests: The wound culture showed no bacterial growth; blood glucose was 7.08 mmol/L, albumin was 35.5 g/L,

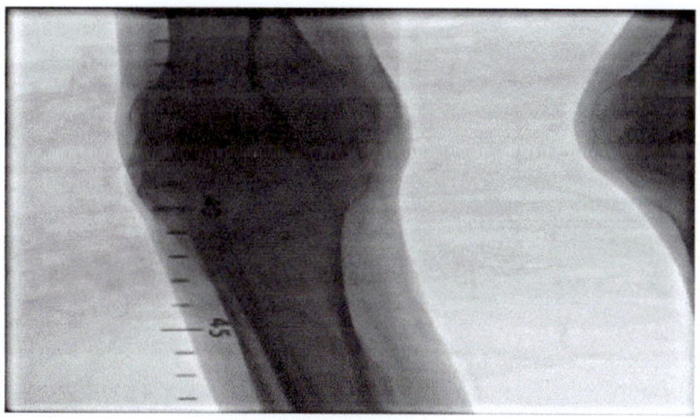

Fig. 8.6 Intraoperative angiography showing arterial occlusion

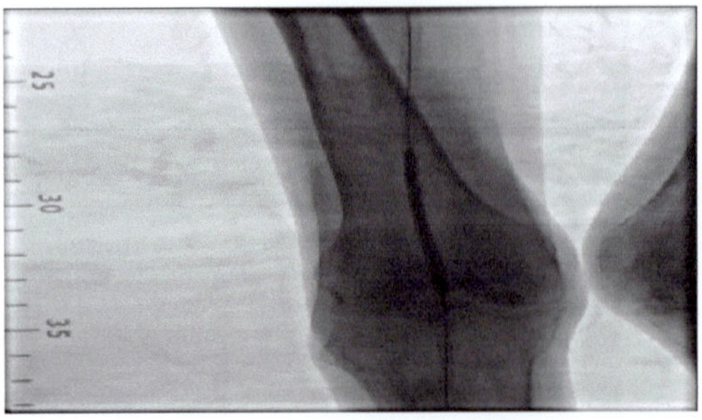

Fig. 8.7 Balloon dilation and stent implantation during surgery

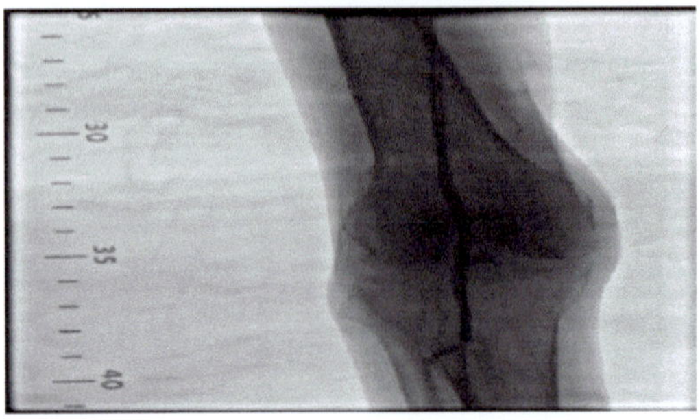

Fig. 8.8 Postoperative angiography showing patent artery

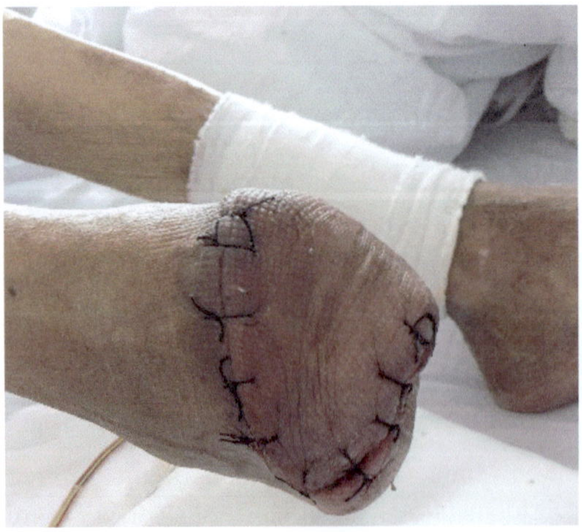

Fig. 8.9 Good flap blood circulation after intervention

WBC was 6.14×10^9/L, neutrophil percentage was 79.5%, neutrophils were 4.9×10^9/L, CRP was 6.05 mg/L.

8.2 Case Analysis

Diabetic foot gangrene is a serious complication of diabetes, with a high rate of disability. The timing of interventional surgery for diabetic foot gangrene caused by lower limb vascular disease is crucial. For patients with diabetic foot gangrene combined with chronic infection, it is advisable to first perform debridement surgery, and then perform vascular recanalization surgery after the wound infection is controlled, to avoid sudden improvement of limb blood supply aggravating foot infection. This preserves the limb for patients with impaired blood supply.

Bibliography

1. Wahbi ALA. Autoamputation of diabetic toe with dry gangrene: a myth or a fact? Diabetes Metab Syndr Obes. 2018;11:255–64.
2. Peeters P, Verbist J, Keirse K, et al. Endovascular procedures and new insights in diabetic limb salvage. J Cardiovasc Surg. 2012;53(1):31–7.
3. Jiangning W, Lei G, Tiangui C, et al. Professor Wang Jiangning's team's comprehensive diagnosis and treatment of diabetic foot cases. Beijing: Science and Technology Literature Publishing House; 2018.
4. Mills JL. Lower limb ischaemia in patients with diabetic foot ulcers and gangrene: recognition, anatomic patterns and revascularization strategies. Diabetes Metab Res Rev. 2016;32(Suppl 1):239–45.
5. Allen LL, Kalmar G, Driver VR. Treatment of a high-risk diabetic patient with peripheral vascular disease and osteomyelitis. Tech Vasc Interv Radiol. 2016;19(2):96–100.

A Case of Difficult-to-Heal Pressure Sore Wound Repair

9

Lei Gao and Jiangning Wang

9.1 Case Summary

The patient, a 35-year-old male, was admitted to the hospital due to a skin rupture in the chest and back for more than 3 months and a rupture in the right buttock for 1 month.

[Present Illness] The patient had been bedridden for a long time due to paralysis. Three months ago, skin ulcers appeared on the chest and back. After self-medication, there was no significant improvement, so the patient came to our hospital for treatment. After routine dressing changes and symptomatic treatment, the patient was discharged. One month ago, a skin ulcer appeared on the right buttock, about the size of a broad bean at the beginning. Despite self-medication, there was no improvement, and the depth of the wound increased. The patient came to our hospital again for further treatment and was admitted to our department with a diagnosis of "soft tissue infection." Since the onset of the disease, the patient had been clear-minded, with normal spirit, diet, and sleep, and had no significant weight loss.

L. Gao · J. Wang (✉)
Department of Orthopedics, Beijing Shijitan Hospital, Capital Medical University, Beijing, China
e-mail: gaolei3337@bjsjth.cn; wangjn@bjsjth.cn

[Past History] The patient had a history of hypertension for 7 years, with the highest reaching 180/110 mmHg, controlled by oral nifedipine. The patient was diagnosed with neurospinal sheath tumor 20 years ago and underwent neurospinal sheath tumor resection surgery at a tertiary hospital in Beijing 7 years ago, and had been bedridden since the surgery. The patient denied a history of diabetes, hyperlipidemia, coronary heart disease, and stroke, denied a history of hepatitis, tuberculosis, and close contact history, and denied a history of trauma. The patient had a history of blood product transfusion and had undergone "necrotic tissue debridement surgery on the left buttock" and "necrotic tissue debridement surgery on the right buttock." The patient was allergic to cephalosporins and anesthetics (specifics unknown), with no food allergy history. Vaccinations had been carried out as planned.

[Admission Examination]

1. Specialist examination. A wound about 2.0 cm × 2.0 cm × 4.0 cm in size could be seen on the right buttock, reaching the muscle layer, with red and swollen skin around it, reduced sensation, and secretion exudation; on the chest and back, there was a wound about 3.0 cm × 2.0 cm in size, with black scabs in the center, red and swollen skin around the wound, reduced sensation, and secretion exudation (Figs. 9.1 and 9.2).

J. Wang, L. Gao (eds.), *Refractory Wounds*, Experts' Perspectives on Medical Advances,
https://doi.org/10.1007/978-981-96-2067-8_9

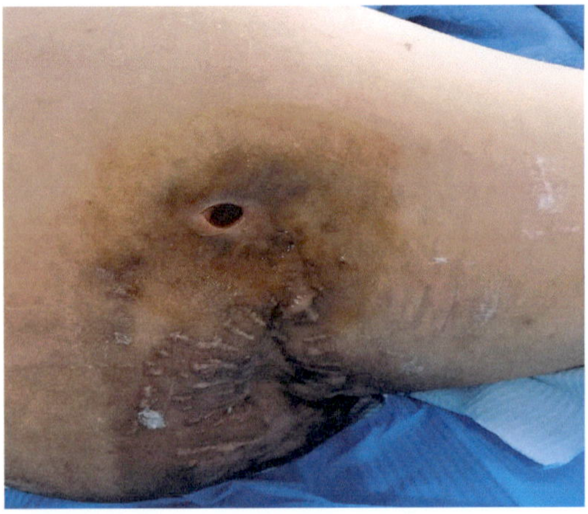

Fig. 9.1 Patient's right buttock

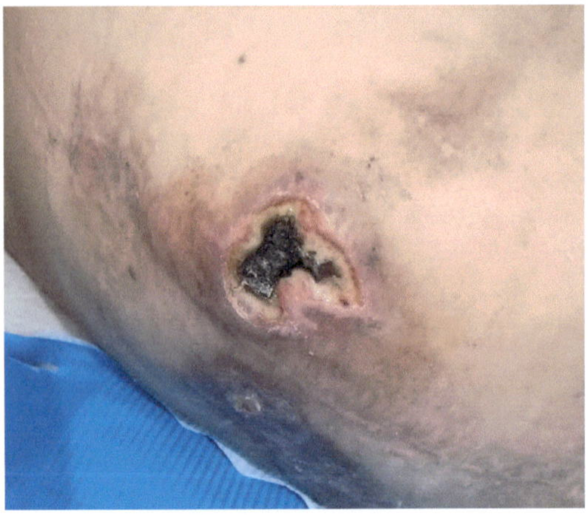

Fig. 9.2 Patient's back wound upon admission

2. Routine examination. ① Biochemical profile: alanine aminotransferase 16 U/L, aspartate aminotransferase 13 U/L, total bilirubin 11.6 μmol/L, direct bilirubin 3.2 μmol/L, indirect bilirubin 8.4 μmol/L, total protein 73.4 g/L, sodium 141 mmol/L, chloride 102 mmol/L, calcium 2.42 mmol/L, phosphorus 1.2 mmol/L, serum iron 2.9 μmol/L, serum magnesium 0.89 mmol/L, potassium 3.57 mmol/L, creatinine 34 μmol/L, uric acid 298 μmol/L, serum glucose 8.55 mmol/L, creatine kinase 25 U/L, lactate dehydrogenase 137 U/L, globulin 29.4 g/L, albumin 44.0 g/L, alkaline phosphatase 67 U/L, urea nitrogen 5.58 mmol/L. ② Routine blood test (venous blood): WBC 6.72 × 10^9/L, neutrophil percentage 71%, PLT 405 × 10^9/L, HGB 105 g/L. ③ CRP 74.35 mg/L. ④ PCT 0.02 ng/mL.
3. Imaging examination. Pelvic CT scan and three-dimensional reconstruction: Both hip joints are in place, joint space is narrowed, acetabular rim osteophyte formation, bilateral iliac bone osteophyte formation. Bone density is reduced. High-density shadow of soft tissue mass in the right buttock and local gas shadow can be seen. Bilateral femoral lateral strip-like soft tissue shadow (Fig. 9.3).

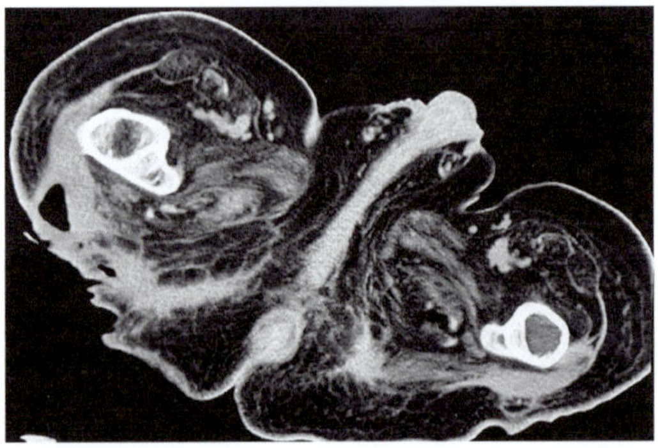

Fig. 9.3 Pelvic CT scan shows soft tissue infection in the right buttock

[Preliminary Diagnosis] Soft tissue infection in the buttock (right), back soft tissue infection, thoracolumbar spinal cord sheath tumor, paraplegia (bilateral lower limb paralysis), grade 3 hypertension (extremely high risk).

[Treatment and Outcome] After admission, the patient was given anti-infection, swelling reduction, and symptomatic treatment with nutritional nerve drugs. Alginate dressing was used for drainage in the wound cavity, and growth factor repair dressing was changed. After the preoperative examination was completed, on the third day of admission, exploration of blood vessels, nerves, and tendons in the right buttock and necrotic tissue debridement were performed under local anesthesia. During the operation, a 2.0 cm × 2.0 cm × 4.0 cm wound in the right buttock was completely excised. A 5.0 cm × 5.0 cm cystic cavity was found at the bottom of the wound, which was completely excised, and all necrotic tissue and inflammatory granulation tissue were scraped off. Hemostasis was thoroughly achieved with absorbable hemostatic gauze, the wound cavity was repeatedly rinsed with hydrogen peroxide and sterile saline, a drainage tube was placed, and the wound was sutured layer by layer. Postoperative anti-infection treatment was given; the patient was instructed to turn over regularly to avoid pressing on the wound. The necrotic scab and necrotic fascia tissue on the chest and back wounds were removed. Due to the patient's previous thoracic metal implant internal fixation surgery, the skin tension of the back wound was relatively large, the wound was not closed, and it was covered with medical gauze. One week after the operation, the wound healed well (Figs. 9.4 and 9.5).

In order to facilitate the rapid healing of the wound on the right buttock, the patient spent a long time in a left-side inclined position after surgery. Ten days post-surgery, due to pressure, two ulcers formed again on the left buttock (previous surgical site). Upon examination, a wound about 1.5 cm × 1.0 cm in size was observed near the anus at the 8 o'clock position on the left buttock. This wound was formed due to pressure on the scar tissue from previous surgery, with inflammatory granulation tissue growth, reduced sensation, and a small amount of exudate (Fig. 9.6). An ulcer wound about 2.5 cm × 3.0 cm in size was observed near the left hip on the outer side of the left buttock. The wound reached about 3.0 cm deep into the muscle layer, with a 4.0 cm × 5.0 cm wound cavity formed under the purulent fascia tissue, with a large amount of purulent secretion (Fig. 9.7).

Three days after changing the dressing of the wound, a surgical debridement was performed under local anesthesia on the wound near the left hip on the outer side of the left buttock. During the surgery, the ulcer wound was completely cleaned, necrotic fascia tissue was excised, forming a 4.0 cm × 5.0 cm wound (Fig. 9.8). After pressing and suturing the ischial tuberosity that could be probed deep into the wound, the wound cavity was rinsed three times with hydrogen peroxide and saline, but exudate was still observed. The wound was not closed. Post-surgery, the wound dressing was changed once daily, using

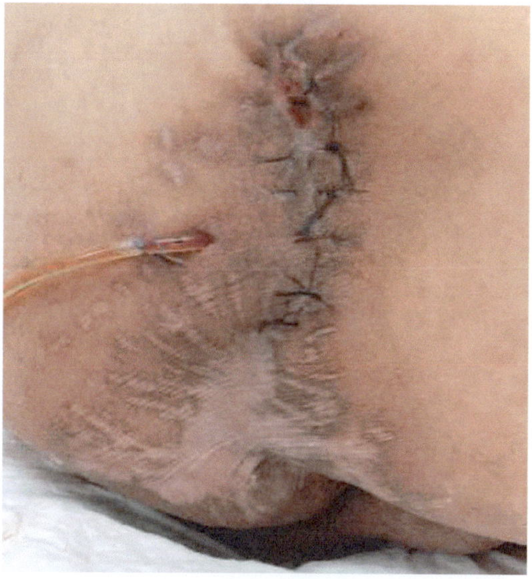

Fig. 9.4 Condition of the wound on the right buttock 1 week after surgery

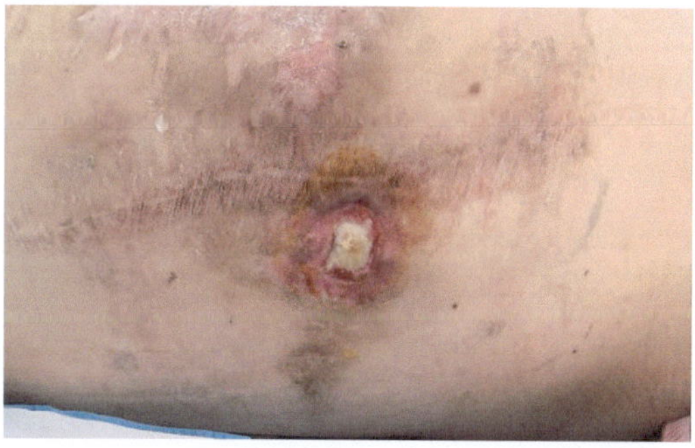

Fig. 9.5 Condition of the wound on the chest and back 1 week after surgery

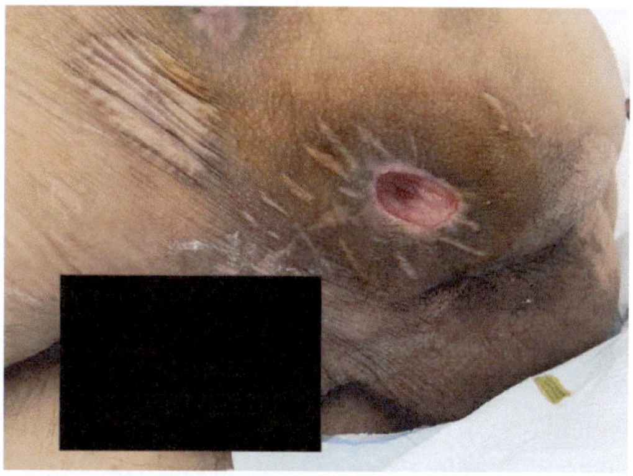

Fig. 9.6 Ulcer wound formed on the left buttock due to pressure

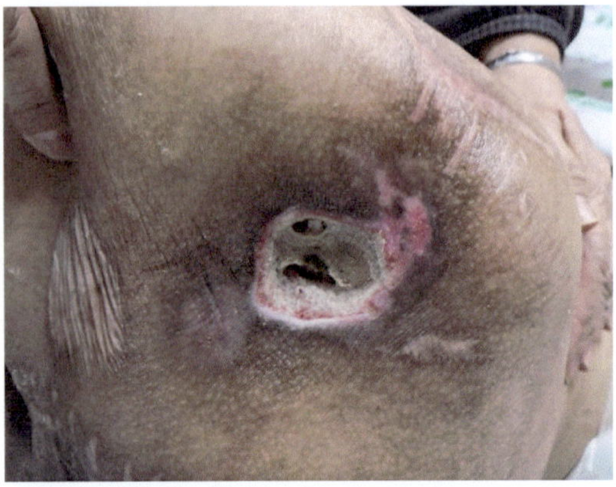

Fig. 9.7 Ulcer wound formed near the left hip on the outer side of the left buttock due to pressure

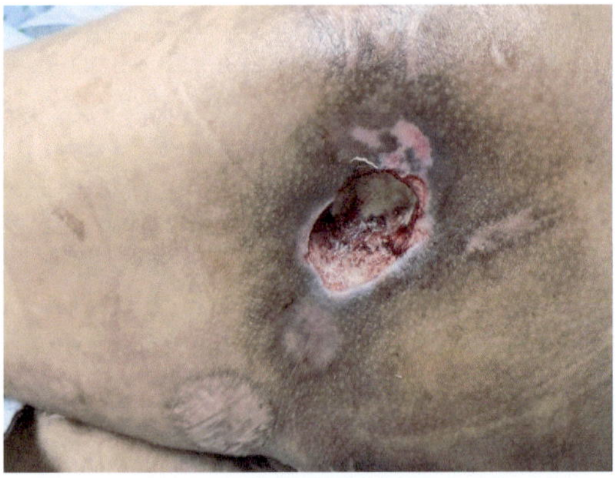

Fig. 9.9 Postoperative wound dressing condition (left lateral buttock near the left hip wound)

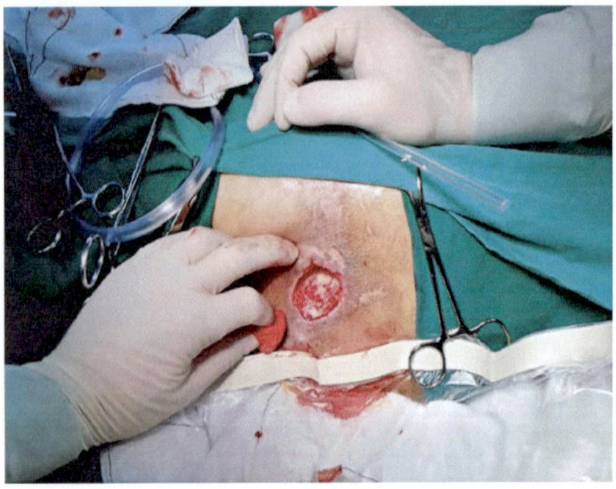

Fig. 9.8 Intraoperative wound condition

alginate for drainage and silver ion gel dressing for treatment (Fig. 9.9).

After the operation, the patient was given symptomatic anti-infection medication, and the wound was regularly dressed. After 2 weeks of dressing, due to the patient's special position, the wound was inevitably compressed. Although the granulation tissue grew well, it did not show a healing trend (Fig. 9.10). At this time, the original sutured wound on the right buttock was compressed due to the patient's long time lying on the right side, causing it to crack again, forming a wound about 1.0 cm × 1.0 cm deep to the fascia layer, with more exudate (Fig. 9.11). The wound on the chest and back improved after dressing, but it was difficult to heal because it was near the protrusion of the internal metal object (Fig. 9.12).

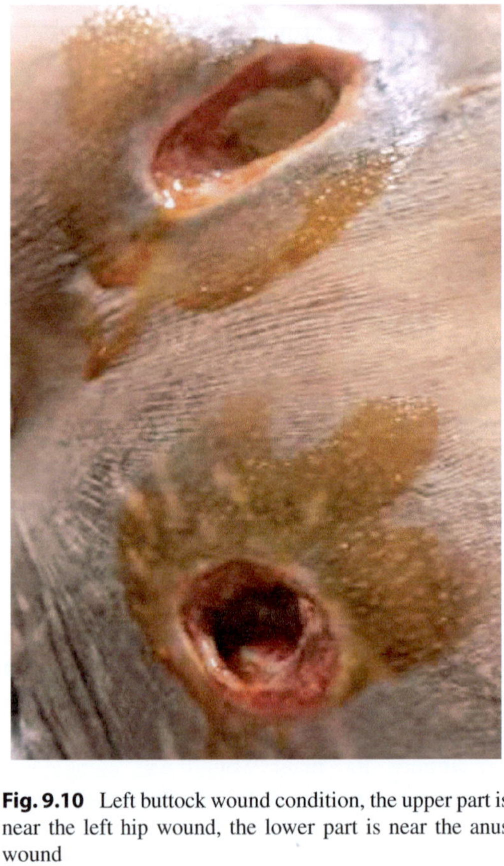

Fig. 9.10 Left buttock wound condition, the upper part is near the left hip wound, the lower part is near the anus wound

In order to promote wound healing, necrotic tissue debridement was performed again under local anesthesia. After thorough debridement of the wound on the left lateral buttock near the left hip, it was closed with tension reduction

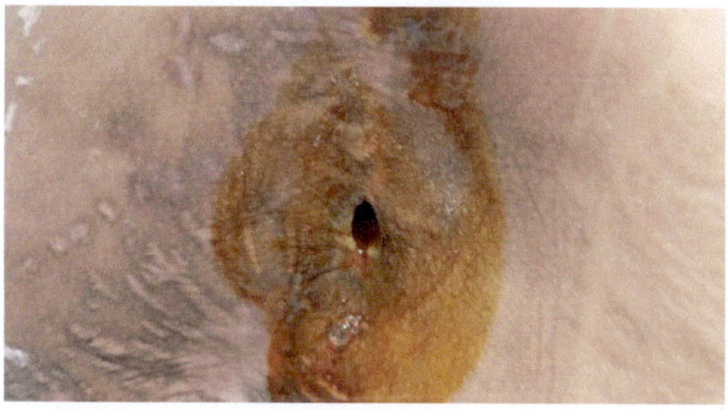

Fig. 9.11 The original wound on the right buttock cracked again to form a wound

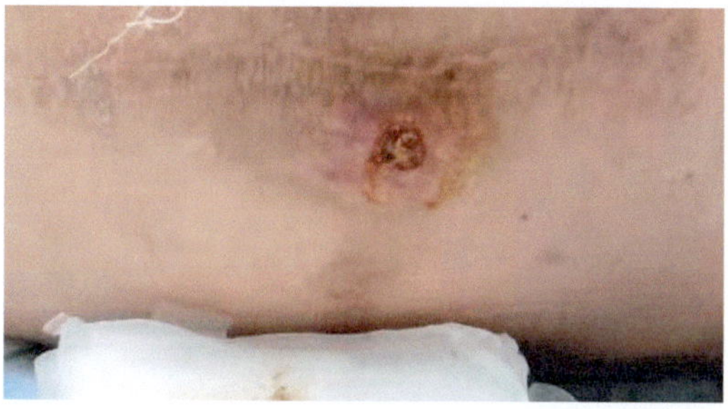

Fig. 9.12 Chest and back wound

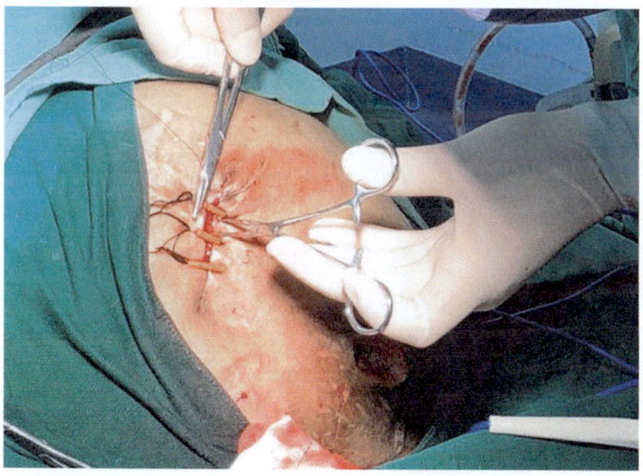

Fig. 9.13 The wound on the left lateral buttock near the left hip was closed with tension reduction after debridement

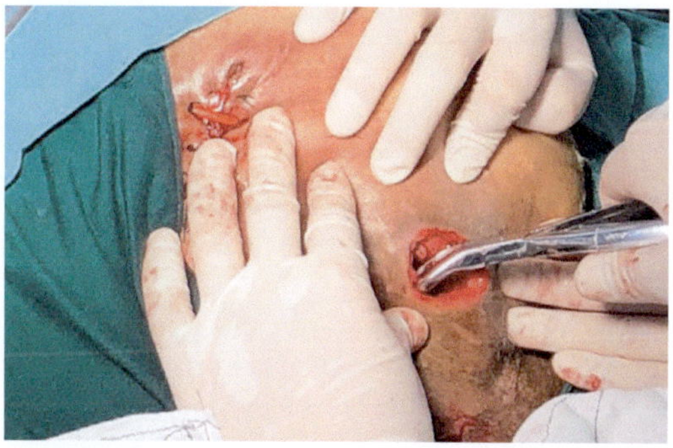

Fig. 9.14 Thorough debridement of the wound near the anus on the left buttock

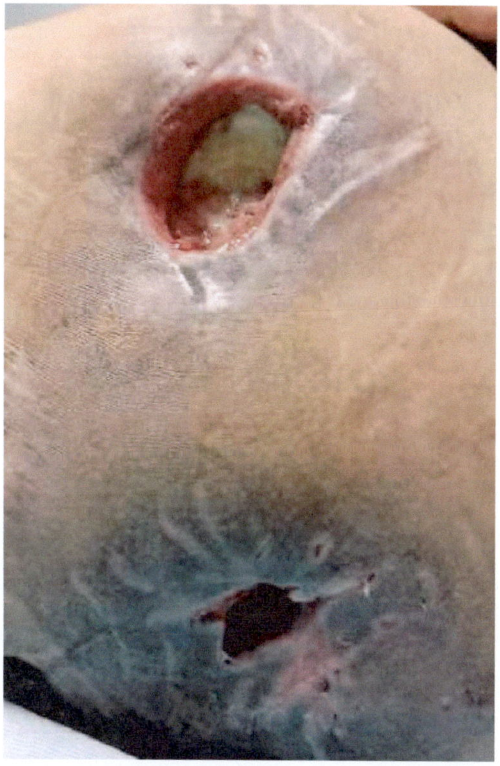

Fig. 9.15 The condition of the wound on the left buttock 2 weeks after the dressing change, the upper part is near the left hip wound, and the lower part is near the anal wound

(Fig. 9.13), the wound near the anus on the left buttock was thoroughly debrided (Fig. 9.14), and wound dressing treatment was continued after the operation.

Due to the high tension of the wound, severe edema occurred around the wound on the third day after the surgery. The tension-reducing line was removed, and the two wounds on the left buttock continued to be treated with dressing changes (Fig. 9.15).

Due to the patient's position, frequent turning and the use of air cushion beds and other pressure reduction measures did not achieve good results. Therefore, after the wound met the closure condi-

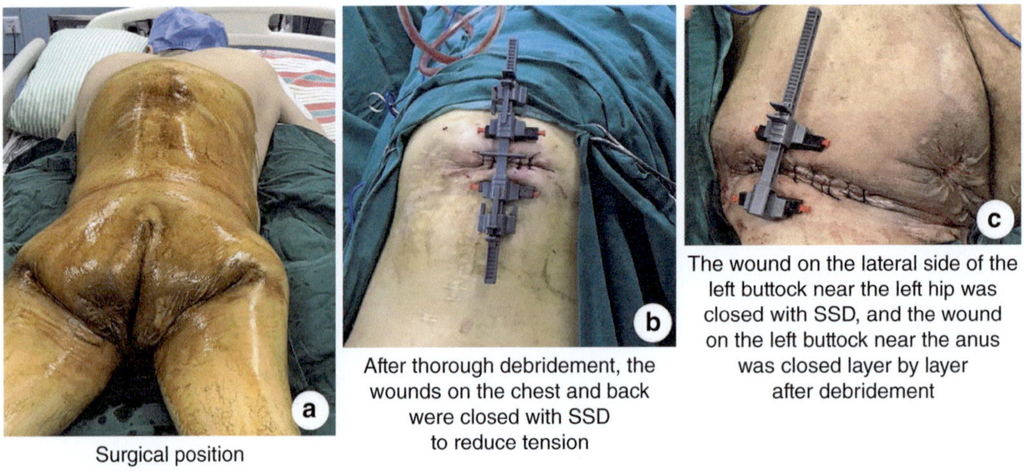

Fig. 9.16 Skin stretching device. (**a**) Surgical position. (**b**) After thorough debridement, the wounds on the chest and back were closed with SSD to reduce tension. (**c**) The wound on the lateral side of the left buttock near the left hip was closed with SSD, and the wound on the left buttock near the anus was closed layer by layer after debridement

tions 2 weeks after the dressing change, necrotic tissue debridement and skin soft tissue closure device closure surgery were performed on the left buttock. At the same time, thoracic and back necrotic tissue debridement + *skin stretching device* closure surgery was performed (Fig. 9.16). During the surgery, a 2.0 cm × 2.0 cm wound was visible after thorough debridement of the back. Necrotic soft tissue and exudate could be seen in the wound. A fusiform incision was made, and the necrotic tissue in the wound was completely removed until fresh bloody fluid was seen. After repeatedly rinsing the incision with hydrogen peroxide and saline, the incision was sutured layer by layer. The skin tension was high, and a *skin stretching device* was installed at the incision to relieve the skin tension of the incision. After the operation, the surgical incision was slowly stretched to reduce tension.

For the lateral wound of the left buttock, a large amount of fresh granulation tissue formation and necrotic tissue were visible. A fusiform incision was made to remove the necrotic tissue inside and around the wound.

Until there was complete healing, active bleeding could be seen in the wound. An electric knife was used to stop the bleeding and the wound was repeatedly rinsed with hydrogen peroxide and sterile saline. If active bleeding could be seen in the wound, absorbable hemostatic gauze is used to stop the bleeding and the incision is sutured layer by layer. When the skin tension is high, a *skin stretching device* is installed at the incision edge to relieve the skin tension of the incision, and the surgical incision is slowly stretched after the operation to reduce tension.

The patient continued to maintain an absolute prone position after the operation, the wound was dressed every other day, and the *skin stretching device* was dynamically adjusted according to the skin tension of the wound (Fig. 9.17).

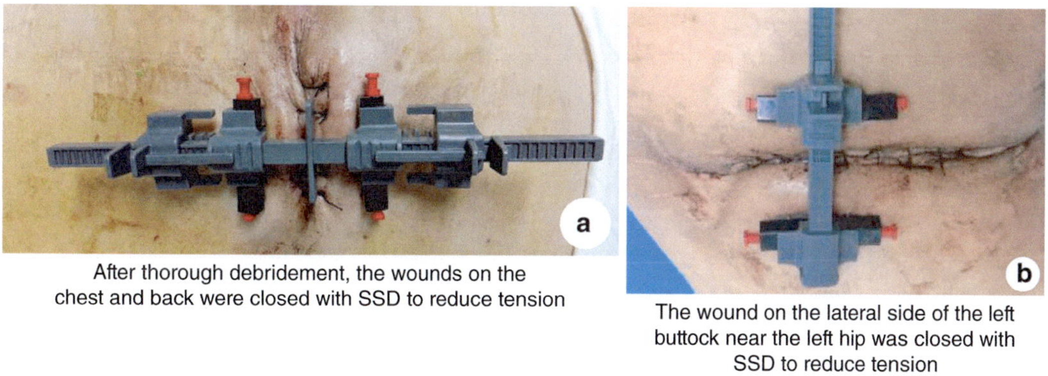

Fig. 9.17 The *skin stretching device* was dynamically adjusted according to the skin tension of the wound. (**a**) After thorough debridement, the wounds on the chest and back were closed with SSD to reduce tension. (**b**) The wound on the lateral side of the left buttock near the left hip was closed with SSD to reduce tension

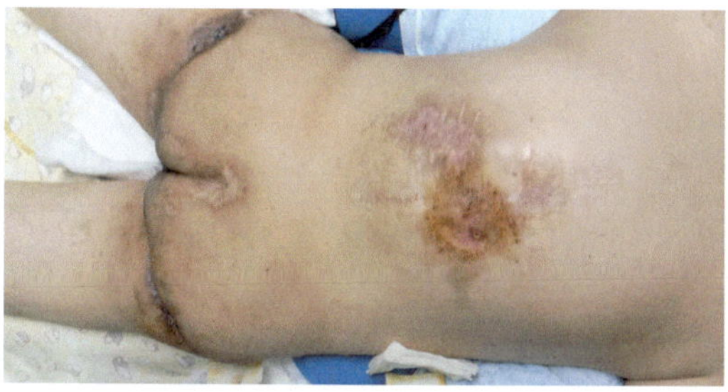

Fig. 9.18 Patient's prone position and the healing of all wounds

Two weeks after the surgery, the *skin stretching device* on the chest, back, and left buttock were removed. The wounds in these two areas healed. At the same time, the wound on the right buttock was cleaned.

The patient was kept in a prone position after the surgery, and all wounds eventually healed (Fig. 9.18).

9.2 Case Analysis

9.2.1 The Importance of Postoperative Position for the Healing of Pressure Sores

Pressure sores refer to soft tissue damage caused by local tissue being under pressure for a long time, leading to persistent local ischemia, hypoxia, and malnutrition, such as ulcers and necrosis. The most basic and important factor causing pressure sores is pressure, so it is now preferred to rename pressure sores as "pressure ulcers" or "pressure wounds."

Intermittent pressure relief is the key to effectively preventing pressure sores. Depending on the condition, turn over regularly, change position every hour when sitting, lift the body every 15 minutes, and change position every 1–2 h when lying down. Guttmamx first proposed in 1995 that when lying on the side, the body is at a 30-degree angle with the bed, and the pressure borne by the pressure area is half of the body weight. This has now been used as an effective method to prevent pressure sores. Therefore, it can be seen that after the debridement of the pressure sore, it should be kept absolutely decompressed. The zero load of the wound is the prerequisite for healing. The fundamental reason why the patient in this case repeatedly debrided but the wound did not heal was that the wound was under load or intermittent load after debridement, and the wound was difficult to heal under pressure. Finally, the patient was in a prone position, which ensured zero load and created favorable conditions for wound healing.

9.2.2 The Application of *Skin Stretching Device* in the Repair of Difficult-to-Heal Pressure Sores

In the clinical treatment of pressure sores, especially in the repair of large-area pressure sores, it is found that the principle of slowly closing the wound using *skin stretching device* technology. After installing the skin stretching device in the first stage of surgery, the maximum tension of the wound edge is pulled (transitioned from the minimum tension to the maximum tension), and the skin around the wound forms new skin due to tension, thereby gradually reducing the tension. After a certain period of time, the skin stretching device is used again to stretch the skin, so that the wound is closed under reduced tension.

In order to allow the skin around the wound to stretch sufficiently, we believe the following points are worth noting: ① Maintaining a constant tension is very important, especially when the skin is mechanically stretched over a certain period of time (8–12 h) during the non-acute stretching process due to the collagen fibers of the skin. After this, the tension at the wound edge will decrease, not enough to reach the maximum tension of the skin, so it is necessary to perform cyclic stretching again to keep the wound edge at the maximum tension state.

② This technique is a holistic stretching method that substitutes points for surfaces. For local skin, it is a line formed by connecting three points. The impact on skin microcirculation is small. After stretching, the skin around the wound edge maintains a good transcutaneous oxygen pressure, so the new skin formed by stretching can obtain sufficient microcirculation blood supply. ③ Since the *skin stretching device* requires chronic stretching and needs to be fixed around the wound edge, the device and the needle path need to be regularly cared for to keep them in a relatively clean environment and avoid contamination.

9.2.3 Surgical Treatment of Pressure Sores

Although pressure sores can be cured through nonsurgical treatment, it takes a long time. Therefore, for those who do not heal for a long time with nonsurgical treatment, the wound granulation is old, scar tissue forms at the edge, and there is bone joint infection or sinus formation, surgical treatment should be actively adopted. During the operation, the cystic tissue formed by long-term pressure sores should be completely removed, and at the same time, ensure that the surgical area is not compressed after the operation.

The tissue of the pressure sore wound and the scar at the base should all be removed. If it involves the bone surface, part of the bone should be chiseled off; those with osteomyelitis should be treated with anti-infection treatment for at least 6 weeks before surgery. Depending on the location of the pressure sore, design different skin flaps or musculocutaneous flaps, the blood supply should be good, and the suturing tension should be small. If the diameter is less than 3 cm after removal, it can be directly sutured. If the tension is too large, a tension-reducing incision can be made. For larger pressure sores, transfer flaps can be used, such as S-shaped and VY flaps.

9.2.4 Conclusion

After the pressure sore wound is debrided, active and effective measures should be taken to reduce the burden. At the same time, for pressure sore wounds that are large in area and cannot be directly sutured with low tension, *skin stretching device* can be used for slow closure.

Bibliography

1. Barwick A, Tessier J, Mirow J, et al. Computed tomography derived bone density measurement in the diabetic foot. J Foot Ankle Res. 2017;10(11):1–5.
2. Uzun G, Mutluo G, Lu M, Karag ZH, et al. Pitfalls of intralesional ozone injection in diabetic foot ulcers: a case study. J Am Coll Clin Wound Spec. 2014;4(4):81–3.
3. Chinese Medical Association Diabetes Branch. Screening and management guidelines for lower extremity arterial disease in patients with type 2 diabetes. Chin J Diabet. 2013;5(2):82–8.
4. Toprak O, Cirit M, Yesil M, et al. Impact of diabetic and pre-diabetic state on development of contrast-induced nephropathy in patients with chronic kidney disease. Nephrol Dial Transplant. 2007;22(3):819–26.
5. Pendsey S. Management of modern diabetic foot. Translated by Wang Jiangning. Beijing: People's Health Publishing House; 2017.
6. Jiangning W, Lei G. New progress in the treatment of chronic wounds of diabetic foot. Chin J Repair Reconstruct Surg. 2018;32(7):832–7.

Case of Hip Nonhealing Wound Repair

10

Lei Gao and Jiangning Wang

10.1 Case Summary

Patient, male, 54 years old. Admitted to the hospital due to nonhealing wounds on both hips for over 4 months.

[Present Illness History] Four months before admission, the patient developed abscesses on both hips and underwent surgery at a local hospital. After the operation, symptomatic treatments such as dressing changes were given, but the wounds did not heal. He was discharged from the hospital 5 days ago and came to our hospital for treatment. The outpatient department admitted him with "skin and soft tissue infection of both hips." Since the injury, the patient's diet, sleep, and bowel movements had been normal, and there had been no significant change in weight.

[Past History] History of dermatomyositis; history of scoliosis. Denied history of hepatitis B, tuberculosis, and close contact history, denied history of trauma, denied history of blood product transfusion, denied history of drug and food allergies, vaccinations were carried out as planned.

L. Gao · J. Wang (✉)
Department of Orthopedics, Beijing Shijitan Hospital, Capital Medical University, Beijing, China
e-mail: gaolei3337@bjsjth.cn; wangjn@bjsjth.cn

[Admission Examination]

1. Specialized physical examination. A wound about 12.0 × 6.0 cm in size could be seen on the right hip, the wound edge was not blackened, granulation tissue could be seen on the wound surface, purulent secretions were exuding, and the smell was foul. A wound about 2.0 cm in diameter could be seen on the left hip; the wound edge was not blackened, granulation tissue could be seen on the wound surface, purulent secretions were exuding, and the smell was foul, forming a cavity toward the periphery, with a minimum depth of about 5.0 cm, with the deepest part about 7.0 cm (Figs. 10.1 and 10.2).
2. Laboratory examination. ① Biochemical full item: alanine aminotransferase 19 U/L, aspartate aminotransferase 30 U/L, total bilirubin 7.3 μmol/L, direct bilirubin 3.4 μmol/L, indirect bilirubin 3.9 μmol/L, total protein 60.6 g/L, sodium 135 mmol/L, chloride 104 mmol/L, calcium 2.16 mmol/L, phosphorus 1.17 mmol/L, serum iron 6.1 μmol/L, serum magnesium 0.93 mmol/L, potassium 4.05 mmol/L, creatinine 61 μmol/L, uric acid 471 μmol/L, serum glucose 5.06 mmol/L, creatine kinase 72 U/L, lactate dehydrogenase 315 U/L, globulin 26.8 g/L, albumin 33.8 g/L, alkaline phosphatase 64 U/L, urea nitrogen 5.16 mmol/L. ② Blood routine (venous blood): WBC 9.47 × 10^4/L, neutrophil percentage

J. Wang, L. Gao (eds.), *Refractory Wounds*, Experts' Perspectives on Medical Advances,
https://doi.org/10.1007/978-981-96-2067-8_10

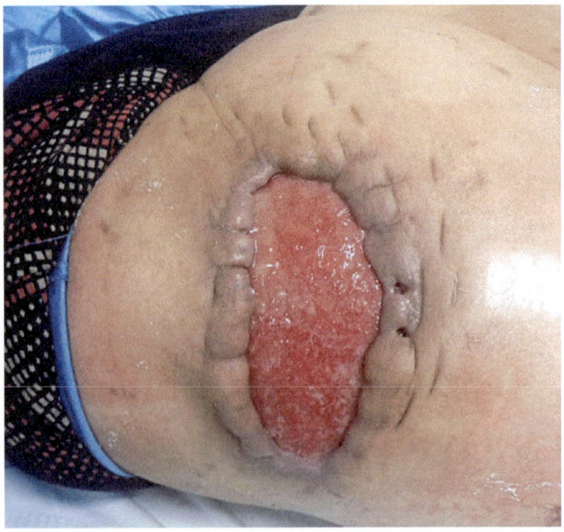

Fig. 10.1 Right hip wound

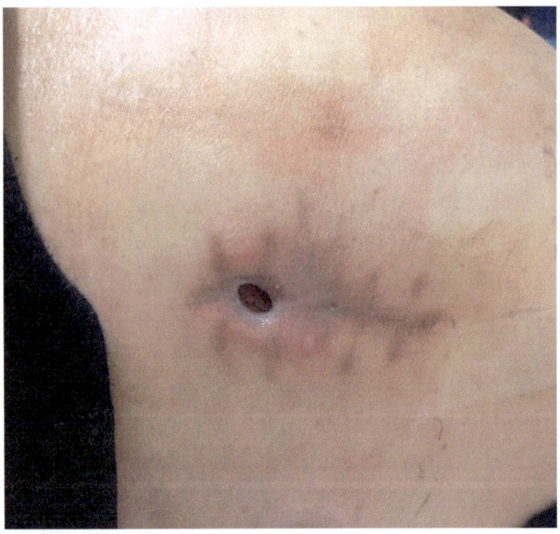

Fig. 10.2 Left hip wound

80.4%, PLT 316 × 10^4/L, HGB 147 g/L. ③ CRP 43.14 mg/L. ④ PCT 0. 03 ng/mL.

[Preliminary Diagnosis] Hip soft tissue infection (bilateral), dermatomyositis, scoliosis.

[Treatment and Outcome] After admission, the patient was given anti-infection, swelling reduction, and symptomatic treatment with nutritional neuro-drugs. After completing the preoperative examination, on the day of admission, the patient underwent bilateral hip debridement + neurovascular tendon exploration surgery + **skin stretching device** closure surgery; during the operation, the tissue scissors moderately trimmed the left hip wound fascia, and then used a curette to scrape off the necrotic tissue, considering the patient's wound condition is good, one-stage wound closure (Figs. 10.3 and 10.4). The curette scraped off the inflammatory granulation tissue of the right hip wound, the tissue scissors trimmed the wound edge, and it was rinsed three times with hydrogen peroxide, 0.9% sodium chloride, and iodine; three sets of rod-type wound **skin stretching device**s were installed at the proximal and distal ends of the wound, about 1.5 cm from the wound edge, moderately tightened the clamp to make the wound edges meet, and sterile dressing was applied (Figs. 10.5 and 10.6).

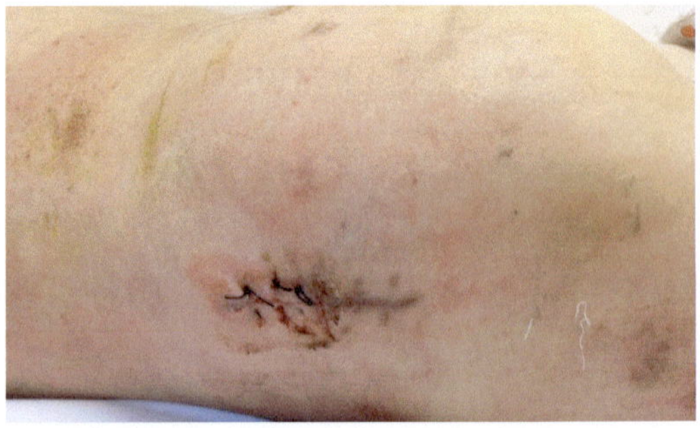

Fig. 10.3 Postoperative day 3, left hip wound

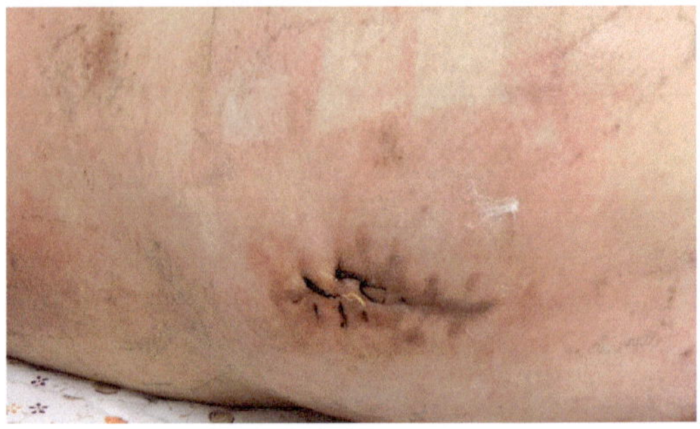

Fig. 10.4 Postoperative day 5, left hip wound

One week after the operation, under local anesthesia, the right hip was debrided + nerve vascular tendon exploration + **skin stretching device** removal + **skin stretching device** closure. After removing the two **skin stretching device**s, it could be seen that the tension on the inner edge of the right hip was smaller, the surrounding skin was relaxed, the wound granulation was fresh,

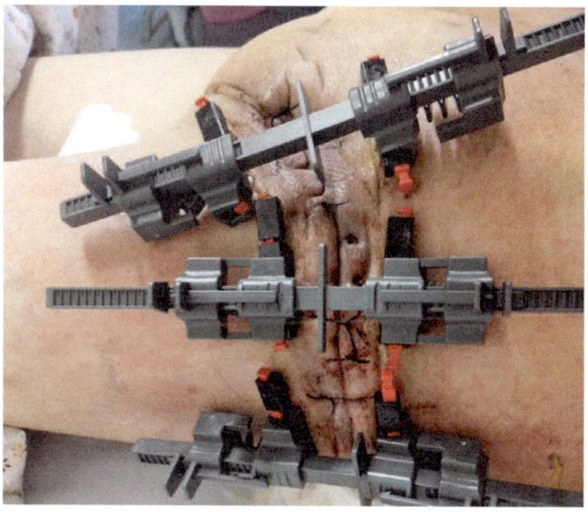

Fig. 10.5 Postoperative day 3, right hip wound

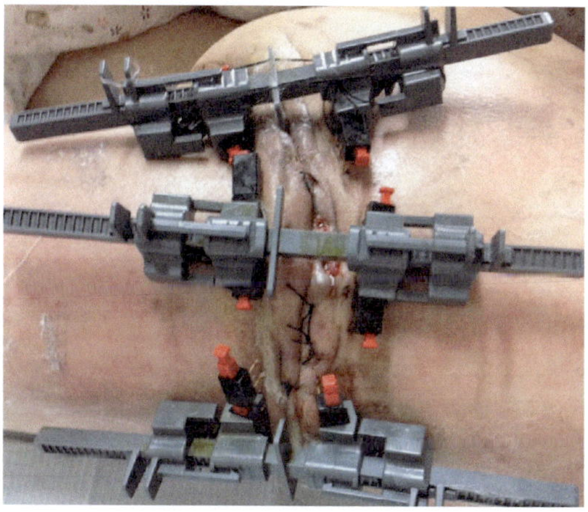

Fig. 10.6 Postoperative day 5, right hip wound

and the tissue was moderately trimmed on the right hip wound fascia; then, the necrotic tissue was scraped off with a spoon, and no important blood vessels and nerves were exposed. Hydrogen peroxide, 0.9% sodium chloride, iodine wash 3 times. Considering the patient's wound condition was good, the inner tension was small, it was considered to close the inner side of the wound with a tension-reducing suture at one time, and there was still tension in the middle part of the right hip wound. Two sets of **skin stretching device**s were installed in the middle part of the wound, about 1.5 cm from the wound edge, by moderately tightening the clamp to make the wound edge match, sterile dressing (Figs. 10.7, 10.8, 10.9, and 10.10)

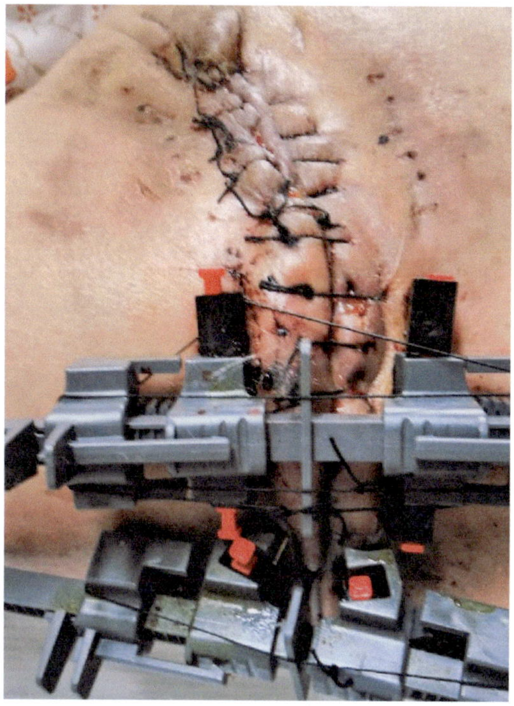

Fig. 10.7 After the second operation: day 1 right hip wound

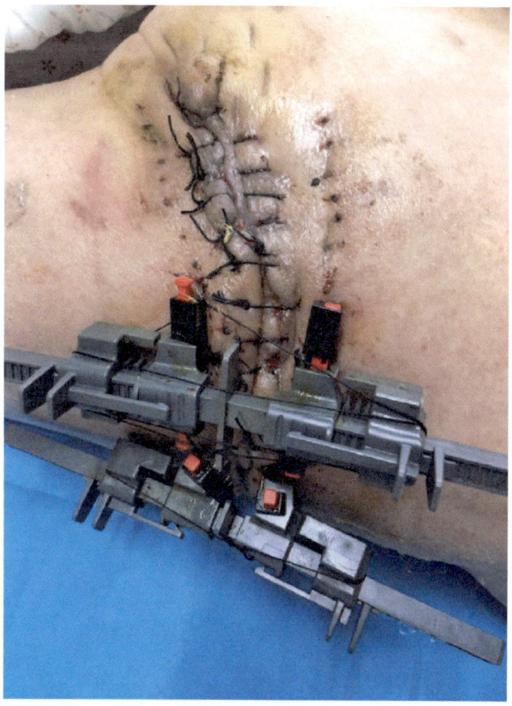

Fig. 10.8 Right hip wound on day 3 after the second surgery

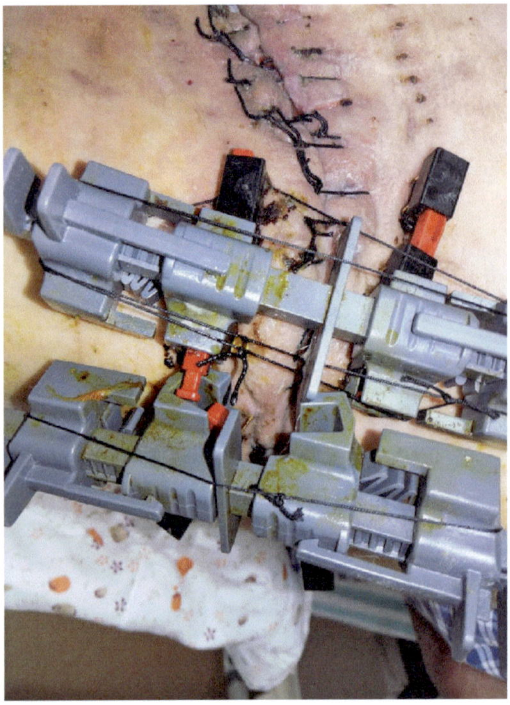

Fig. 10.9 Right hip wound on day 5 after the second surgery

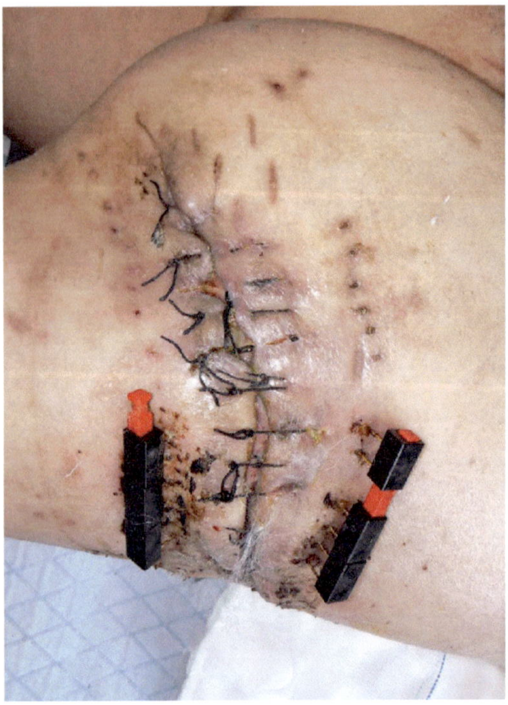

Fig. 10.10 Right hip wound on day 7 after the second surgery

10.2 Case Analysis

10.2.1 Stress Characteristics of the Skin

Human skin has stress relaxation characteristics, creep properties, incomplete recovery after tissue movement, and skin growth characteristics. When we design flaps or use skin stretching closure technology to calculate the area of new skin, we will comprehensively calculate the area of new skin produced by these four skin characteristics. Because the skin soft tissue is stretched and maintains a constant length, the tension of the skin gradually decreases; under a fixed tension, the length of the skin gradually increases within a certain range; the skin soft tissue has a tendency to reset after being moved and healed, but it cannot fully recover; the skin shows limited tissue growth under tension.

10.2.2 Application of Skin Stretching Device

For large skin defects, a skin stretching device can close the wound at once. If the wound cannot be closed after thorough debridement due to trauma, a skin stretching device can be used during surgery. This method of immediate wound closure is used in the technology of skin stretching devices. In addition, our team found in the clinical treatment of pressure sores, especially in the repair of large pressure sores, that the second function of the skin stretching device technology, namely the principle of slow wound closure, can be used. After the installation of the skin stretching device in one surgery, the maximum tension of the wound edge is applied (from the minimum tension to the maximum tension in a cycle), the wound is not closed in one stage and a gap is left. At this time, the secretions in the wound can be better drained, and the reduction of the wound can reduce protein loss. At the same time, the skin around the wound forms new skin after stretching, which gradually reduces the tension. After a certain period of time, the skin stretching device is used again to stretch the skin, and the wound defect area is gradually reduced under the premise of maintaining the maximum tension of the skin. This cycle continues until the wound is finally closed.

10.2.3 Conclusion

The **skin stretching device** is an auxiliary material that can gradually close the wound under reduced tension. It has been applied to the repair of limb trauma wounds and diabetic foot ulcer wounds. The gluteus maximus flap technique is used for the repair of pressure sore wounds. The results confirm that the patient's postoperative wound heals and closes, but the patient's hospital stay is longer, the hospitalization cost is higher, and it brings economic life pressure to the patient. The **skin stretching device** makes the repair of pressure sore wounds simpler and more convenient to a certain extent, and can shorten the wound healing time.

Bibliography

1. Lei G, Tianbo L, Yanling L, et al. Application of skin tension closure device in the repair of difficult-to-heal pressure sore wounds. Chin J Microsurg. 2018;41(1):80–3.
2. Lei G, Shuo W, Lei W, et al. Application of skin tension closure device in the repair of diabetic foot wounds. Chin J Repair Reconstr Surg. 2018;32(5):591–5.
3. Song M, Zhang Z, Liu T. EASApprox® SymbolProp BTRCp skin-stretching system: a secure and effective method to achieve wound closure. Exp Ther Med. 2017;14(1):531–8.
4. Jiangning W, Lei G, Tiangui C, et al. Professor Wang Jiangning's team's comprehensive diagnosis and treatment of diabetic foot cases. Beijing: Science and Technology Literature Publishing House; 2018.
5. Jiangning W, Gengjia T, Zhaofan X, et al. Comprehensive treatment of pressure sores. Beijing: People's Health Publishing House; 2018.

11 Case of Buttock Purulent Hidradenitis Wound Repair

Lei Gao and Jiangning Wang

11.1 Case Summary

Patient, male, 45 years old. The main cause of hospitalization was buttock skin rupture with purulent exudation for 1 year, and increased secretion for more than 1 month.

[Present Illness History] The patient underwent bilateral buttock, posterior thigh, and perineal sweat gland resection due to hidradenitis 4 years ago. One year ago, skin rupture occurred at the 3 o'clock and 7 o'clock positions around the anus (knee-chest position). There was a fecal-like secretion oozing out, and the secretion gradually increased a month ago. The local hospital diagnosed it as anal fistula. The wound around the anus was treated with dressing changes, but there was no sign of improvement. Therefore, the patient came to our hospital for treatment. The outpatient department admitted the patient with "peri-anal soft tissue infection." Since admission, the patient's diet and sleep have been normal, and there had been no significant change in weight.

[Past History] The patient had generally poor health, with sequelae of poliomyelitis for 42 years. The patient had a history of vasculitis and hidradenitis for 20 years, and had a history of blood product transfusion. The patient denied a history of hypertension, diabetes, hyperlipidemia, coronary heart disease, and stroke, denied a history of hepatitis, tuberculosis, and close contact history, denied a history of trauma, denied a history of drug and food allergies. Vaccinations had been carried out as planned.

[Admission Examination]

1. Specialist examination. Scars from hidradenitis surgery could be seen on both buttocks, the back of the thighs, and the perineum. The local skin was hard and thickened, with multiple scar tissue protrusions. Two fistula openings could be probed at the 3 o'clock and 7 o'clock positions of the anus, with fecal-like secretions oozing out. Surgical scars could be seen around the anus. The catheter and bladder fistula tube were well fixed and unobstructed (Figs. 11.1 and 11.2).
2. Laboratory examination. ① Blood routine (venous blood): WBC 5.9×10^9/L, neutrophil percentage 72.3%, neutrophils 4.3×10^9/L, HGB 132 g/L, mean red cell volume 81.7 fL. ② Biochemical examination: globulin 42.8 g/L, albumin 38.5 g/L. ③ CRP 34.13 mg/L. ④ PCT 0.03 ng/mL.
3. Radiological examination. After the injection of contrast agent through the anal catheter, a pelvic CT scan was performed: After the injection of the anal contrast agent, the anterior part of the anus and the soft tissue of

L. Gao · J. Wang (✉)
Department of Orthopedics, Beijing Shijitan Hospital, Capital Medical University, Beijing, China
e-mail: gaolei3337@bjsjth.cn; wangjn@bjsjth.cn

J. Wang, L. Gao (eds.), *Refractory Wounds*, Experts' Perspectives on Medical Advances,
https://doi.org/10.1007/978-981-96-2067-8_11

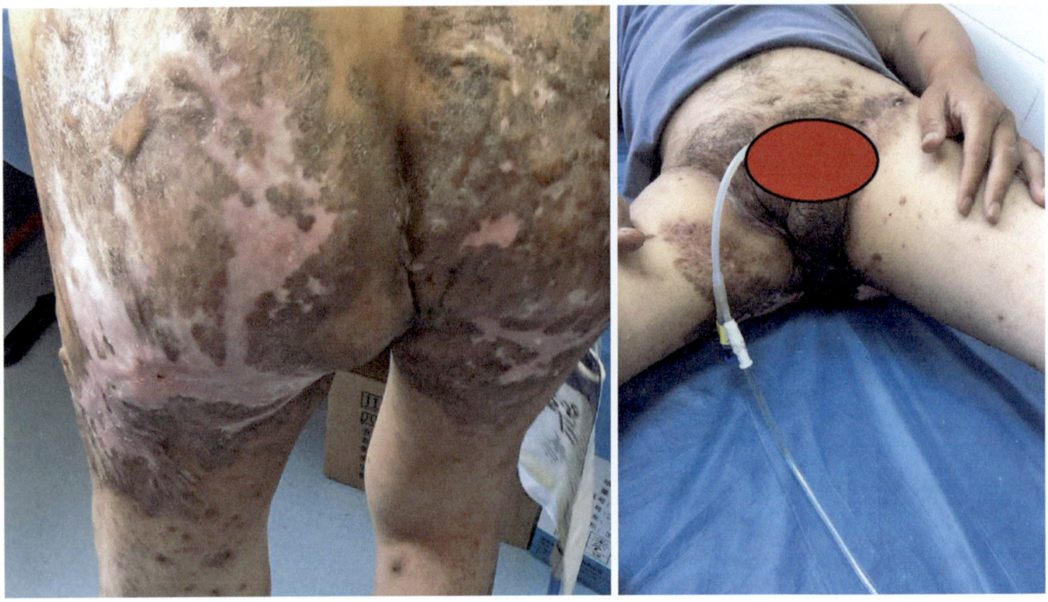

Fig. 11.1 Patient's condition upon admission (scars after hidradenitis surgery on both buttocks, back of thighs, perineum)

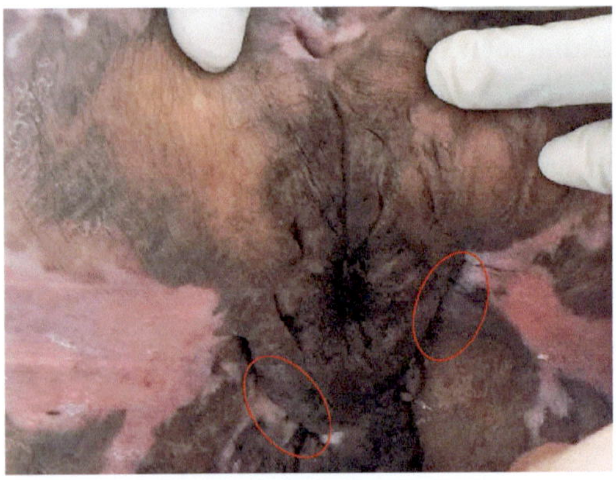

Fig. 11.2 Patient's fistula wound condition upon admission

the buttocks could be seen. The contrast agent leaked through the right levator ani muscle to the subcutaneous area behind the sacrococcygeal, the corresponding subcutaneous fat gap was blurred, the density was increased, and a high-density shadow could also be seen on the left rear (Figs. 11.3 and 11.4). Diagnosis: The findings in the pelvis are consistent with changes in anal fistula, multiple lymph nodes in both groins, and thickening of the skin of both buttocks and testicles.

[Preliminary Diagnosis] Skin infectious sinus, bladder stoma status, suppurative hidradenitis (postoperative), vasculitis (phlebitis), sequelae of poliomyelitis.

[Treatment and Outcome] After admission, the patient was given anti-infection, swelling reduction, circulation improvement, and symptomatic treatment for nutritional nerves, and wound dressing treatment. After preoperative examination and intestinal preparation, necrotic tissue debridement around the anus + adjacent muscle flap transfer to repair the anal fistula was performed under general anesthesia.

The patient was in the prone position, and after satisfactory anesthesia, iodophor was disinfected three times, and a sterile sheet was laid. Exploration revealed postoperative scars of hidradenitis on both buttocks, the back of the thighs, and the perineum, with multiple gaps formed by scar tissue. Two fistula openings could be probed at the 3 o'clock and 7 o'clock positions of the anus, with the fistula at the 3 o'clock position being deeper. The two fistula openings were scraped with a curette until bleeding. Intraoperative exploration confirmed that both the 3 o'clock and 7 o'clock positions were fistula

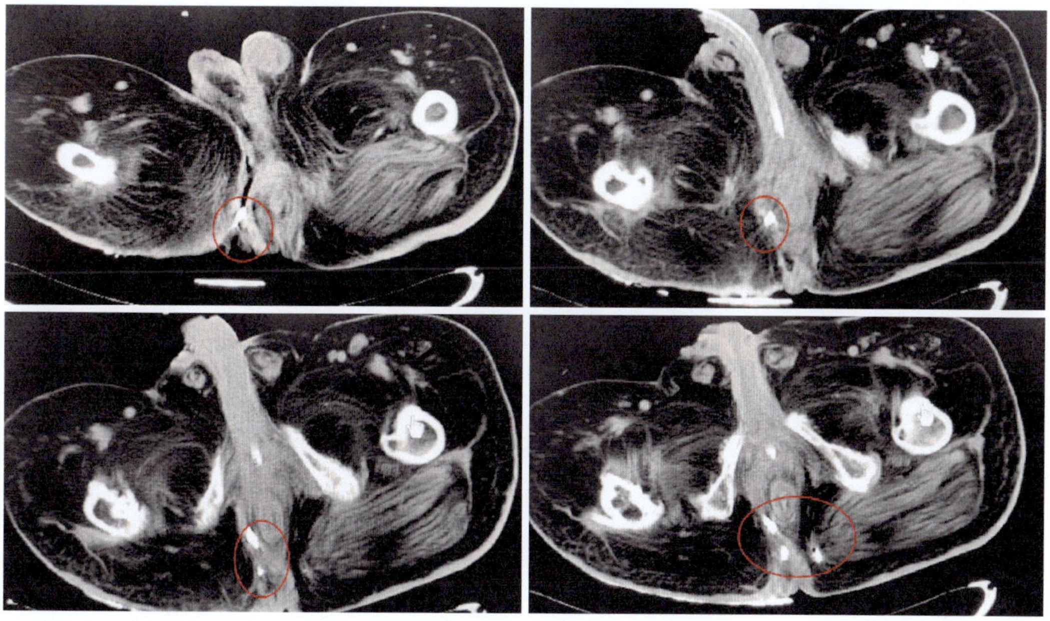

Fig. 11.3 Pelvic CT scan after injection of contrast agent through the anal catheter

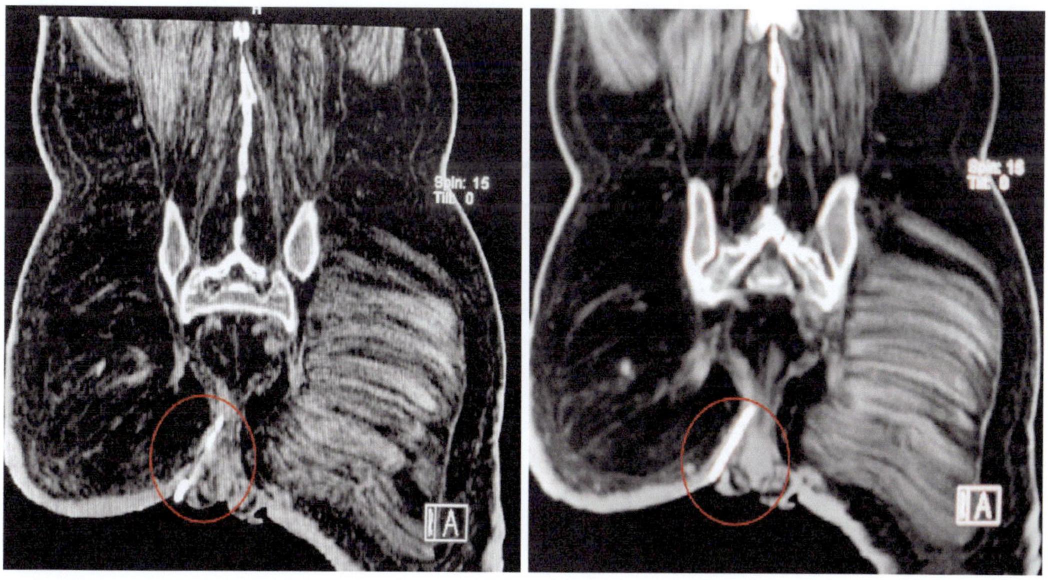

Fig. 11.4 Pelvic CT scan after injection of contrast agent through the anal catheter

openings, communicating with the anus. The fistula openings were rinsed three times with hydrogen peroxide, saline, iodophor, and saline. The tissues around the fistula openings at the 3 o'clock and 7 o'clock positions of the anus were freed, and a pedicled muscle flap was taken, which was completely filled into the fistula opening, sutured layer by layer, and a drainage tube was left in the anus (Figs. 11.5, 11.6, 11.7, and 11.8).

After the operation, continued to use anti-infection, swelling reduction, circulation improvement, and nutritional nerve drugs for symptomatic treatment, and change the dressing every other day. The patient was strictly forbid-

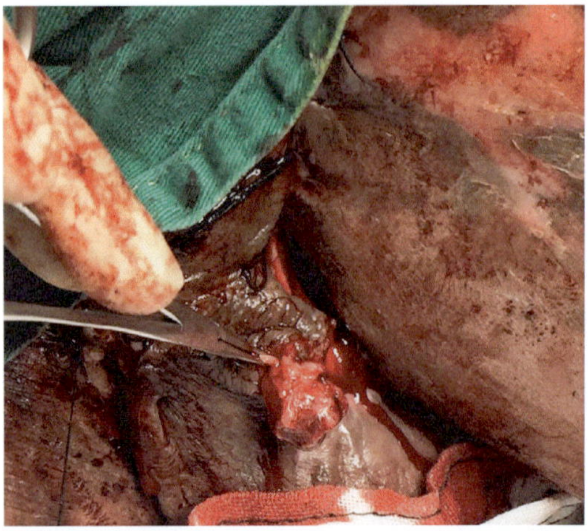

Fig. 11.5 Free three-point muscle flap

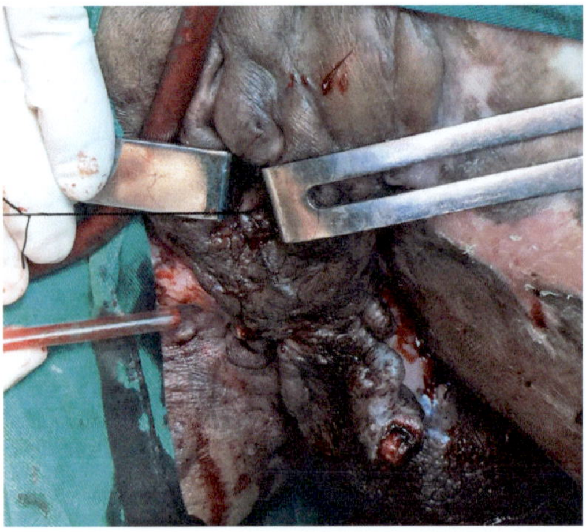

Fig. 11.6 The distal end of the three-point muscle flap was completely filled in the three-point sinus under the pull of the guide wire, and the guide wire was passed from the near-end opening of the anal rectal fistula to the rectum and out of the anus

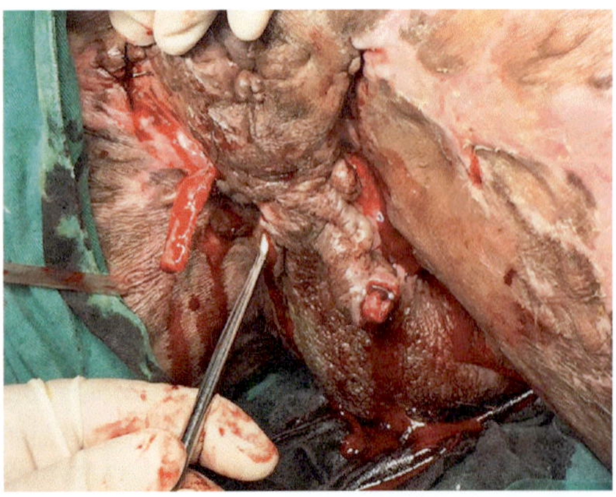

Fig. 11.7 Free seven-point muscle flap

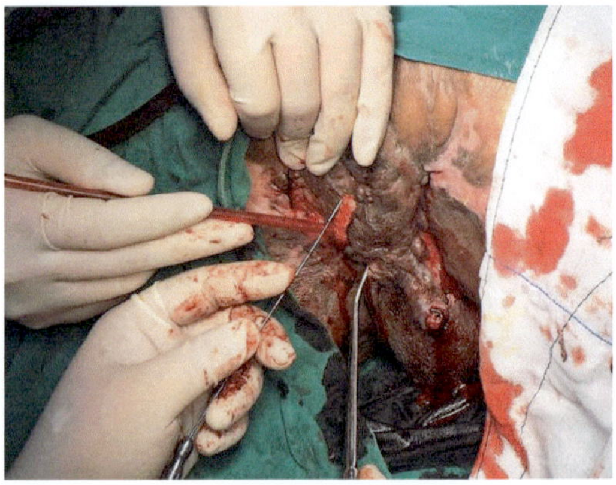

Fig. 11.8 With the assistance of a vascular probe, the distal end of the muscle flap with a guide wire was completely filled in the seven-point anal rectal fistula

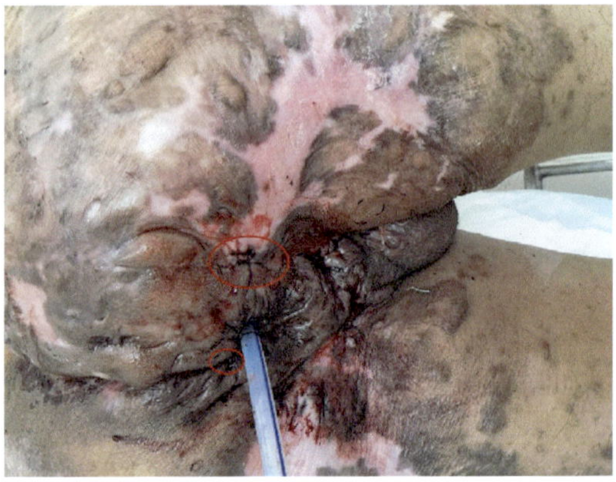

Fig. 11.9 Dressing change on the first day after surgery

den to eat or drink, and the intestinal secretions flow out from the anal drainage tube (Figs. 11.9, 11.10, and 11.11). On the tenth day after the operation, the wound healed, the sutures were removed, the anal rectal drainage tube was removed, and no secretions were seen at the original fistula site during normal defecation (Fig. 11.12).

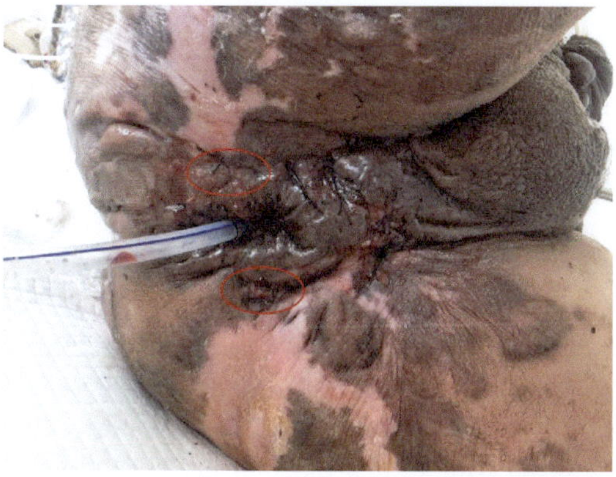

Fig. 11.10 Dressing change on the third day after surgery

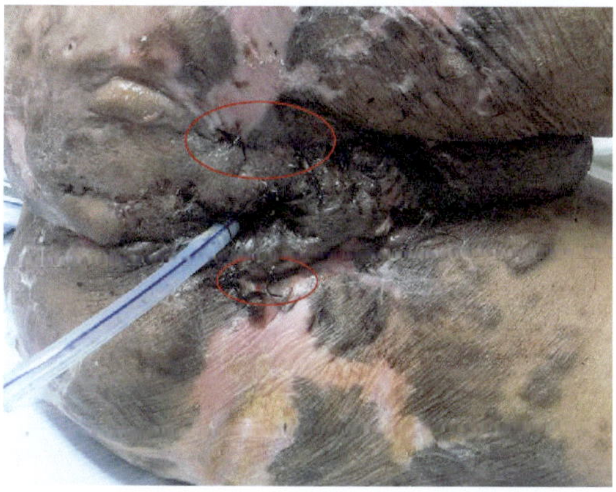

Fig. 11.11 Dressing change on the seventh day after surgery

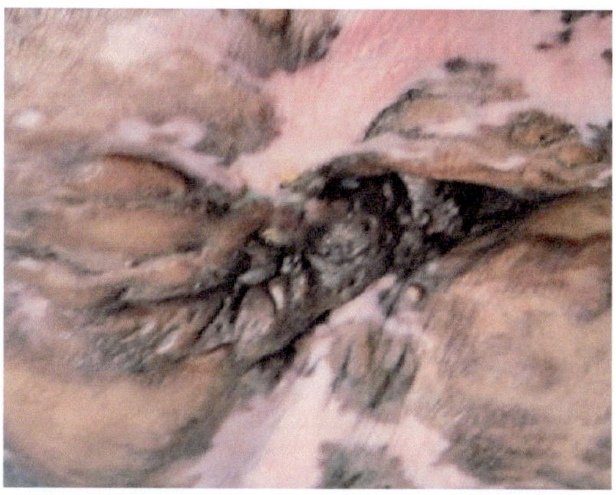

Fig. 11.12 Wound on the tenth day after surgery

11.2 Case Analysis

11.2.1 Fistula Wound Formed by Hidradenitis

Infections of the sweat glands can lead to recurrent infections in the adjacent skin and subcutaneous soft tissues, resulting in a wide range of chronic inflammation. Sometimes, small abscesses or complex sinuses and fistulas may form, known as suppurative hidradenitis. The disease often occurs in areas where sweat glands are concentrated, such as the buttocks, anus, genitals, and buttocks. When it occurs around the anus, it is called perianal suppurative hidradenitis. In traditional Chinese medicine, it falls under the category of cellulitis and buttock fistula. Jackman reported that four out of 125 cases of perianal suppurative hidradenitis turned into squamous cell carcinoma, with an incidence rate of 3.2%. It can be seen that this disease has the potential to turn malignant if it does not heal over a long period, mostly occurring 10–20 years after the onset of the disease.

The patient had a history of hidradenitis in the buttocks for over 20 years, and underwent bilateral buttocks, posterior thighs, and perineal sweat gland removal surgery 4 years ago. Three years after the surgery, a rectal anal fistula formed around the anus. Over the past year, the wound had been repeatedly infected due to fecal contamination, with a tendency to form purulent ulcers. Such wounds were difficult to heal. Once formed and if the fistula was not treated in time, many sinuses will form in succession, merge into a piece, and cause extensive subcutaneous necrosis, skin ulceration, and can extend to the area around the anus. Therefore, thorough debridement of necrotic tissue in the sinus was particularly important.

11.2.2 Differential Diagnosis of Hidradenitis Fistula Wound in the Buttocks

This disease first presents with recurrent unhealed purulent infections under the skin around the anus, with a long course of disease and slow onset. With long-term recurrent attacks, it gradually spreads widely. It should be differentiated from the following two easily confused diseases:

1. Low complex anal fistula: There is one or more than two internal openings in the anal crypt, two or more than two channels communicating with the external opening, and the fistula channel is below the deep layer of the external sphincter. The fistula is deep, with granulation tissue inside, often with an internal opening communicating with the anal rectum, generally with a history of anal rectal abscess.
2. Sacrococcygeal teratoma: This disease is a congenital disease caused by abnormal embryonic development, often occurring in young and middle-aged people, with an external opening in front of the sacrum behind the anus. Digital rectal examination often reveals a lump or fullness in front of the sacrum. Barium enema lateral view can show a widened gap between the rectum and sacrum, a semicircular filling defect or impression in the rectum, and surgery can reveal hair, teeth, and bone in the cavity. Mucus can also be seen in the cavity.

11.2.3 Treatment of Hidradenitis Wound

The cause of purulent hidradenitis of the buttocks lies in the blockage and infection of the large sweat gland outlets in the buttocks, resulting in the rupture of the gland duct and the formation of recurrent inflammation in the skin and even under the skin, eventually forming abscesses, sinus tracts, skin fistulas, and scars.

Early treatment of hidradenitis with local and systemic antibiotics is effective. If surgical treatment is performed, simple incision and drainage can help control local infection, but recurrence is inevitable after surgery; radical surgery requires the removal of all skin and subcutaneous fat layers, and depending on the range of the lesion, one-stage suturing, open wound dressing after excision, or adjunctive skin flap transfer, musculocutaneous flap suturing, skin grafting repair, etc. For patients with purulent hidradenitis of the buttocks with a large range of lesions and fused infection foci, the lesion of purulent hidradenitis of the buttocks can be removed in combination with postage stamp skin grafting.

11.2.4 Conclusion

Perianal purulent hidradenitis is a chronic inflammation of the large sweat glands in the anal skin. Repeated swelling of the infected pus forms chronic cellulitis. It causes a wide range of complex sinus tracts and fistulas under the skin of the anus, perineum, and buttocks. Thorough debridement and application of musculocutaneous flaps to fill the fistula is an effective treatment for this disease.

Bibliography

1. Kong Lingzhuo W, Xinfeng. Surgical treatment of a case of refractory purulent hidradenitis. Chin J Leprosy Skin Dis. 2019;35(2):99–101.
2. Mi C, Wei Z, Hongyan Y, et al. Surgical treatment of purulent hidradenitis. Chin J Aesthet Med. 2018;27(9):45–8.
3. Jemec GB. Clinical practice. Hidradenitis suppurativa. N Engl J Med. 2012;2(2):158–64.
4. Hui Z, Zhimin W. A case of complex perianal and buttock apocrine gland suppurative infection. Chin J Colorectal Dis. 2018;38(5):78.
5. Thorlacius L, Garg A, Ingram JR, et al. Towards global consensus on core outcomes for hidradenitis suppurativa research: an update from the HISTORIC consensus meetings I and II. Br J Dermatol. 2018;178(3):715–21.

12 Three Cases of Large Area Pressure Injury

Lei Gao, Tiangui Chen, Xinyuan Qin, and Jiangning Wang

12.1 Case Summary

12.1.1 Case 1

The patient, female, 38 years old was admitted to the hospital due to sacrococcygeal and right buttock soft tissue injury caused by a car accident 20 days ago.

[Present Illness History] The patient was involved in a car accident 20 days ago, injuring the pelvic area. After the accident, there was no loss of consciousness, but she felt pain in the injured area and could not walk. She was rescued and sent to a local hospital, where she was given blood transfusion, fluid replacement, anti-infection treatment, and other treatments, the specific medication was unknown; she underwent sigmoid colon single-cavity fistula + sacrococcygeal debridement + right tibial node traction + VSD suction surgery. Later, it was found that the soft tissue of the right buttock was infected with secretion exudation for more than 8 days, and routine dressing changes were given. The patient and her family came to our hospital for further treatment, and the outpatient department admitted her to our department with "soft tissue infection." Since the onset of the disease, the patient had been conscious, in good spirits, and had a normal diet; she had symptoms of fever, but no chills.

[Admission Examination]

1. Specialist examination. The sigmoid colon stoma was discharging gas and feces normally; a urinary catheter was in place, draining yellow urine; there was no edema in both lower limbs; there was an irregular wound from the labia majora to the anus, which had been sutured, without redness or bleeding; there was a yellowish-white necrotic tissue with black eschar about 15.0 × 15.0 cm in size in the sacrococcygeal and right buttock area; there was a wound about 7.0 × 7.0 cm × 3.0 cm in size around the anus, the wound was bright red, with fresh blood oozing out, the pain was obvious on touch, and there were potential cavities about 7.0 × 15.0 cm and 2.0 × 7.0 cm in size on the right side and above the wound, the pain was obvious on touch; there was no deformity in the pelvic area, the right hip was obviously tender, and the pelvic squeeze.

   Positive compression separation test; limited mobility in the right lower limb and mild limitation in the left lower limb. Normal pulsation of bilateral femoral arteries, dorsal foot arteries, and posterior tibial arteries; normal

L. Gao · T. Chen · X. Qin · J. Wang (✉)
Department of Orthopedics, Beijing Shijitan Hospital, Capital Medical University, Beijing, China
e-mail: gaolei3337@bjsjth.cn; csy800808@163.com; doctorqin1987@163.com wangjn@bjsjth.cn

J. Wang, L. Gao (eds.), *Refractory Wounds*, Experts' Perspectives on Medical Advances,
https://doi.org/10.1007/978-981-96-2067-8_12

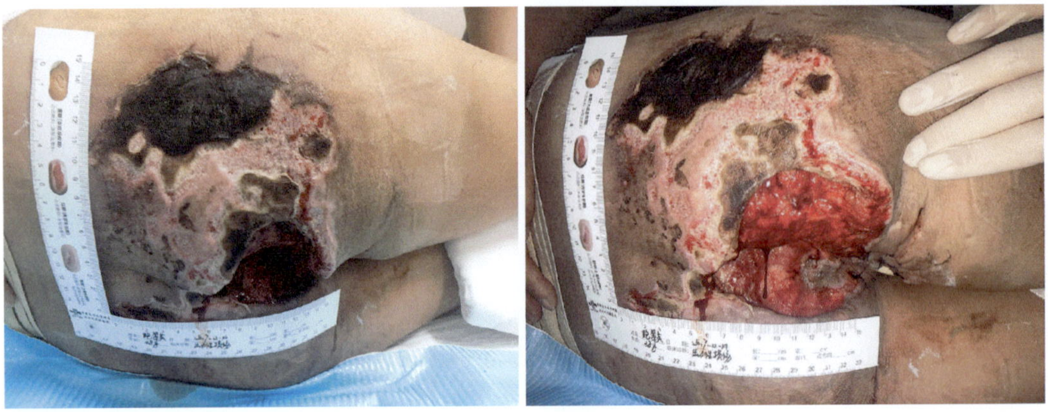

Fig. 12.1 Sacrococcygeal and right buttock wound

sensation in both lower limbs; normal muscle strength and muscle tone. Anorectal sensation is present, anorectal reflex is absent, digital examination reveals relaxed anal sphincter, no fresh blood on the glove upon withdrawal (Fig. 12.1).

2. Laboratory examination. ① Blood test: WBC 6.85×10^9/L, neutrophil percentage 80%, HGB 105 g/L, albumin 34.6 g/L. ② Deep wound bacterial culture result: *Escherichia coli*

[Treatment and Outcome] After admission, the patient was given symptomatic supportive treatment such as anti-infection, improving circulation, correcting hypoalbuminemia, and nutritional support. After ruling out surgical contraindications, necrotic tissue debridement of the sacrococcygeal and right buttock, vascular nerve tendon exploration, **skin stretching device** installation, and VSD suction were performed under general anesthesia. Postoperatively, skin expanders were used to help reduce the tension of the sutured wound, and the wound was regularly dressed (Fig. 12.2).

The wound healed well after tension treatment and VSD negative pressure treatment, and the patient was discharged smoothly. The follow-up results after discharge were good (Fig. 12.3).

12.1.2 Case 2

The patient is a 62-year-old male.

[Present Illness History] Three years ago, he was diagnosed with "spinal cord cavity" in a tertiary hospital in Beijing.

He gradually developed sensory and motor disorders in both lower limbs, along with incontinence of stool and urine, and has been using a wheelchair for a long time; 15 months ago, three pressure injuries broke out on his buttocks, two of which healed after symptomatic treatment with Kangfuxin liquid, iodophor, etc., but the ulcer on the right buttock did not heal, and there was no obvious infection; 12 months ago, due to contamination after defecation, the infection worsened, with local redness, swelling, heat, and pain in the right buttock and thigh, edema in both lower limbs, elevated body temperature, and he went to the hospital. The patient visited multiple hospitals without receiving treatment. Two weeks after the infection worsened, the patient underwent a right buttock and thigh incision and drainage procedure at another top-tier hospital in Beijing. After treatment, the infection in the buttock and thigh was controlled, the lower limb edema subsided, and only a wound of about 5.0 × 5.0 cm in the buttock remained unhealed. Despite continuous dressing changes, there were still no obvious signs of healing (and no obvious symptoms of infection). The patient's vital signs were stable, he was conscious, and his spirits were good.

[Admission Examination]

1. Spsecialist examination. Sensation in both lower limbs completely disappeared, movement disappeared, about 3.0 cm from the anus

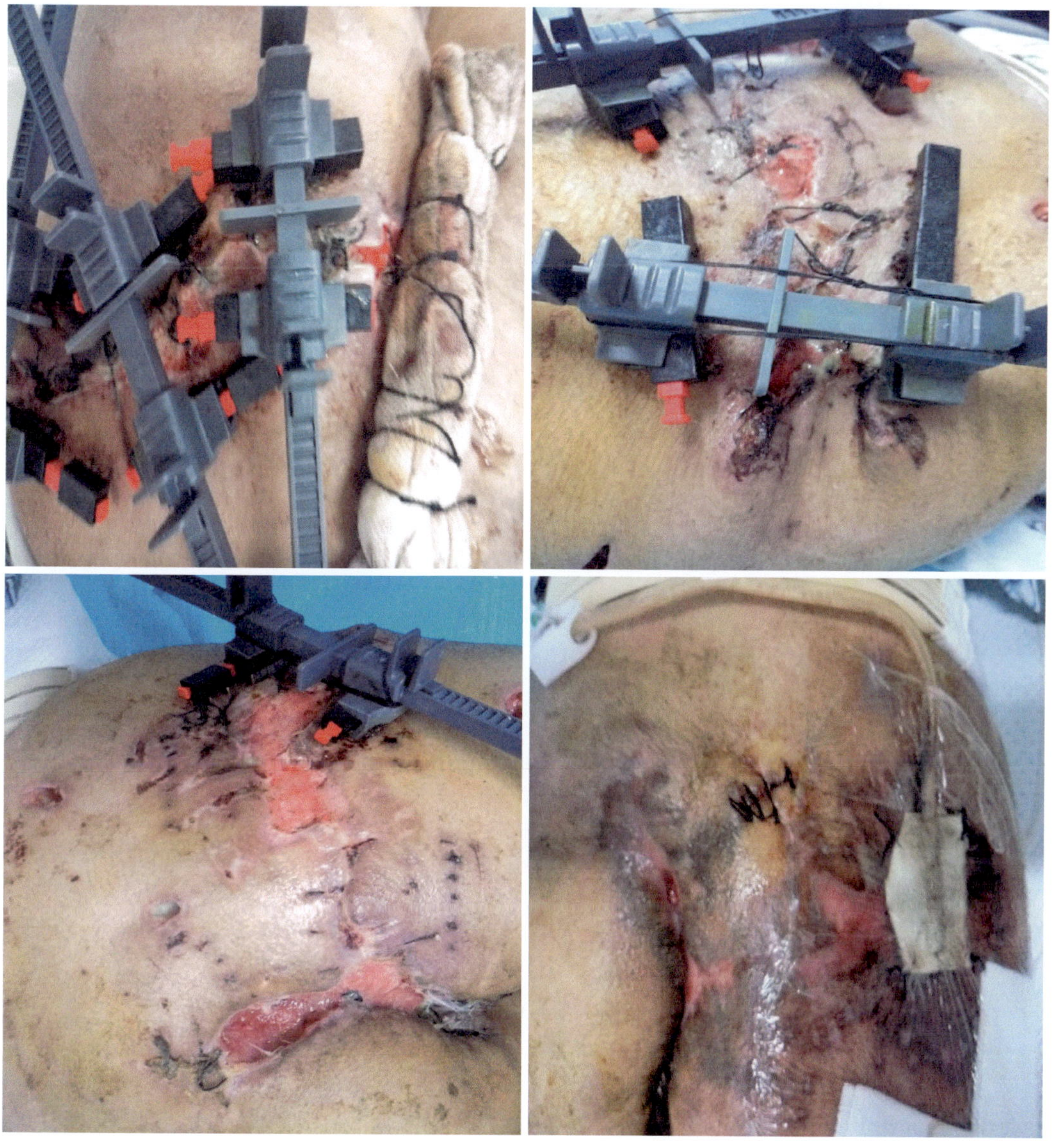

Fig. 12.2 Postoperative skin expander to help reduce suture wound tension

on the right buttock, a wound of 5.0×6.0 cm could be seen, a large number of "tadpole-like" hyperplasias could be seen in the wound, no obvious purulent secretion and active bleeding were found, no redness and swelling around, no edema in both lower limbs, muscle strength 0 level (Fig. 12.4).

3. Imaging examination. No obvious abnormalities were seen in the chest X-ray. The pelvic X-ray showed that the structure of the right ischial bone was unclear due to external pseudoshadow. No obvious abnormalities were found in the color Doppler ultrasound of both lower limb vessels and the heart.
4. Laboratory examination. No obvious abnormalities were found in various indicators. No obvious bacterial growth was found in the culture of wound secretions.

[Treatment and Outcome] After admission, the patient was given symptomatic supportive treatment such as anti-infection, circulation improvement, and nutritional support. After excluding surgical contraindications, debridement and suturing of necrotic tissue in the right buttock + Vacuum Sealing Drainage (VSD) suction surgery + vascular nerve tendon exploration were performed under general anesthesia. During the operation, it was found that the wound reached the sacrum, there was a black shadow of about 2.0 × 1.0 cm at the sacrum, and a cavity of about 1.0 × 0.5 cm could be explored, with no obvious purulent secretion (Fig. 12.5). The wound was regularly dressed after the operation (Fig. 12.6).

The wound underwent debridement surgery and VSD treatment, the stitches were removed 24 days after the surgery, and the healing was good and the patient was discharged smoothly (Fig. 12.7). Long-term follow-up after discharge (Fig. 12.8).

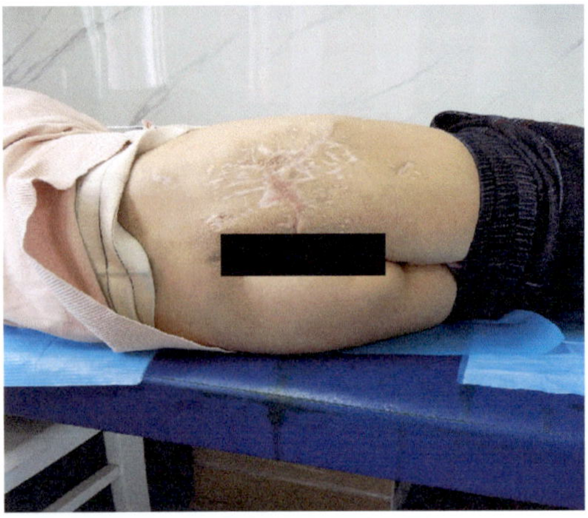

Fig. 12.3 Follow-up after discharge

12.1.3 Case 3

Patient, female, 99 years old. Admitted to the hospital due to necrosis and exudation in the sacrococcygeal area for more than 2 months.

[Present Illness History] The patient has been bedridden for a long time, ignored the rupture and exudation in the sacrococcygeal area that appeared 2 months ago. Ten days ago, she found necrotic tissue in the sacrococcygeal area, the rupture deepened, and she was treated at a certain emergency rescue center in Beijing, where she was given wound dressing changes (specific drugs unknown) and symptomatic treatment such as anti-infection, but the symptoms did not improve significantly. The symptoms of necrotic infection in the sacrococcygeal wound worsened, and she came to our hospital for further treatment. She was admitted to the hospital with the diagnosis of "soft tissue infection."

[Past History] Hypertension for more than 30 years, highest 160/90 mmHg, controlled by 1 tablet of Shihuida (1 time/day); bedridden due to cerebral infarction, usually taking aspirin enteric-coated tablets 100 mg (1 time/day), clopidogrel bisulfate 75 mg (1 time/day), atorvastatin calcium 20 mg (1 time/day) for control; history

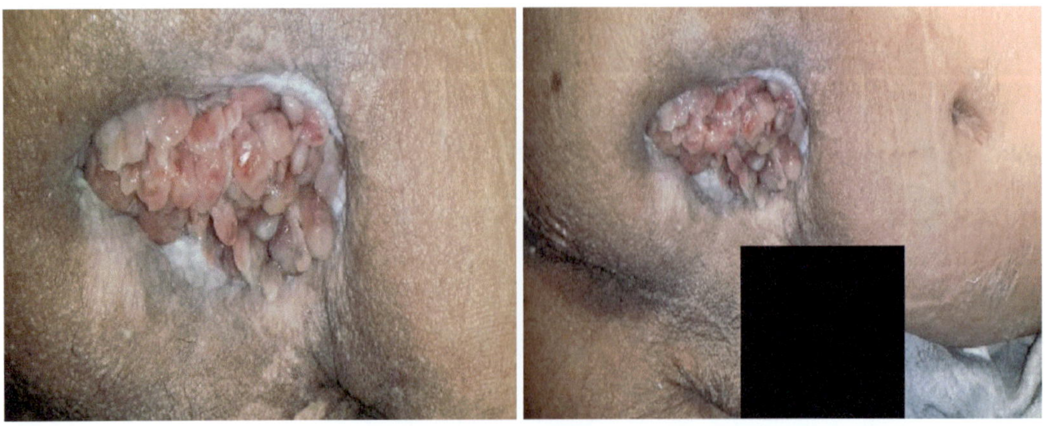

Fig. 12.4 A large number of "tadpole-like" hyperplasias can be seen in the wound

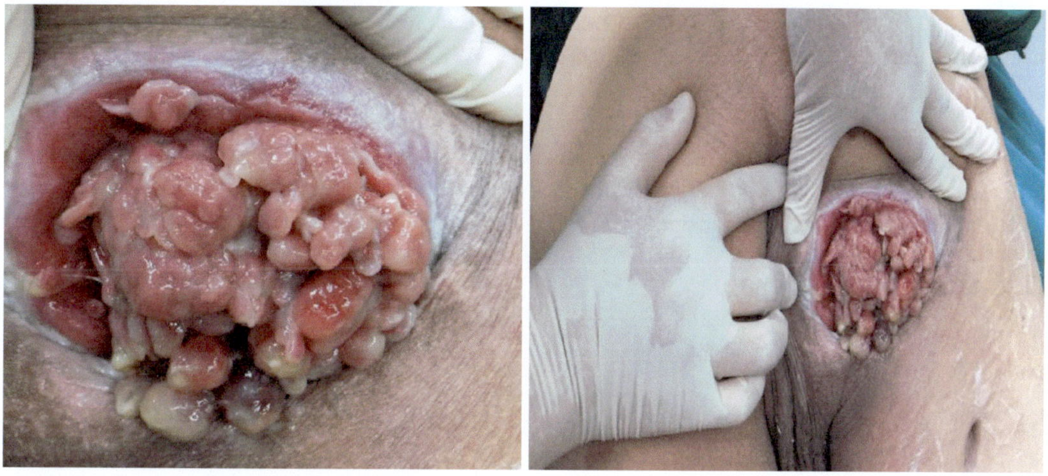

Fig. 12.5 No obvious purulent secretion seen in the wound

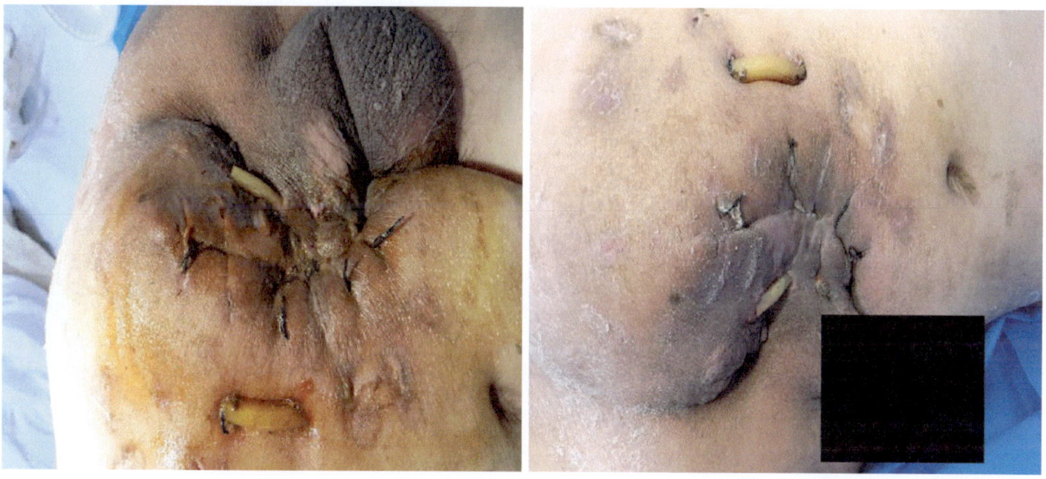

Fig. 12.6 Postoperative wound

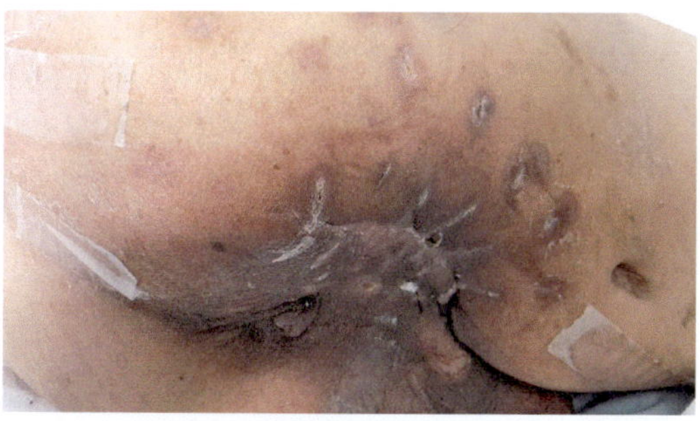

Fig. 12.7 Good wound healing 24 days after surgery

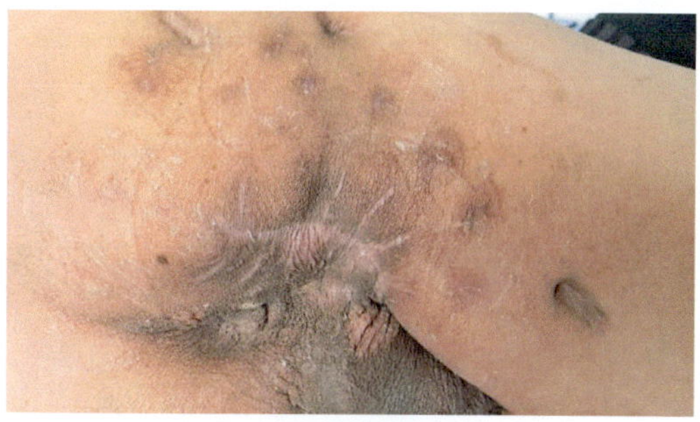

Fig. 12.8 Postoperative follow-up

of heart failure and chronic bronchitis. Denies history of chronic diseases such as diabetes; denies history of hepatitis B, tuberculosis and close contact history; denies surgical history, trauma history, blood product transfusion history; denies drug and food allergy history. Vaccination was carried out as planned.

[Admission Examination]

1. Specialist examination. Bedridden; sacrococcygeal area can be seen about 15.0 cm × 5.0 cm in size.

    The wound, with a large amount of purulent necrotic tissue attached to it, reaches the depth of the sacrum, has a strong odor, and is surrounded by redness and tenderness. On the left hip, there is a wound about 2.0 cm in diameter, with black scabs attached, surrounded by redness and tenderness (Fig. 12.9).
2. Laboratory examination. ① Blood routine: WBC 15.03 × 10^9/L, neutrophil percentage 86.6%, HGB 105 g/L. ② Blood biochemistry: albumin 28.2 g/L. ③ CRP 31.46 mg/L. ④ESR 57 mm/h. ⑤Deep wound bacterial culture results: *Enterococcus faecalis*, *Escherichia coli* subspecies.
3. Imaging examination. Sacrococcygeal MRI: Sacrococcygeal soft tissue infection, rough sacrococcygeal bone cortex, local sinus formation.

[Treatment and Outcome] After admission, the patient was given symptomatic treatment such as anti-infection, improving circulation, correcting hypoalbuminemia, and nutritional support. After excluding surgical contraindications, sacrococcygeal ulcer resection and repair surgery + skin expander implantation were performed under intravenous general anesthesia.

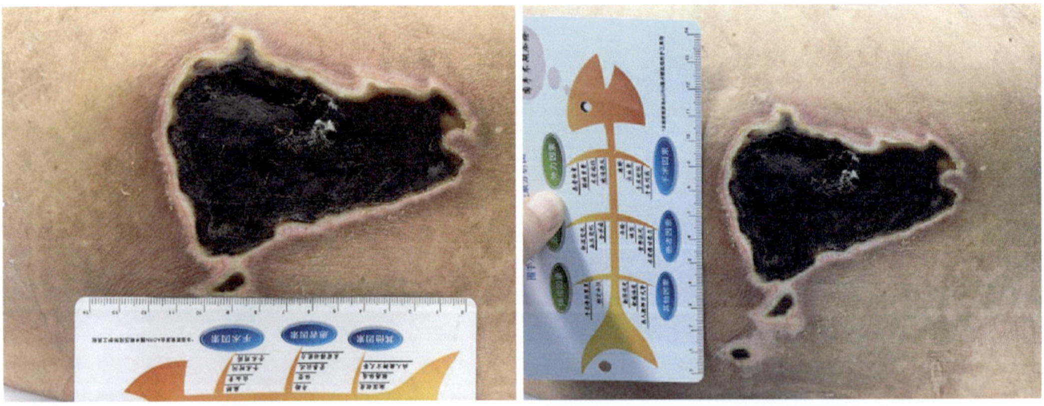

Fig. 12.9 Preoperative wound

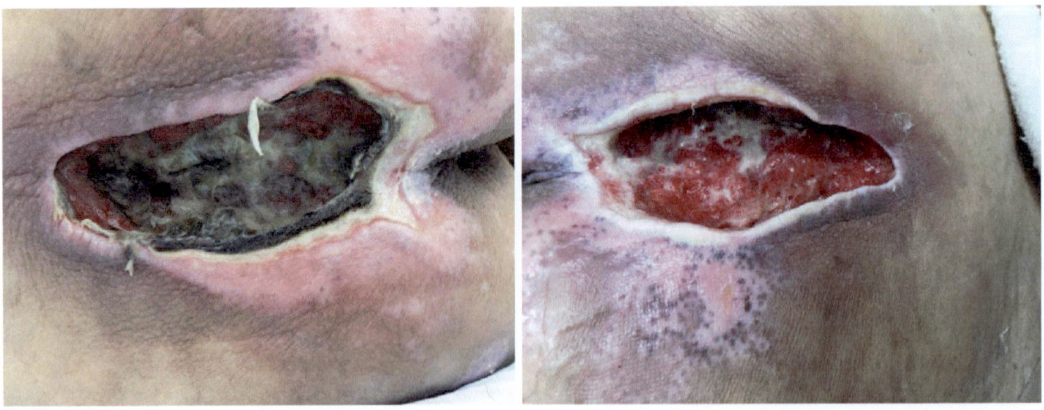

Fig. 12.10 Postoperative ulcer repair

After the operation, the skin expander was pulled to help reduce the tension of the sutured wound, and the wound was regularly dressed (Figs. 12.10 and 12.11).

The wound was treated with traction, and the sutures were removed 3 weeks after the operation, and the healing was good. However, due to the patient's old age and long-term bed rest, gravity-induced pneumonia formed. Before discharge, high fever occurred, with the highest temperature of 40.2 °C, blood culture showed *Staphylococcus epidermidis*, and fungal culture showed *Candida albicans*. After cooperation with the intensive care unit, pharmacy, cardiovascular medicine, respiratory medicine, and other disciplines, according to the drug sensitivity results, antibacterial drugs were used, frequent turning and back patting, active atomization and sputum suction, strengthening of overall nutrition, after 2 weeks of effort, the patient finally turned from danger to safety, all inflammation indicators returned to normal, and the patient was discharged smoothly (Fig. 12.12).

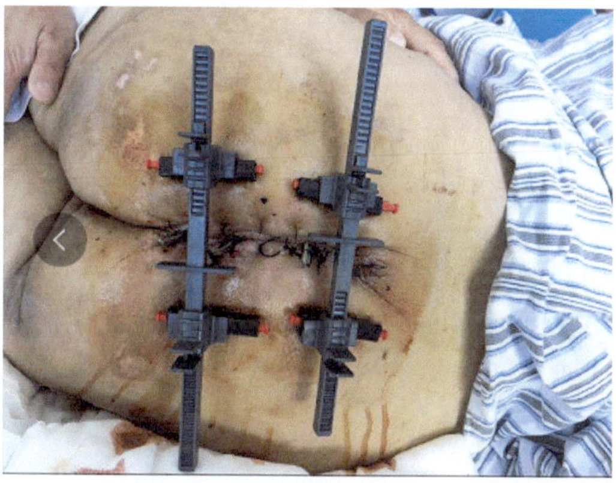

Fig. 12.11 Skin expander implantation

12.2 Case Analysis

12.2.1 Diagnosis and Treatment of Pressure Injuries (Pressure Sores/Bedsores)

Pressure injuries, formerly known as "bedsores" or "pressure sores" are caused by long-term bedridden patients experiencing local pressure, leading to nerve nutrition disorders and blood circulation disorders, local tissue continuous ischemia, and then leading to malnutrition and soft tissue necrosis. This disease not only occurs in the lying position but many also occur in the sitting position; so now the term "pressure injury" is more commonly used, which more accurately summarizes the essence of the disease from the pathological and physiological perspectives. This disease is one of the common complications in clinical practice, and it is easy to cause infection. Once it worsens, it can cause great pain to the patient, and even lead to sepsis and death, so it is a "stubborn disease" that nursing work needs to overcome. Pressure injuries are more likely to occur in long-term bedridden patients, spinal cord injuries, chronic neurological diseases

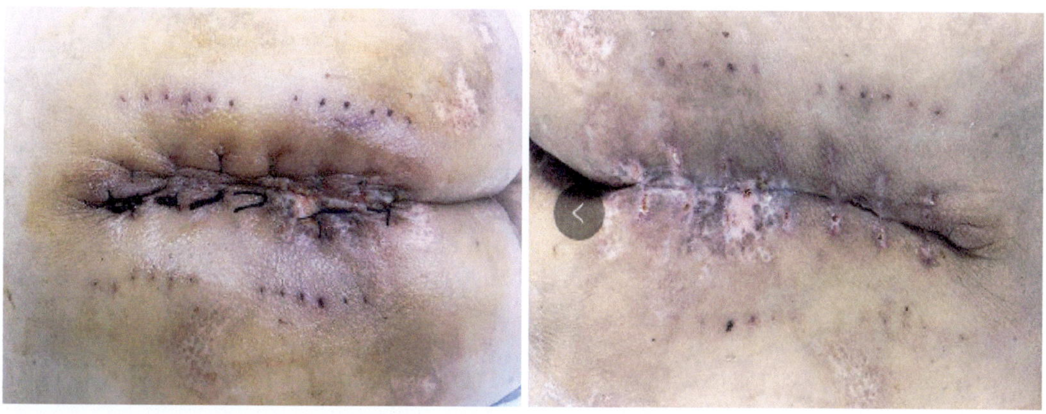

Fig. 12.12 Postoperative wound

(mainly cerebrovascular diseases), physically weak patients, various consumptive diseases, and elderly patients. If there is hypoalbuminemia, incontinence, fractures, malnutrition, lack of vitamins, etc., it is more likely to occur. About 95% of pressure injuries occur in the bony prominences of the lower body, and the most common sites are the sacrococcygeal area, ischial tuberosities, greater trochanters of the femur, medial and lateral malleoli, and heels.

12.2.2 Causes and Risk Factors of Pressure Injuries

Pressure, shear force, friction, and moisture are the main factors causing pressure injuries.

Age, smoking, low blood pressure (especially diastolic pressure), arteriosclerotic heart disease, diabetes, cognitive impairment, malnutrition, anemia, etc., are risk factors. ① Pressure is the vertical force borne on the force-bearing surface, which is the most important pathogenic factor and is closely related to the pressure time. Ulcers form faster under high pressure than under low pressure. When the pressure exceeds the average capillary pressure of 4.27 kPa, it will cause skin blood flow to stop. Due to the accumulation of lymphatic stasis, anaerobic metabolic waste can also easily cause tissue necrosis. Pressure diffuses from the skin from shallow to deep, showing a conical decreasing distribution, and is mostly gathered in the protruding parts of the bone in the deep layer. Muscles and adipose tissue are more sensitive to pressure than skin, and degenerative necrosis appears first. Atrophy, emaciation, scars, and infected tissues increase the sensitivity to pressure. ② Shear force is applied to the surface of adjacent objects, causing progressive parallel sliding in the opposite direction. It acts on the deep layer, causing relative displacement of the tissues, and can cut off the blood supply of a large area, so it is more harmful than vertical pressure. For example, the tendency of the body to slide down when the head of the bed is raised for a supine patient, and the tendency of the body to move forward for a wheelchair patient, can generate a large shear force on the sacrum and ischial tuberosity, often involving the dorsal branch of the lateral sacral artery and the superficial branch of the superior gluteal artery, causing a large area of tissue ischemia and hypoxia in their supply area. Elderly people are susceptible to shear force due to physiological and immune changes in the skin, which reduce their barrier ability and vascular function. ③ Friction is a force that hinders the movement of an object on the surface of another object when it moves or has a relative movement tendency. Friction acts on the epithelial tissue, can remove the outer protective keratinized skin, and increase the susceptibility to pressure injury. Clinically, the surface is wrinkled and uneven, there are scabs or dragging and pulling patients when moving, all of which generate a large friction. ④ Moisture can be caused by incontinence, sweating, etc., causing skin soaking, softening, and easy to be injured by shear and friction forces. Allman pointed out that when there is fecal incontinence, there are more bacteria and toxins, which is more dangerous than urinary incontinence. This kind of pollutant soaking induces infection and makes the situation worse. ⑤ Smoking is an important risk factor for pressure injuries, and the risk of pressure injuries in smokers is significantly increased. The risk of heel pressure injuries in smokers is four times that of non-smokers, and the amount of smoking is positively correlated with the incidence and severity of pressure injuries. However, if smokers quit smoking, their risk of pressure injuries will be significantly reduced, and the adverse effects of smoking can be partially reversed. ⑥ Cognitive impairment is also a significant risk factor for stress injuries. Those with unclear consciousness are significantly more likely to suffer from stress injuries than those who are semi-conscious. Changes in brain alertness levels, history of cerebrovascular accidents, and dementia are all risk factors for stress injuries. ⑦ Malnutrition is one of the most important risk factors for stress injuries. Low hemoglobin (120 g/L) is an excellent predictive indicator. Hypoalbuminemia is a prior cause of stress injuries, not a result of them. People with serum albumin levels <35 g/L are five times more likely to suffer from stress injuries than the control group. ⑧ Anemia is also one of the main risk factors for stress injuries. Hematocrit <0.36 and hemoglobin <120 g/L are good laboratory cut-off points, which have a good screening predictive effect on the occurrence of stress injuries

12.2.3 Complications and Hazards of Stress Injuries

The main complication of stress injuries is infection. Due to the loss of skin barrier function, exposure of the wound, and frequent contamination by feces and urine, the infection rate is extremely high, including abscesses, osteomyelitis, and sepsis. The mortality rate of complications from stress injury infections can reach 50% under hospital conditions, and it is the direct cause of death for 7–8% of spinal cord injury patients. The mortality rate related to stress injuries in the elderly is 23–37%. The mortality rate of elderly people with stress injuries is four times higher than that of elderly people without stress injuries. If the stress injury does not heal, the mortality rate increases by six times.

Bibliography

1. Daifeng H, Chuanan S, Tao L, trans. Basic theory and prevention of pressure sores. Beijing: People's Military Medical Publishing House; 2015.
2. de Azevedo Macena MS, Da Costa Silva RS, Dias Fernandes MIDC, et al. Pressure ulcer risk evaluation in critical patients: clinical and social characteristics. Open Nurs J. 2017;1:91–7.
3. Daifeng H, Wanli C, Hongjie D. Common knowledge of bedsores prevention. Beijing: Jindun Publishing House; 2016.
4. Hongjie D, Jiakai C, Daifeng H, et al. Analysis of factors affecting the healing of stage III and IV pressure ulcers. Chin J Trauma Repair (Electronic Edition). 2015;10(6):466–9.
5. Artmann CW, Solomon J, Palmer JA, et al. Contextual facilitators of and barriers to nursing home pressure ulcer prevention. Adv Skin Wound Care. 2016;29(5):226–38.
6. Goode PS, Burgio KL, Halli AD, Jones RW, Richter HE, Redden DT, Baker PS, Allman RM. Prevalence and correlates of fecal incontinence in community-dwelling older adults. J Am Geriatr Soc. 2005;53(4):629–35.

A Case of Refractory Diabetic Wound

13

Shuo Wang, Jiangning Wang, and Lei Gao

13.1 Case Analysis

Patient, male, 64 years old. The main reason for admission to our department was the non-healing ulceration of the left foot for more than 4 months.

[Present Illness History] The patient found a blister on the sole of the foot that burst after walking 4 months ago. After changing the dressing himself, the wound did not heal and gradually became larger and deeper. He was treated at a local hospital a month ago, considering "diabetic foot," and was given symptomatic dressing change treatment. The wound did not improve significantly, so he visited our outpatient clinic.

[Past History] History of type 2 diabetes for more than 20 years, no regular treatment, blood sugar not tested.

[Admission Examination]

1. Specialist examination. A 1.0 × 1.0 × 1.0 cm wound can be seen on the sole of the right foot, deep to the fascia layer, with necrotic soft tissue inside, more secretions, no odor, no obvious pain on touch, and poor movement of the five toes (Fig. 13.1). Weak pulse of both feet dorsalis pedis.
2. Laboratory examination. ① Blood routine: WBC 3.63 × 10^{10}/L, neutrophil percentage 46.4%, HGB 148 g/L. ② Blood biochemistry: albumin 35.6 g/L. ③ CRP 23.4 mg/L. ④ Deep wound bacterial culture result: *Escherichia coli*.
3. Imaging examination. Lower limb vascular imaging (CTA): atherosclerosis of both lower limb arteries (Fig. 13.2).

[Preliminary Diagnosis] Type 2 diabetic foot ulcer (right), type 2 diabetic peripheral vascular disease, type 2 diabetic peripheral neuropathy, type 2 diabetes, hypertension level 3 (very high risk).

[Treatment and Outcome] After admission, the patient was given symptomatic treatment with anti-infection, swelling reduction, circulation improvement, and neurotrophic and anticoagulant drugs. On the fourth day of admission, relevant examinations were completed and debridement and necrotic tissue removal treatment were performed. The granulation tissue in the wound was fresh, and the wound cavity was large, about 3.0 × 4.0 × 3.0 cm. Dressings were changed daily after surgery. On the third day after surgery, a micro-oxygen device was installed (Fig. 13.3), and dressings continued to be changed daily. On the 15th day after surgery, the wound had healed (Fig. 13.4).

S. Wang · J. Wang (✉) · L. Gao
Department of Orthopedics, Beijing Shijitan Hospital, Capital Medical University, Beijing, China
e-mail: shenkemao@qq.com; wangjn@bjsjth.cn; gaolei3337@bjsjth.cn

J. Wang, L. Gao (eds.), *Refractory Wounds*, Experts' Perspectives on Medical Advances,
https://doi.org/10.1007/978-981-96-2067-8_13

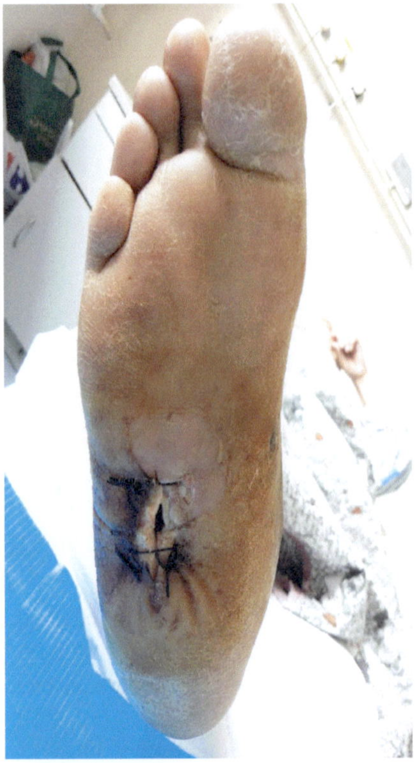

Fig. 13.1 Preoperative

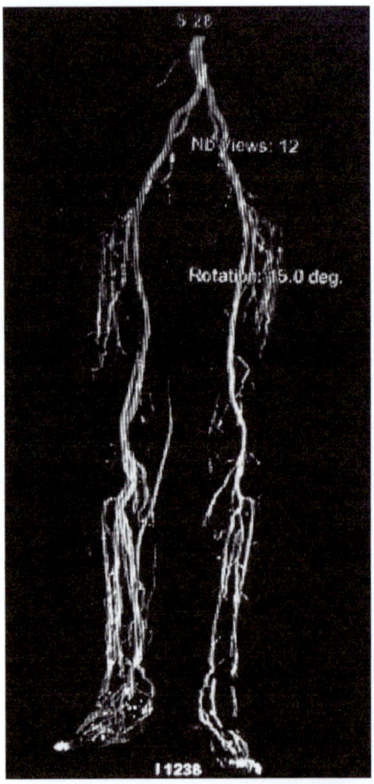

Fig. 13.2 CTA suggests mild lower limb vascular occlusion

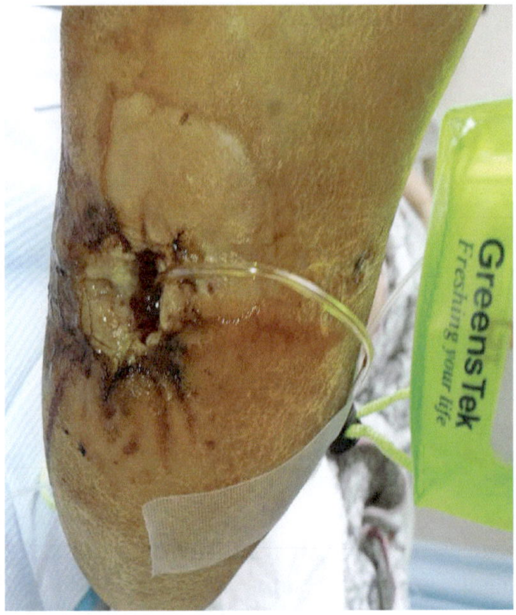

Fig. 13.3 Micro-oxygen treatment started on the third day after surgery

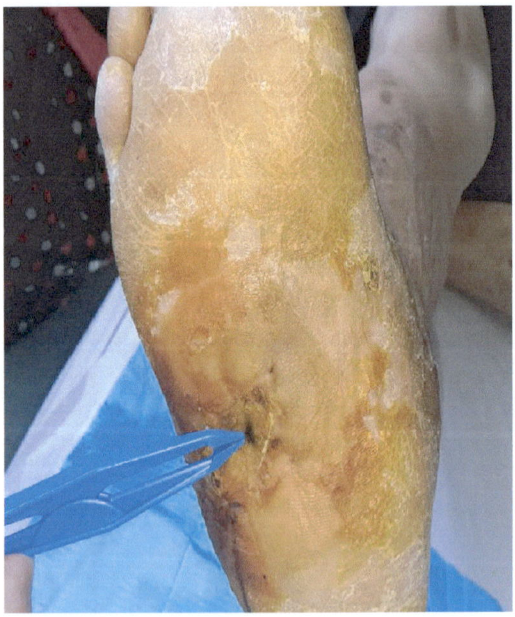

Fig. 13.4 On the 15th day of using micro-oxygen, the wound completely healed, no further surgery required

13.2 Case Analysis

13.2.1 Diabetic Foot

The wounds of diabetic patients are difficult to heal due to low resistance and susceptibility to infection without medical intervention. This patient's wound deteriorated and expanded over 3 months of changing dressings outside the hospital, resulting in local ulceration and necrosis, diagnosed as a diabetic foot ulcer. CTA suggests that the condition of the lower limb vessels is acceptable. After controlling blood sugar well and thoroughly removing necrotic tissue, the condition of the lower limb vessels is still acceptable, and dressings can be changed regularly, and the wound exudate gradually decreases.

13.2.2 Micro-oxygen Treatment of Wounds

In 2002, the American Wound Certification Association proposed the TIME principle, that is, a complete wound treatment process should include debridement (T), (anti)-infection or inflammation (I), moisture balance (M), and edge trimming (E). However, with the development of the times, experts have a deeper understanding of the nature of wound hypoxia and the pathophysiology of correcting hypoxia, and proposed the TIMEO2 Principle. This emphasizes the role of local wound oxygen. According to a literature search, we found that oxygen is a controlling factor in tissue repair, and it is expected to improve the healing of refractory wounds. The effects of high-purity oxygen on wounds include: ① through the migration and replication of fibroblasts, collagen is produced and its tensile strength is increased; ② promotes angiogenesis and vascular reconstruction; ③ activates the phagocytic function of inflammatory cells through the process of "respiratory burst," thus playing an anti-infection role; ④ produces analgesic effects. However, it is worth noting that an important premise for the treatment of wounds with micro-oxygen is that the granulation tissue of the wound must be fresh.

13.2.3 Conclusion

For diabetic foot ulcers, timely medical intervention is needed, to assess the blood supply of the lower limbs, remove necrotic tissue through surgery, and promote wound healing through micro-oxygen therapy after surgery, which can make local tissues easier to heal.

Bibliography

1. Shah JB. Correction of hypoxia, a critical element for wound bed preparation guidelines: TIMEO 2 principle of wound bed preparation. J Am Col Certif Wound Spec. 2011;3(2):26–32.
2. Gilligan AM, Waycaster CR, Motley TA. Cost-effectiveness of becaplermin gel on wound healing of diabetic foot ulcers. Wound Repair Regen. 2015;23(3):353–60.
3. Knighton DR, Silver IA, Hunt TK. Regulation of wound-healing angiogenesis- effect of oxygen gradients and inspired oxygen concentration. Surgery. 1981;90(2):262–70.
4. Bosco MC, Delfino S, Ferlito F, et al. The hypoxic synovial environment regulates expression of vascular endothelial growth factor and osteopontin in juvenile idiopathic arthritis. J Rheumatol. 2009;36(6):1318–29.
5. Dhamodharan U, Viswanathan V, Krishnamoorthy E, et al. Genetic association of IL-6, TNF-α and SDF-1 polymorphisms with serum cytokine levels in diabetic foot ulcer. Gene. 2015;565(1):62–7.
6. Sen CK. Wound healing essentials: let there be oxygen. Wound Repair Regen. 2009;17(1):1–18.
7. Tandara AA, Mustoe TA. Oxygen in wound healing - more than a nutrient. World J Surg. 2004;28(3):294–300.
8. Gordillo GM, Roy S, Khanna S, et al. Topical oxygen therapy induces vascular endothelial growth factor expression and improves closure of clinically presented chronic wounds. Clin Exp Pharmacol Physiol. 2008;35(8):957–64.
9. Jiangning W, Gengjia T, Zhaofan X, authors. Comprehensive treatment of pressure sores. Beijing: People's Health Publishing House; 2018.

10. Xin Y, Zhongguo L, Likun H, et al. Clinical observation of oxygen generator promoting non-primary wound healing. Chinese Drugs and Clinics. 2014;14(2):226–8.
11. Blackman E, Moore C, Hyatt J, et al. Topical wound oxygen therapy in the treatment of severe diabetic foot ulcers: a prospective controlled study. Ostomy Wound Manage. 2010;56(6):24–31.
12. Hayes PD, Alzuhir N, Curran G, et al. Topical oxygen therapy promotes the healing of chronic diabetic foot ulcers: a pilot study. J Wound Care. 2017;26(11):652–60.
13. Yu J, Lu S, Mclaren AM, et al. Topical oxygen therapy results in complete wound healing in diabetic foot ulcers. Wound Repair Regen. 2016;24(6):1066–72.
14. Jiangning W, Lei G, Tiangui C, et al. Professor Wang Jiangning's team's comprehensive diagnosis and treatment of diabetic foot cases. Beijing: Science and Technology Literature Publishing House; 2018.

A Case of Refractory Wound Combined with Peripheral Vascular Disease in Diabetes

14

Shuo Wang, Jiangning Wang, and Lei Gao

14.1 Case Summary

Patient, female, 57 years old. The main reason for admission is that the left foot's big toe was amputated 3 months ago, and the external ankle has been ulcerated for more than 2 months.

[Present Illness History] The patient's left big toe ulcerated and turned black 3 months ago. She was treated at a local hospital and was considered to have "diabetic foot." She underwent distal amputation of the big toe. After symptomatic treatment, the wound gradually turned black. She was treated at a provincial hospital with symptomatic, anti-infective, analgesic, and hypoglycemic treatments. The symptoms did not significantly alleviate, and the second toe gradually turned black. She came to our outpatient clinic for further treatment and was admitted to our department with "diabetic foot." Since the onset of the disease, the patient has had no fever, normal bowel movements, good sleep and spirit, and no significant weight loss.

[Past History] Hypertension for 24 years, treated with oral valsartan, blood pressure controlled at 130/70 mmHg; diabetic for 22 years, currently on insulin treatment, blood sugar not regularly monitored; hyperlipidemia for 20 years.

[Admission Examination]

1. Specialist examination. Both feet skin color basically normal, no obvious swelling, the first toe of the left foot can see skin necrosis, the second toe can see skin black necrosis, no sensation, no obvious odor, pressing pain is obvious, left ankle can see local skin defect, local tissue whitening, no obvious bone exposure (Fig. 14.1). The movement of the affected foot is limited. Both feet skin temperature is okay, dorsalis pedis artery pulse not touched.
2. Laboratory examination. WBC 8.4×10^9/L, neutrophils 6.4×10^9/L, ESR 79 mm/h, amylase 30 U/L, serum iron 7.4 μmol/L, uric acid 373 μmol/L, blood glucose 10.67 mmol/L, γ-glutamyl transferase 77 U/L, CRP 22.51 mg/L, glycated hemoglobin 6.6%. Bacterial culture results from the outside hospital: *Pseudomonas aeruginosa*, sensitive to levofloxacin, gentamicin, meropenem, amikacin.
3. Imaging examination. CTA showed almost complete occlusion of the middle segment of the femoral artery, slow blood flow, severe occlusion of the distal femoral artery and artery, complete occlusion of the anterior tibial artery and posterior tibial artery, slight contrast of the peroneal artery (Fig. 14.2). Imaging diagnosis: Multiple atherosclerotic

S. Wang · J. Wang (✉) · L. Gao
Department of Orthopedics, Beijing Shijitan Hospital, Capital Medical University, Beijing, China
e-mail: shenkemao@qq.com; wangjn@bjsjth.cn; gaolei3337@bjsjth.cn

J. Wang, L. Gao (eds.), *Refractory Wounds*, Experts' Perspectives on Medical Advances,
https://doi.org/10.1007/978-981-96-2067-8_14

changes in the lower extremities CTA. Defect of the distal phalanx of the left big toe.

[Preliminary Diagnosis] Type 2 diabetic foot gangrene, type 2 diabetic retinopathy, type 2 diabetic peripheral vascular disease, type 2 diabetic peripheral neuropathy, grade 2 hypertension (very high risk).

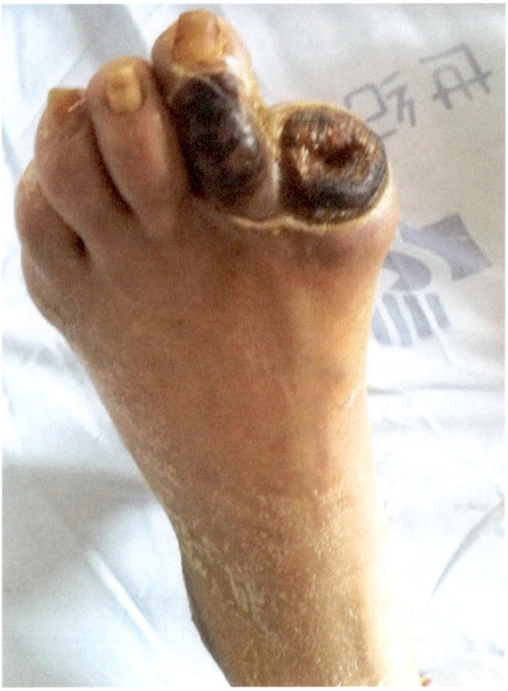

Fig. 14.1 Patient's first time admission with left foot

[Treatment and Outcome] After admission, the patient was given symptomatic treatment with anti-infection, swelling reduction, circulation improvement, neuro-nutrition, and anticoagulant drugs. On the fourth day of admission, bilateral femoral artery puncture and pressurized perfusion surgery were performed under local anesthesia (Fig. 14.3), and on the sixth day, left lumbar sympathetic ganglion destruction surgery was performed under local anesthesia. After the surgery, the skin temperature of the lower limbs increased, and the dorsal artery pulse of the foot improved. On the seventh day, left lower limb arterial balloon dilatation surgery was performed under local anesthesia, after which the dorsal artery pulse of the left foot was strong and the skin temperature increased. On the 14th day of admission, the first and second toes of the left foot were amputated under spinal anesthesia, and after the surgery, symptomatic treatment was given with anti-infection, pain relief, microcirculation improvement, and neuro-nutrition. The wound was regularly dressed, and it healed seven days later (Fig. 14.4).

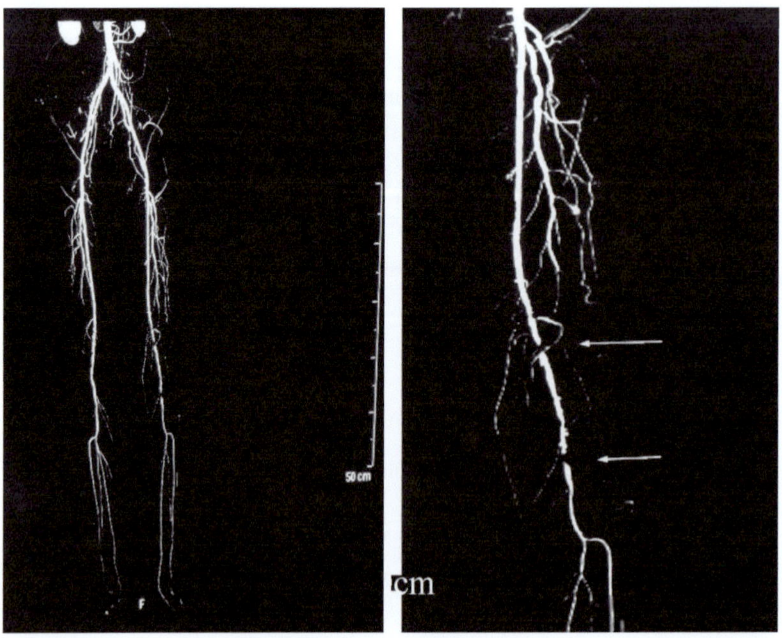

Fig. 14.2 Lower limb arterial angiography shows interruption of the left femoral artery

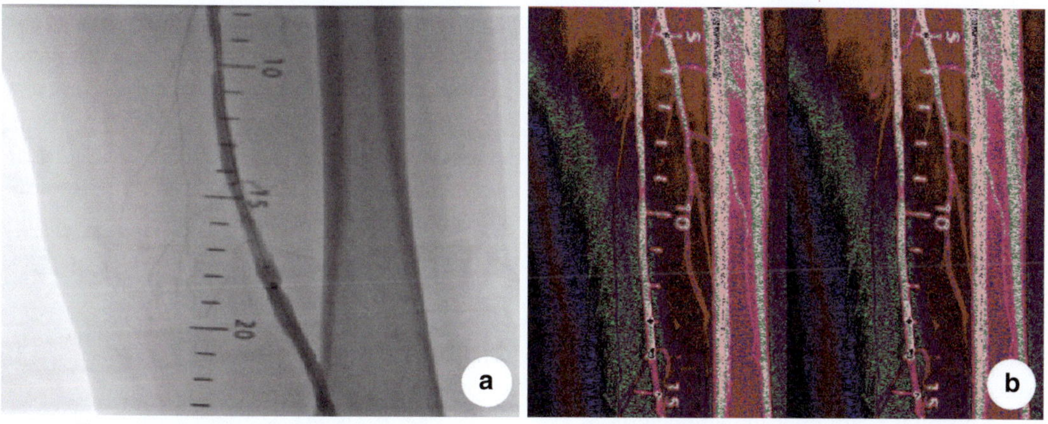

The upper segment of the femoral artery was patent at the stenosis

Patency at the stenosis of the lower segment of the femoral artery

Fig. 14.3 During the intervention, the balloon dilatation of the femoral artery defect area was successful, and the contrast agent passed smoothly. (**a**) The upper segment of the femoral artery was patent at the stenosis. (**b**) Patency at the stenosis of the lower segment of the femoral artery

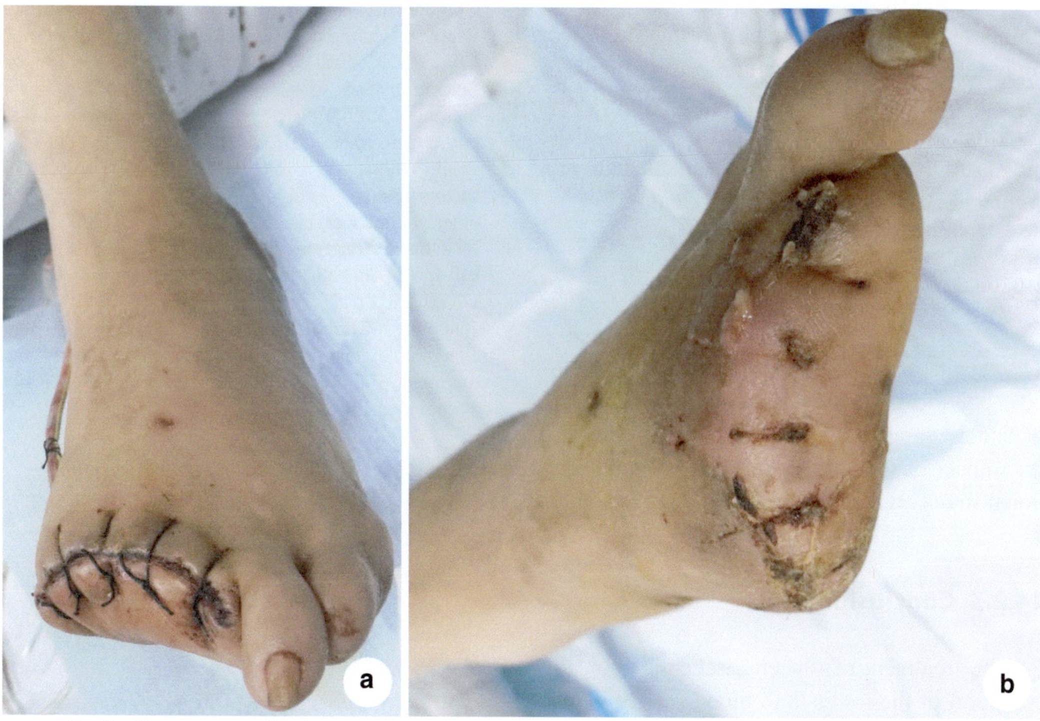

On the first postoperative day

On the 23rd postoperative day

Fig. 14.4 After toe amputation. (**a**) On the first postoperative day. (**b**) On the 23rd postoperative day

14.2 Case Analysis

14.2.1 Diabetic Ischemic Lesions

Patients with diabetic ischemic disease experience significant pain, with most patients suffering from tissue necrosis and exudation due to trauma or uncomfortable shoes. The subcutaneous tissue turns dark red or black, leading to ulceration and necrosis, and in severe cases, it dries up and turns black, leading to purulent infections. The patient in this case was admitted to the hospital again after the amputation of the left big toe due to it turning black. At the local hospital, the distal first toe was removed due to ulceration, but the postoperative wound still did not heal, and the second toe gradually turned black and necrotic, diagnosed as diabetic foot with vascular disease. Combined with the lower limb arterial CTA, it is suggested that the lower limb blood vessels are significantly blocked. Pressurized perfusion and lumbar sympathetic ganglion destruction were used to improve the blood supply to the lower limbs, and the patient's wound healed smoothly after amputation.

14.2.2 Amputation

The repair of the wound requires various methods, but the basic requirement for closing the wound is good local blood supply. In addition, the impact of the patient's vital signs and nutritional status on the wound should be noted.

14.2.3 Conclusion

For the treatment of diabetic ischemic foot, the condition of the lower limb blood supply is particularly important. Simply dealing with the wound cannot heal the wound. Conditions must first be created for wound healing. Pressurized perfusion and lumbar sympathetic surgery can promote the improvement of lower limb blood supply. Using lower limb vascular shaping surgery can further improve the blood supply of the affected limb, greatly increasing the probability of local wound healing after surgery.

Bibliography

1. Barwick A, Tessier J, Mirow J, et al. Computed tomography derived bone density measurement in the diabetic foot. J Foot Ankle Res. 2017;10(11):1–5.
2. Uzun G, Mutluoğlu M, Karagöz H, et al. Pitfalls of intralesional ozone injection in diabetic foot ulcers: a case study. J Am Coll Clin Wound Spec. 2014;4(4):81–3.
3. Jiangning W, Gengjia T, Zhaofan X, et al. Comprehensive treatment of pressure sores. Beijing: People's Health Publishing House; 2018.
4. Chinese Medical Association Diabetes Branch. Screening and management guidelines for lower extremity arterial disease in patients with type 2 diabetes. Chin J Diab. 2013;5(2):82–8.
5. Deng Wuquan Y, Qiongwu CB, et al. Analysis of factors related to amputation of diabetic foot in the elderly. Pract Geriatrics. 2009;23(3):183–6.
6. Xiaohui L, Yonghong Z. Treatment strategy for limb salvage in diabetic foot. World Latest Med Inform Digest. 2018;5:57–8.
7. Jiangning W, Lei G, Tiangui C, et al. Professor Wang Jiangning's team's comprehensive diagnosis and treatment of diabetic foot cases. Beijing: Science and Technology Literature Publishing House; 2018.

15 Comprehensive Treatment of a Patient with Difficult-to-Heal Pressure Injury Combined with Pneumonia

Lei Gao and Jiangning Wang

15.1 Case Summary

Patient, male, 89 years old. Admitted to the hospital due to skin ulceration in the left buttock for over 9 months.

[Medical History] The patient had been bedridden for a long time due to sequelae of cerebral infarction 5 years ago. He developed skin ulceration in the left buttock 9 months ago. Despite regular dressing changes, the wound did not improve, and the area and depth increased. He sought treatment at a local tertiary hospital. Although the wound in the buttock shrank after regular dressing changes, there was no healing trend. In order to seek further diagnosis and treatment, he came to our hospital. The outpatient department admitted him to our department with "soft tissue infection." Since the onset of the disease, the patient's general condition had been good, with normal spirit, diet, sleep, and no weight loss.

[Past History] The patient's usual health was average; denied history of hypertension, diabetes, hyperlipidemia, and coronary heart disease; denied history of hepatitis, tuberculosis, and close contact history; denied surgical history, trauma history, and blood product transfusion history; denied drug and food allergy history; vaccinations were carried out as planned.

[Admission Examination]

1. Specialized physical examination. Two wounds of approximately 3.5 × 2.5 cm (perineal area) and 1.0 × 0.5 cm (outer upper side) could be seen on the left buttock. The two wounds were connected and formed a cavity. Inflammatory granulation tissue could be seen in the wound, with secretion exudation (Figs. 15.1 and 15.2).
2. Laboratory examination. ① Routine blood test (venous blood): WBC 10.74 × 10^9/L, neutrophil percentage 85.9%, HGB 123 g/L, hematocrit 0.37 L/L, red blood cell volume distribution width 15.6%, neutrophils 6.6 × 10^9/L. ② Coagulation four items + D-dimer (D-D) + Fibrin degradation products (FDP) + Antithrombin III (AT-III): Antithrombin III quantitative 78%, prothrombin time 13.2 seconds, prothrombin activity 74%, international normalized ratio 1.23, fibrinogen 4.93 g/L, D dimer 334 ng/mL DDU. ③ Biochemical full item: alanine aminotransferase 8 U/L, aspartate aminotransferase 12 U/L, serum iron 9.2 μmol/L, creatinine (creatinine oxidase method) 44 μmol/L, serum glucose 7.43 mmol/L, creatine kinase 46 U/L, A/G 1.1,

L. Gao · J. Wang (✉)
Department of Orthopedics, Beijing Shijitan Hospital, Capital Medical University, Beijing, China
e-mail: gaolei3337@bjsjth.cn; wangjn@bjsjth.cn

J. Wang, L. Gao (eds.), *Refractory Wounds*, Experts' Perspectives on Medical Advances,
https://doi.org/10.1007/978-981-96-2067-8_15

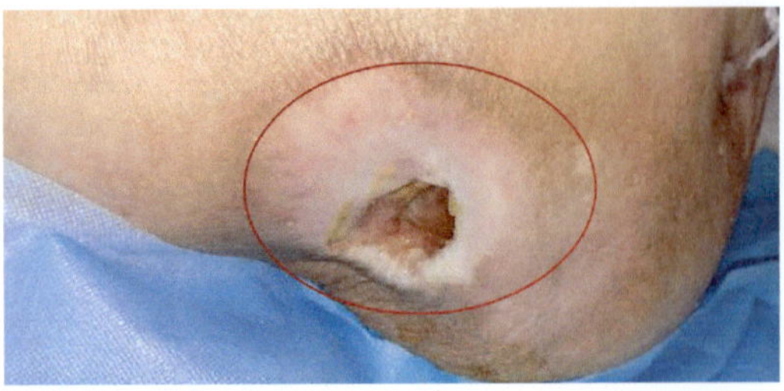

Fig. 15.1 Wound on the left buttock (perineal area) of the patient at admission

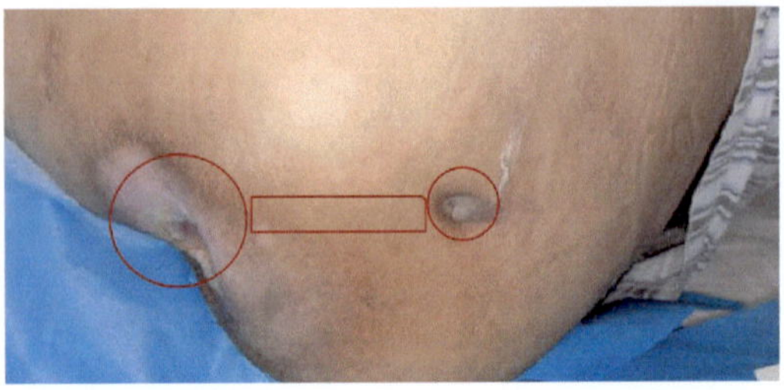

Fig. 15.2 Patient's left buttock upper outer wound at admission, two wounds penetrating, forming a cavity

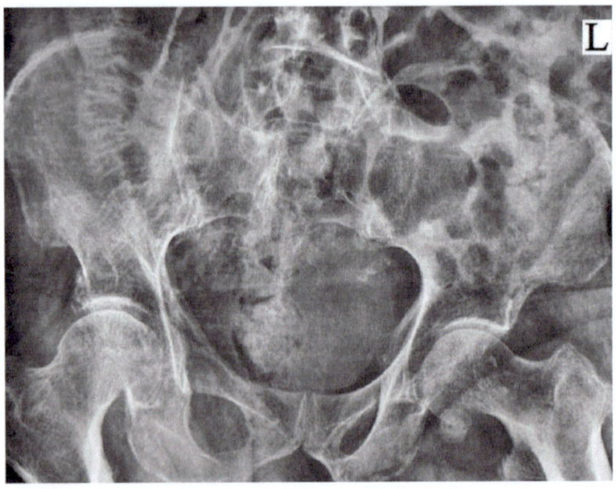

Fig. 15.3 Pelvic X-ray

albumin (bromocresol green method) 31.4 g/L. ④ CRP 30.14 mg/L. ⑤ PCT 0.09 ng/mL.

3. Imaging examination. ① Cranial CT (external hospital) shows multiple lacunar cerebral infarctions, some softening foci formation, brain white matter demyelination, brain atrophy. ② Chest X-ray examination: chronic bronchitis, lower lung infection, enlarged heart shadow, aortic sclerosis. ③ Pelvic X-ray examination: severe osteoporosis, bilateral sacroiliac joints, hip joint degeneration (Fig. 15.3). ④ Pelvic MRI shows a slightly long T2 abnormal signal in the left buttock soft tissue, the distal local soft tissue structure is disordered, slightly high signal in T2 fat suppression sequence, no clear abnormal signal in DWI sequence; adjacent left ischial tuberosity bone marrow cavity shows a patchy long T1, long T2 abnormal signal, the boundary is unclear, high signal in T2 fat suppression sequence. Consider: left buttock soft tissue infection and left ischial tuberosity osteomyelitis possible (Fig. 15.4). ⑤ Vascular examination: lower limb vascular ultrasound shows left calf intermuscular vein thrombosis, bilateral lower limb artery sclerosis. ⑥ Cardiac ultrasound examination: left atrial enlargement, left ventricular wall thickening, ascending aorta widening, aortic valve, mitral valve, tricuspid valve regurgitation (small amount), left ventricular diastolic function decreased, ejection fraction 67%.

[Preliminary Diagnosis] Perineal soft tissue infection, buttock soft tissue infection (left), lung infection, multiple lacunar cerebral infarctions, cerebral atrophy, cerebral white matter demyelination, hypoalbuminemia, left calf intermuscular venous thrombosis.

[Treatment and Outcome] Considering the patient's advanced age, large buttock wound, accompanied by lung infection, lower limb venous thrombosis, hypoalbuminemia, symptomatic treatment with broad-spectrum anti-infection, swelling reduction, circulation improvement, nutritional nerve and anticoagulant drugs were given. Chest X-ray suggested bilateral lower lobe pneumonia, considered to be aspiration pneumonia, a complication caused by long-term bed rest; actively performed back patting to promote sputum discharge, nebulized inhalation of expectorant drugs. At the same time, sputum culture examination was carried out, sensitive antibiotics were selected, wound bacterial culture, combined use of antibacterial drugs. The wound near the perineum on the left buttock was locally treated with silver ion hydrogel, alginate dressing was used to fill the cavity, the wound on the upper outer part of the buttock

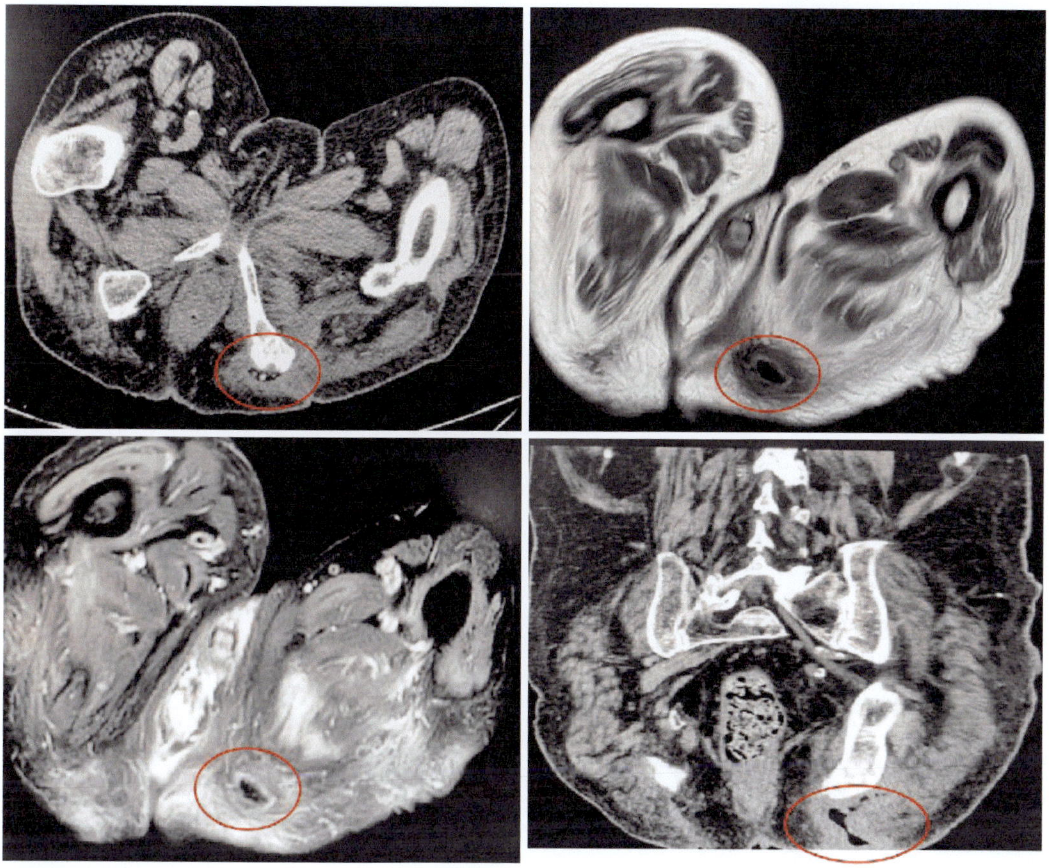

Fig. 15.4 Pelvic MRI

was covered with silver ion alginate dressing, and sterile dressing was used for bandaging and fixation. After the preoperative examination was completed and the condition was stable, exploration of blood vessels, nerves, and tendons in the left buttock + necrotic tissue debridement + sequestrum removal + skin traction closure were performed under general anesthesia. During the operation, a 3.0 × 3.0 cm wound was visible in the perineal area of the left buttock, with a cavity inside the wound, about 14.0 cm deep. After repeatedly rinsing the wound with hydrogen peroxide, sterile saline, and dilute iodophor, the wound was incised, the scar tissue at the edge of the perineal wound was removed, and it was visible that the gluteus maximus and gluteus medius were separated from the ischium, forming a closed cavity, about 14.0 × 8.0 × 6.0 cm in size. Inflammatory granulation tissue formation was visible inside the wound. After thoroughly scraping off the inflammatory granulation tissue on the surface of the wound with a curette, a large amount of bleeding was visible on the wound surface. After thoroughly stopping the bleeding with a surgical hemostatic device, the necrotic fat, muscle, and tendinous tissue inside the wound were removed. Necrotic bone was visible at the lower edge of the ischium, which was completely removed with a bone rongeur. The wound was repeatedly rinsed with hydrogen peroxide, sterile saline, and dilute iodophor. The tension of primary wound closure was high, so a **skin stretching device** was used to stretch the skin around the wound to its maximum extent. Two drainage tubes were placed; 2–0 absorbable sutures were used to sew the muscles and subcutaneous tissues, and size 7 sutures were used to sew the skin. After the operation, there was a blood loss of 300 mL, and 2 U of suspended red blood cells were transfused during the operation (Figs. 15.5, 15.6, 15.7, 15.8, 15.9, and 15.10). Continue to provide symptomatic treatment such as anti-infection, cough suppression, expectoration, and asthma relief, change the dressing regularly, and closely observe the changes in the patient's condition (Figs. 15.11 and 15.12).

On the sixth day after the patient's surgery, the patient suddenly felt suffocated at noon, had difficulty breathing, and turned pale with cyanotic lips. The patient was given continuous nasal cannula oxygen at 2 L/min. The electrocardiogram monitor showed an oxygen saturation of 42%, heart rate of 117 beats/min, blood pressure of 177/88 mmHg, and respiratory rate of 23 breaths/min. The patient's arterial pulse and breathing were weak, and the pupils were dilated. After consulting with the senior attending physician, the patient was given assisted breathing with a simple respirator, suctioned to remove a small amount of brown food residue, suggesting aspiration. An intravenous line was established, and the patient's family was notified by phone that the patient's condition was critical. The family expressed a willingness to actively resuscitate. After intubation, a large amount of pasty food residue gushed out of the tube. After intermittently suctioning out

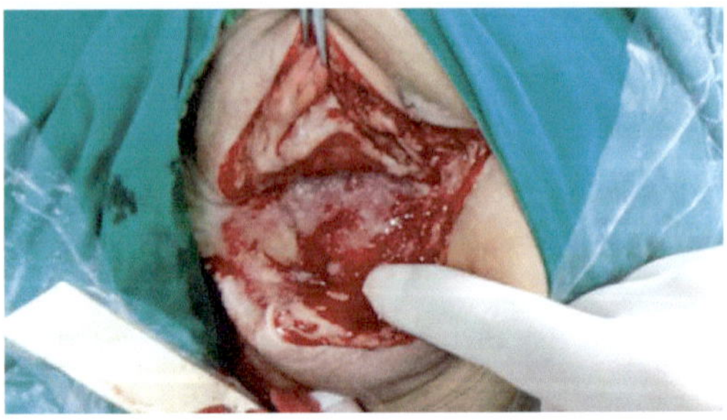

Fig. 15.5 Intraoperative complete opening of the sinus tract reveals the formation of inflammatory granulation tissue within the wound

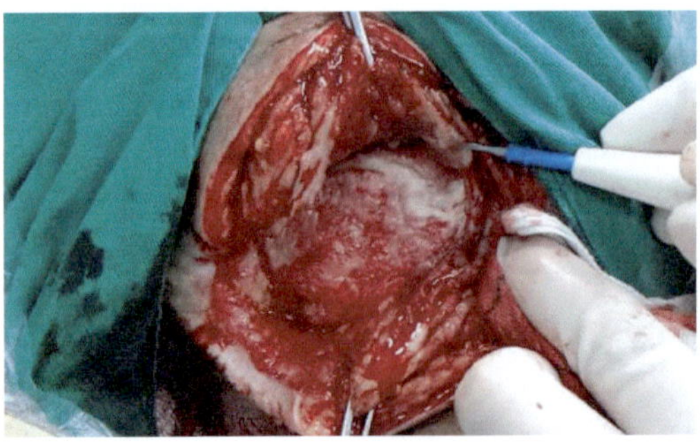

Fig. 15.6 Intraoperative complete opening of the sinus tract reveals the separation of the gluteus maximus and gluteus medius from the ischium

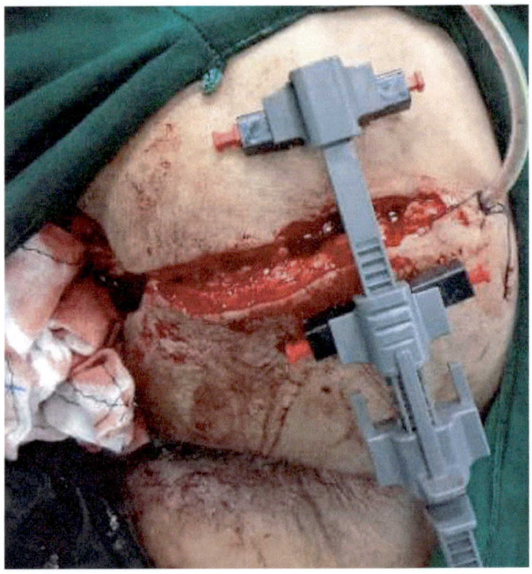

Fig. 15.7 Using a closure device to close the wound

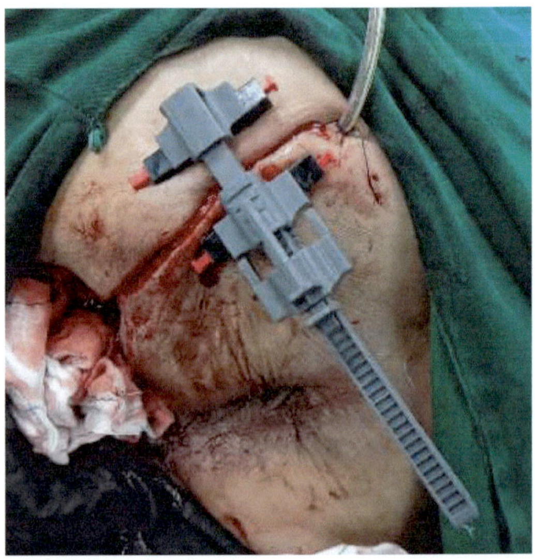

Fig. 15.8 Using a closure device to close the wound

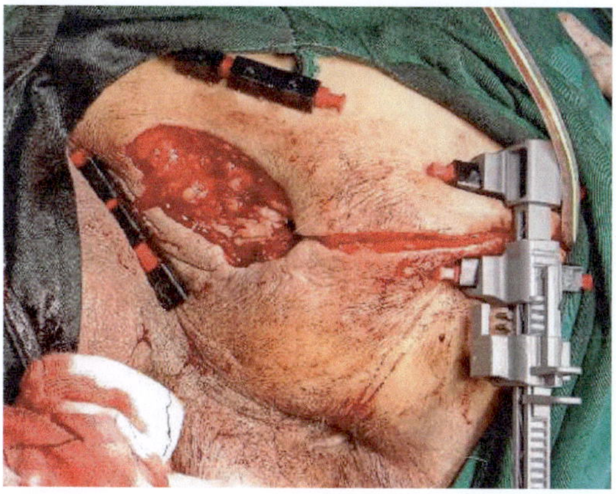

Fig. 15.9 Using a closure device to close the wound

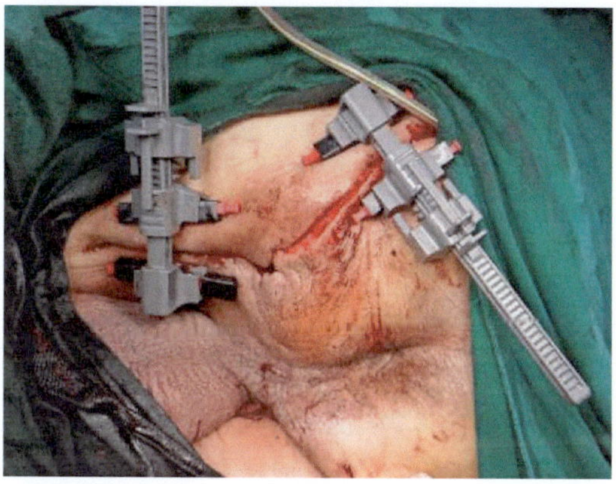

Fig. 15.10 Using a closure device to close the wound

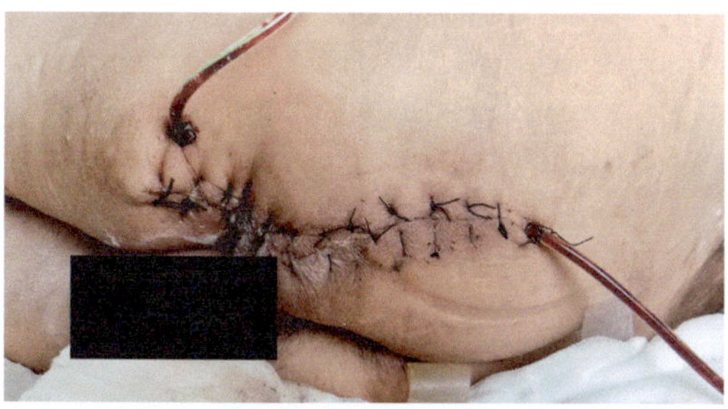

Fig. 15.11 Condition of wound dressing change 3 days after surgery

a large amount of food residue, the electrocardiogram monitor showed a heart rate of 125 beats/min, oxygen saturation of 86%, and blood pressure of 168/82 mmHg. The patient's condition was explained to the family again, and resuscita-

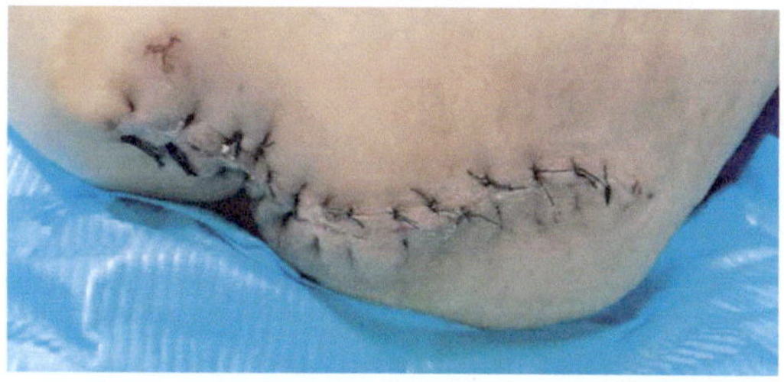

Fig. 15.12 Condition of wound dressing change 5 days after surgery, removal of drainage tube

tion continued with assisted breathing from a respirator. The electrocardiogram monitor showed a heart rate fluctuating between 96 and 102 beats/min, oxygen saturation of 100%, and blood pressure of 157/72 mmHg. The patient's condition was explained to the family again, and they signed an informed consent form. The patient was given continuous assisted breathing from a respirator, the pupils were equal in size, and the light reflex was present. The resuscitation was successful. After active resuscitation, the patient was given continuous assisted breathing from a respirator. The patient's vital signs were stable, with a heart rate of 78 beats/min, oxygen saturation of 100%, blood pressure of 132/67 mmHg, and respiratory rate of 27 breaths/min. Wet rales and wheezing could be heard in both lungs, and the breath sounds in the right lower lung were reduced. The patient's condition was stable 24 h later, and the endotracheal tube was removed at the strong request of the family.

Subsequent treatment: ① The patient was put on a no-food or water diet. ② Nutritional support, anti-infection, cough suppression, and expectorant symptomatic treatments were given. ③ The patient and family were informed of the patient's condition, which was currently critical, and a gastric tube placement procedure was needed to provide nasal feeding. The risks and complications of gastric tube placement were also explained. ④ The wound was regularly dressed. ⑤ The patient's condition was closely monitored. After five more days of treatment, the sutures on the wound were intermittently removed. One week later, the wound was completely healed and the patient was discharged (Figs. 15.13 and 15.14).

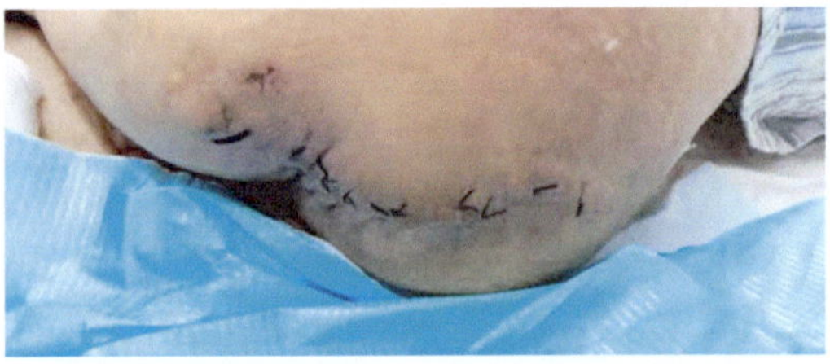

Fig. 15.13 On the 11th day after surgery, the sutures on the wound were intermittently removed

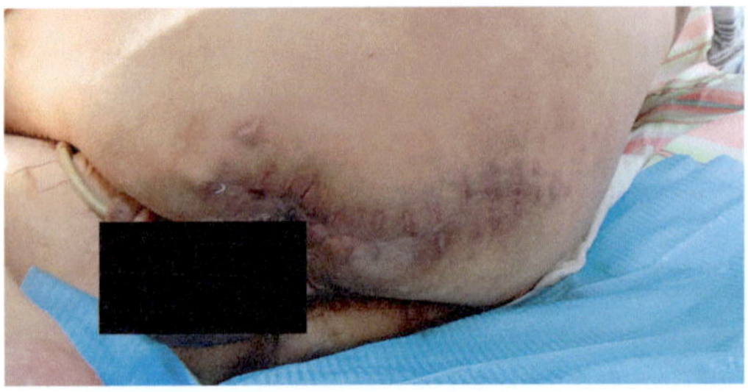

Fig. 15.14 On the 13th day after surgery, the wound healed

15.2 Case Analysis

15.2.1 Handling of Pressure Injury Patients with Pneumonia

Pressure injury is caused by long-term pressure on local tissues, resulting in continuous ischemia, hypoxia, and malnutrition, leading to skin tissue ulceration and necrosis. It often occurs in comatose, paralyzed, or long-term bedridden patients, regardless of season, age, or gender. Pressure injury patients often have concomitant pneumonia due to long-term bed rest, so the treatment of pneumonia is particularly important. Long-term bed rest makes it difficult to cough up respiratory secretions, which accumulate in the bronchioles and become a good culture medium for bacteria, easily inducing lung infection, i.e., pneumonia. Lung infection is extremely dangerous for the elderly. If not controlled, it can cause sepsis, toxemia, respiratory distress, and even increase the burden on the heart, leading to cardiopulmonary disease.

This case was diagnosed with pneumonia due to long-term bed rest upon admission. Anti-infection treatment was given (antibacterial drugs were chosen based on sputum culture results). Postoperatively, aspiration pneumonia occurred due to aspiration, leading to sudden respiratory failure, acute tracheal intubation, and mechanical ventilation. This shows that while surgically treating the wound, if there is multidisciplinary cooperation within the department, it can greatly help the patient's prognosis.

15.2.2 The Necessity of Establishing a Small ICU within the Surgical Department

Currently, our department has dedicated internal medicine physicians, nutritionists, and internal medicine physicians who perform blood purification operations, forming a small Intensive care unit (ICU) within the department. The department can independently complete respiratory support technology, nutritional support technology, and continuous slow blood purification technology. If a patient with diabetic foot or pressure injury suddenly becomes critically ill, they can be immediately rescued within the department and receive critical care. This allows the patient to receive the most effective resuscitation and the most timely life support treatment (Fig. 15.15).

Based on the current situation in Chinese hospitals, most critically ill patients are admitted to the ICU for treatment. Family members cannot provide the final care and attention to the patient before their passing, and are only allowed to visit for 1 h each day. This causes great distress to the family members. Some family members strongly refuse to enter the ICU, insisting on treatment in the general ward, but at the same time do not give up treatment. Our department has implemented Continuous Renal Replacement Therapy (CRRT) technology within the ward, enabling bedside treatment for critically ill patients in the general ward.

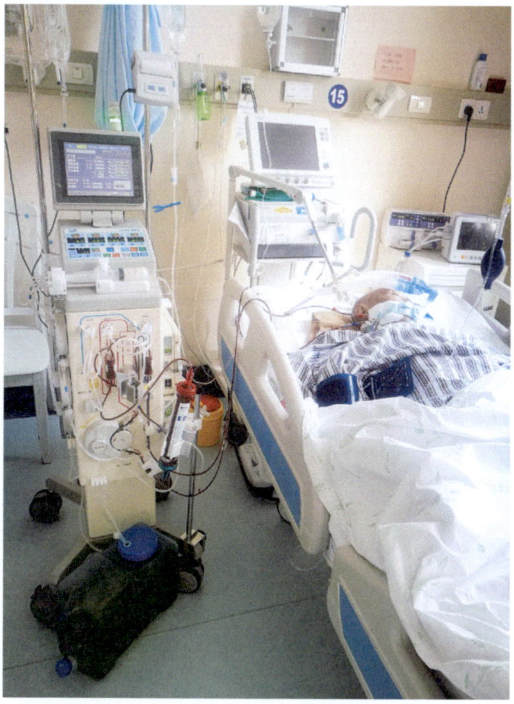

Fig. 15.15 In-department ICU, independently completing nutritional support + respiratory support technology + CRRT technology

Bibliography

1. Jiangning W, Gengjia T, Zhaofan X, et al. Comprehensive treatment of pressure sores. Beijing: People's Health Publishing House; 2018.
2. de Azevedo MMS, da Costa SRS, Dias Fernandes MIDC, et al. Pressure ulcer risk evaluation in critical patients: clinical and social characteristics. Open Nurs J. 2017;1:91–7.
3. Artmann CW, Solomon J, Palmer JA, et al. Contextual facilitators of and barriers to nursing home pressure ulcer prevention. Adv Skin Wound Care. 2016;29(5):226–38.

16 Two Cases of Difficult-to-Treat Cancerous Wounds in the Groin Area

Yefeng Yin, Jiangning Wang, and Lei Gao

16.1 Case Summary

16.1.1 Case 1

Patient, male, 57 years old. Admitted to the hospital due to a rupture in the right groin area after surgery and radiation therapy for squamous cell carcinoma, which had lasted for over 5 months.

[Medical History] The patient discovered a lump on the inner side of his right thigh in July 2017, the size of a peanut, which gradually enlarged. In January 2018, he underwent surgery to remove it at another hospital. In February, due to recurrence, he underwent surgery again. Postoperative pathology indicated highly differentiated squamous cell carcinoma. After radiation therapy, the local area ruptured and did not heal, accompanied by a foul smell. He came to our hospital for further treatment, and was admitted to our department with the diagnosis of "cancerous ulcer in the right groin."

[Past History] History of hypertension for over 10 years, highest 150/100 mmHg, without regular treatment.

In 1999, a high-altitude fall resulted in multiple fractures throughout the body, including a pelvic fracture, right tibia fracture, and thoracic vertebral compression fracture, along with a shattered right testicle. The patient was treated with external fixation for the fractures at another hospital.

[Admission Examination]

1. Specialist examination. A 6.0 × 6.0 cm ulcerative wound was observed on the inner side of the right thigh near the groin. The wound depth reached the fascia, with a large amount of yellow necrotic tissue attached, foul-smelling and dirty, with obvious tenderness. A 1.0 × 1.0 cm hard, immobile lump was visible on the inner side of the wound. The skin around the wound was dark red (Fig. 16.1).
2. Laboratory examination. ① Wound bacterial culture: *Pseudomonas aeruginosa* and *Staphylococcus aureus*. ② Blood routine: WBC 11.61 × 10^9/L, neutrophil percentage 90.3%, neutrophils 10.5 × 10^9/L. ③ Ward biochemistry: albumin 30.2 g/L. ④ Routine pathology: Highly differentiated cells seen in the background of inflammatory cells.
3. Imaging examination. ① Chest CT: Multiple small nodules in both lungs, lung bullae, and follow-up suggested. ② Right thigh MRI: Changes after surgery and radiotherapy for highly differentiated cancer of the right thigh, irregular serrated changes in the anterior skin margin soft tissue defect, close to the femoral artery, localized swelling of the adjacent rec-

Y. Yin · J. Wang (✉) · L. Gao
Department of Orthopedics, Beijing Shijitan Hospital, Capital Medical University, Beijing, China
e-mail: yefeng541009@163.com; wangjn@bjsjth.cn; gaolei3337@bjsjth.cn

J. Wang, L. Gao (eds.), *Refractory Wounds*, Experts' Perspectives on Medical Advances,
https://doi.org/10.1007/978-981-96-2067-8_16

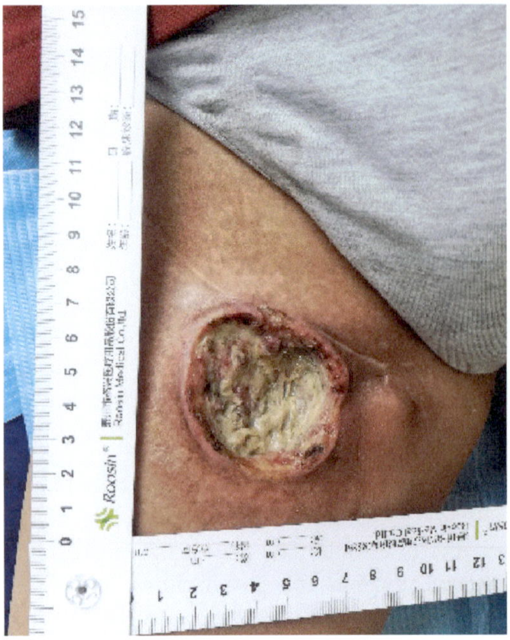

Fig. 16.1 Wound in the right groin area

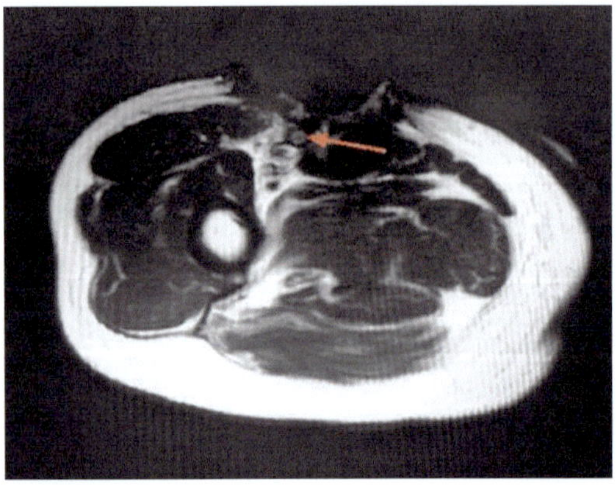

Fig. 16.2 Right leg MRI shows cancerous ulcer close to the femoral vein

tus femoris, iliopsoas, and pubic muscle, slightly high signal on STIR, considering recurrence (Fig. 16.2).

[Preliminary Diagnosis] Malignant tumor in the groin (right), lower limb soft tissue infection (right), chronic bronchitis, lung bullae, testicular injury (right), anemia.

[Treatment and Outcome] After the patient was admitted, various auxiliary examinations were actively completed. On April 25, 2019, the patient underwent iliac artery balloon occlusion + right inguinal debridement + squamous cell carcinoma radical surgery under spinal anesthesia. During the surgery, the balloon occluded the blood supply of the right iliac artery, carefully separated the femoral artery/vein and femoral nerve, and performed locally isolated perfusion chemotherapy (Figs. 16.3, 16.4, 16.5, and 16.6).

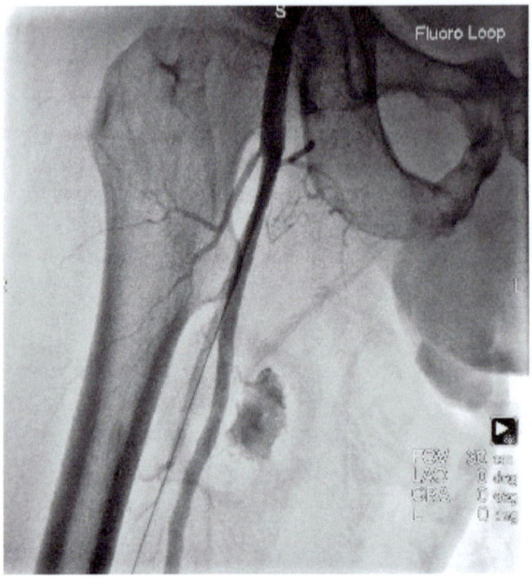

Fig. 16.3 Tumor and femoral artery position

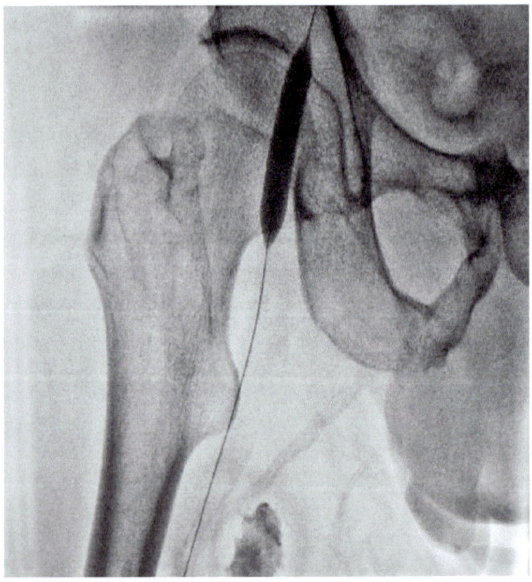

Fig. 16.4 Balloon occlusion of the iliac artery isolates high-dose perfusion chemotherapy

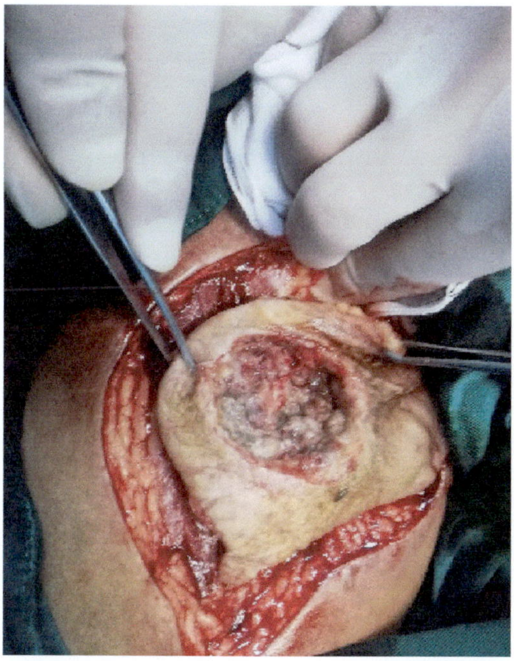

Fig. 16.5 Cancerous wound extended radical resection

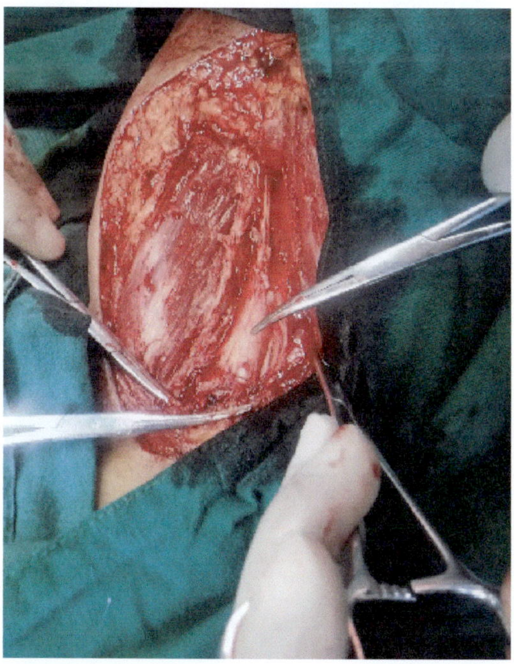

Fig. 16.6 No obvious bleeding during surgery

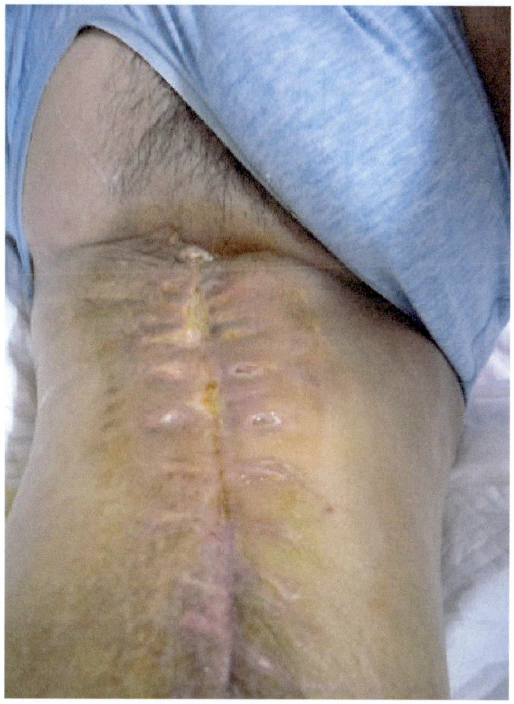

Fig. 16.7 Stitches removed 2 weeks after surgery

Regular wound dressing changes were performed postoperatively.

A re-examination was conducted 5 days after the surgery. ① Wound bacterial culture: no bacterial growth. ② Routine blood test: WBC 5.14×10^9/L, neutrophil percentage 67.3%, neutrophils 3.5×10^9/L. ③ Ward biochemistry: albumin 39 g/L. The postoperative wound healed well, and the stitches were removed 2 weeks after the surgery (Fig. 16.7).

16.1.2 Case 2

The patient, a 59-year-old male, was admitted to the hospital due to a nonhealing skin ulcer with exudate in the left inguinal area for 2 months after penile cancer surgery 2 years ago.

[Present Illness History] The patient was diagnosed with penile cancer 2 years ago and underwent surgery at a local hospital. Three months ago, a lump was palpable in the left inguinal area without any obvious cause. The patient underwent lump incision and drainage biopsy surgery at a local hospital. The postoperative pathology showed squamous cell carcinoma. The incision in the left groin area did not heal, with necrotic tissue exudate and odor. The patient came to our hospital for treatment, and was admitted to our department with the outpatient diagnosis of "metastatic cancer with necrotizing fasciitis."

[Past Medical History] The patient has a 10-year history of cervical lymph node tuberculosis and underwent surgery for penile cancer at another hospital in 2017.

[Admission Examination]

1. Specialist examination. A wound approximately 5.0 × 2.0 cm in size can be seen in the left inguinal area, with a depth of 5.0 cm. The skin around the wound is red and swollen; the soft tissue inside the wound is dark in color, partially grayish-white, with unclear structure. Squeezing reveals necrotic tissue resembling rotten flesh, accompanied by a foul smell. A hard lump approximately 2.0 × 3.0 cm in size can be seen on the left scrotal wall, with a wound approximately 0.5 × 1.0 cm in size on the surface, which is noticeably painful to touch (Fig. 16.8).
2. Laboratory examination. C-Reactive Protein (CRP) 32.76 mg/L, Procalcitonin (PCT) 0.07 ng/L, neutrophil percentage 89.5%. Pathology of necrotic tissue in the wound: squamous cell carcinoma.
3. Imaging examination. Both PET/CT and pelvic MRI showed a small nodule in the anterior part of the urethral sponge, enlarged lymph nodes in the left inguinal area, suggesting metastasis.

[Preliminary diagnosis] Metastatic squamous cell carcinoma, necrotizing fasciitis, soft tissue infection, postoperative malignant tumor of the penis, secondary malignant tumor of the inguinal lymph nodes.

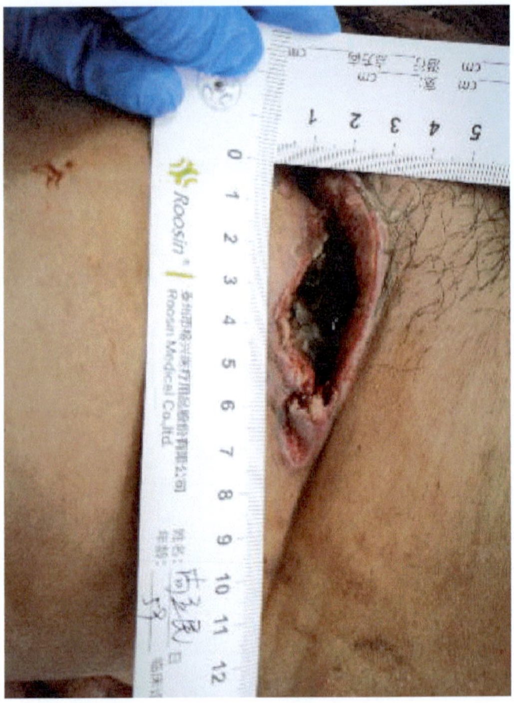

Fig. 16.8 Frontal view of the inguinal wound

[Treatment and outcome] After the patient was admitted to the hospital, relevant auxiliary examinations were completed. There were no obvious contraindications for surgery. On January 15, 2019, the patient underwent muscle vascular nerve exploration surgery + debridement of necrotic skin and subcutaneous tissue + radical surgery for squamous cell carcinoma under spinal anesthesia. During the operation, local isolation and high-dose perfusion chemotherapy were performed (Figs. 16.9, 16.10, and 16.11). Regular dressing changes were performed postoperatively.

Two weeks postoperation laboratory test results: CRP 2.78 mg/L, PCT 0.03 ng/L, neutrophil percentage 65.3%. The post-operative wound recovery is good (Fig. 16.12).

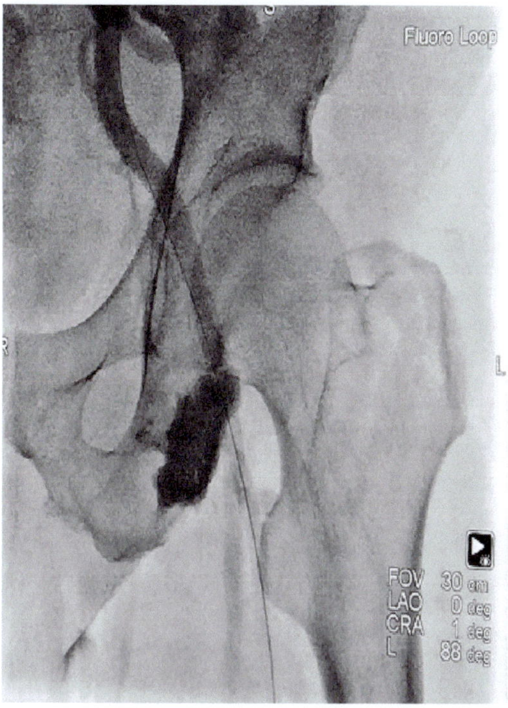

Fig. 16.9 Intraoperative angiography showing the position of the tumor and blood vessels

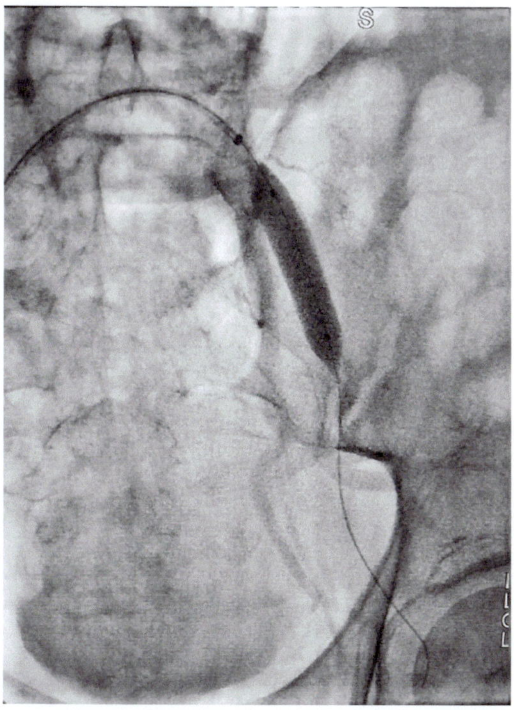

Fig. 16.10 Blood flow in the balloon segment of the iliac artery

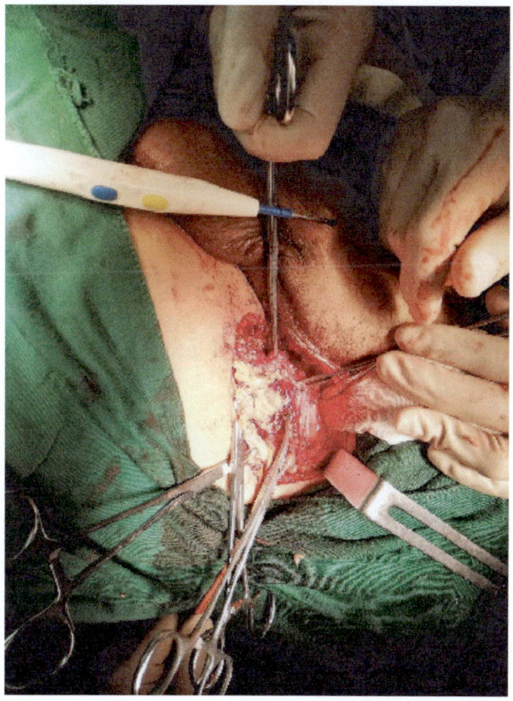

Fig. 16.11 Intraoperative enlargement of tumor ulcer resection

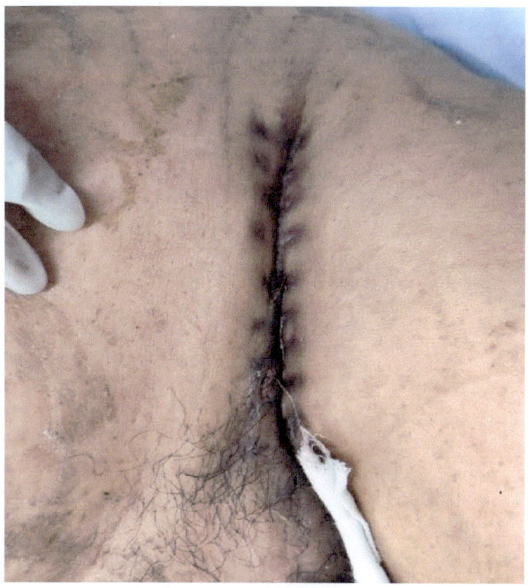

Fig. 16.12 Two-week postoperation disassembly

16.2 Case Analysis

After local radiotherapy of the tumor, the tissue fibrosis is severe, and once ulceration occurs, the treatment will be very tricky. For large area defects, skin flaps can be used for repair. The inguinal cancerous ulcer is close to the large blood vessels, the surgical risk is high, and the recurrence rate is high. The use of interventional surgery to block the upstream large blood vessels in the surgical area can: ① greatly reduce the surgical risk, create conditions for surgical operations, and avoid irreversible consequences; ② reduce bleeding during surgery and save clinical blood use; ③ during the operation, local tumor blood vessels can be perfused with high-dose isolated chemotherapy, which can increase the effect of chemotherapy drugs and reduce the systemic adverse reactions of chemotherapy.

Bibliography

1. Shack RB. Management of radiation ulcers. South Med J. 1982;75(12):1462–6.
2. Erbs G, Muller FE. Permanent closure of radioulcers of the lower abdomen and groin region by abdominal dermolipectomy with displacement plastic surgery. Z Plast Chir. 1981;5(3):150–7.
3. Leard T, Barrett C. Successful management of severe unilateral lower extremity lymphedema in an outpatient setting. Phys Ther. 2015;95(9):1295–306.
4. Tan MKH, Luo R, Onida S, et al. Venous leg ulcer clinical practice guidelines: what is AGREEd? Eur J Vasc Endovasc Surg. 2019;57(1):121–9.
5. Shinjo T, Izawa Y, Watanabe N, et al. The utility of resuscitative endovascular balloon occlusion of the aorta for temporary hemostasis after extensive bilateral lower extremity injuries: a case report. Radiol Case Rep. 2019;14(5):623–6.

Post-Facial Radiotherapy Cancerous Infectious Wound: One Case

17

Yefeng Yin, Jiangning Wang, and Lei Gao

17.1 Case Summary

Patient, female, 26 years old. The main reason for admission was a right facial mass that ulcerated and was accompanied by pain for over a month after radiotherapy.

[Medical History] The patient underwent a right lower concave mass excision surgery + right mandibular block osteotomy on November 17, 2010, due to a mass in the area behind the right upper molar. The postoperative pathological diagnosis was moderately differentiated mucinous epidermoid carcinoma. On December 22, 2010, she underwent postoperative radioactive particle implantation for the mass behind the right upper molar, after which she experienced progressive difficulty in opening her mouth. On August 16, 2017, she underwent scar release for mucinous epidermoid carcinoma in the area behind the right molar and necrotic tissue debridement at another hospital. In October 2018, the right mass recurred and she underwent local radiotherapy again. Since March 2019, she has had a right maxillofacial ulcer, with the ulcerated area and depth gradually increasing. She has sought treatment at several hospitals with poor results and was admitted to our department with a diagnosis of "right facial soft tissue infection." Since the onset of the disease, the patient's spirit, sleep, and diet have been poor. Bowel movements are normal, but she has lost 10 kg in the past 6 months.

[Admission Examination]

1. Specialist examination. The face is asymmetrical, with changes on the right side after radiotherapy. There is a defect about 10.0 × 10.0 cm in size, reaching the bone. The mandible and frontal bone are severely damaged, with a large amount of necrotic tissue attached, dirty and foul-smelling, communicating with the oral cavity, and obvious tenderness on touch. The corner of the mouth is skewed, the right eye cannot open, vision is reduced, and there is a mobile enlarged lymph node with a diameter of about 1.0 cm behind the right sternocleidomastoid muscle (Fig. 17.1).
2. Laboratory examination. ① Wound bacterial culture: *Enterococcus faecalis* + *Pseudomonas aeruginosa*. ② Albumin 29.4 g/L, WBC 11.1 × 10^9/L, neutrophil percentage 87.7%, neutrophils 9.7 × 10^9/L. ③ Tumor markers (April 15, 2019, at another hospital): cytoplasmic keratin fragment 21—1 is 5.82 ng/mL, squamous cell carcinoma antigen 7.2 ng/mL.

Y. Yin · J. Wang (✉) · L. Gao
Department of Orthopedics, Beijing Shijitan Hospital, Capital Medical University, Beijing, China
e-mail: yefeng541009@163.com; wangjn@bjsjth.cn; gaolei3337@bjsjth.cn

J. Wang, L. Gao (eds.), *Refractory Wounds*, Experts' Perspectives on Medical Advances,
https://doi.org/10.1007/978-981-96-2067-8_17

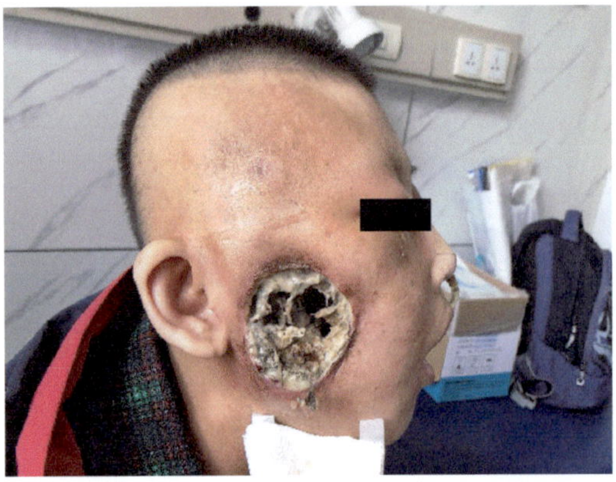

Fig. 17.1 Lateral view of the affected side of the face

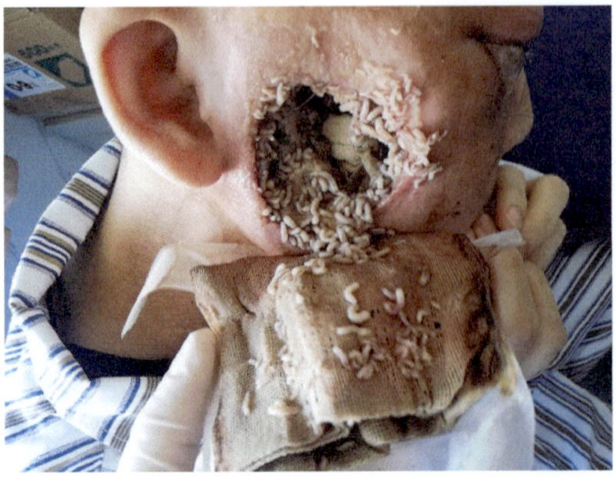

Fig. 17.2 Maggot bio-debridement treatment

3. Imaging examination. ① PET/CT (September 7, 2018, in an external hospital): Right base of the skull, right muscle soft tissue density mass shadow, metabolism increased, considering malignant occupation, right base of the skull bone partially involved. ② Head CT (February 15, 2019, in an external hospital): After right gingival cancer surgery, after particle implantation in the surgical area, there was irregular enhancement in the surgical area and uneven enhancement of the right maxillary sinus mucosa, considering tumor recurrence. Multiple lymph nodes in both sides of the neck, nature to be investigated; destruction of the right maxillary bone and sphenoid bone, considering tumor invasion.

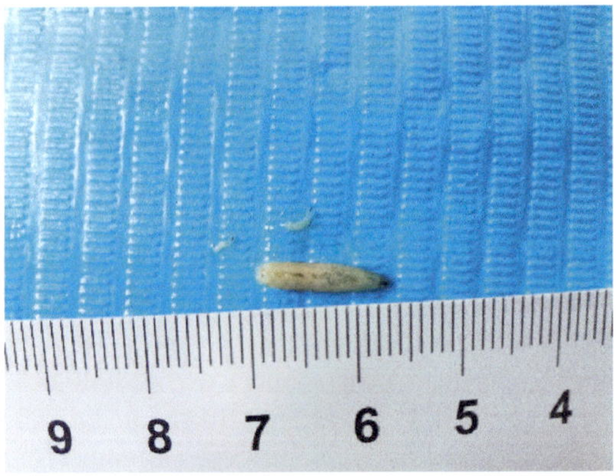

Fig. 17.3 Comparison of maggot size before and after treatment

[Preliminary Diagnosis] Facial squamous cell carcinoma with soft tissue infection, necrotizing fasciitis, base of the skull squamous cell carcinoma.

[Treatment and Outcome] The patient underwent maggot bio-debridement treatment (Fig. 17.2). Five days after maggot bio-debridement treatment, the necrotic tissue of the wound was completely removed, the inflammation index significantly decreased, and the fever subsided; after infection control, the patient underwent facial defect repair treatment and tumor specialist treatment at the oral hospital (Figs. 17.3, 17.4, and 17.5). Laboratory examination: WBC 9.8 × 10^9/L, neutrophil percentage 85.2%, neutrophils 8.4 × 10^9/L.

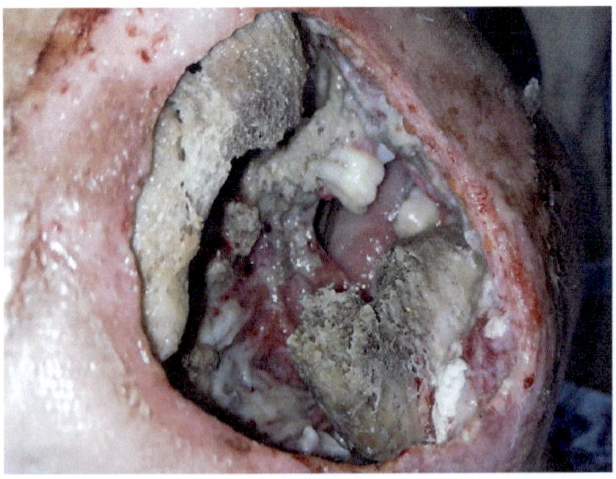

Fig. 17.4 Facial wound after maggot bio-debridement

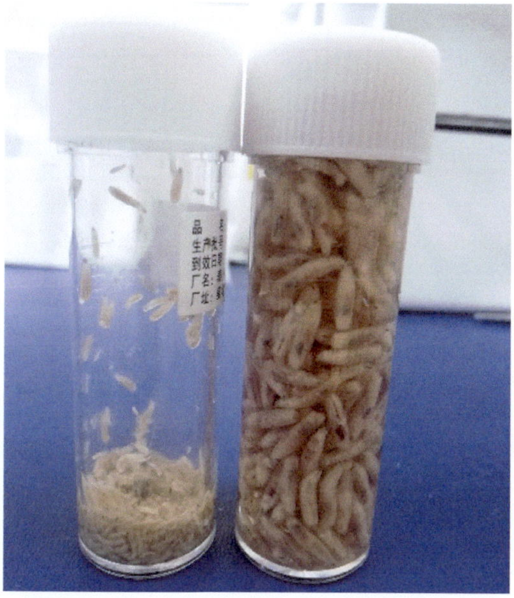

Fig. 17.5 Comparison of maggot volume before and after treatment

17.2 Case Analysis

Cancerous ulcers on the face are relatively rare, local radiotherapy leads to skin soft tissue edema fibrosis; ulcers occur for a long time and cannot heal on their own. The surrounding area of the ulcer is relatively hard, the area is large, and the edges are not neat. The method of diagnosing cancerous ulcers is to take a small piece of diseased tissue for pathological biopsy. For large-area necrotic tissue and deep facial ulcers, surgical operations cannot achieve thorough debridement, and it is impossible to perform flap repair at one stage. Maggot bio-debridement is one of the safe and effective treatment methods and it is worth promoting.

Bibliography

1. Robson V, Cooper R. Using leptospermum honey to manage wounds impaired by radiotherapy: a case series. Ostomy Wound Manage. 2009;55(1):38–47.
2. Borghi A, Gianesini S, Pedriali M, et al. An apparently untreatable ulcer of the face. Int Wound J. 2016;13(5):1084–6.
3. Gupta PJ. Human myiasis in anal carcinomatous ulcer—a case report. Eur Rev Med Pharmacol Sci. 2009;13(6):473–4.
4. Xiaoyong X, Yuanyuan F, Jiangning W, et al. Clinical application of maggot debridement therapy in difficult-to-heal infectious wounds. Advances in Modern Biomedicine. 2014;14(36):7186–9.
5. Lei G, Yefeng Y, Shouyu W, et al. Antibacterial effect of purified maggot secretory antimicrobial peptide on ulcer wounds in diabetic rats. Chinese Journal of Tissue Engineering Research. 2012;16(24):4437–40.

18 Soft Tissue Infection Wound: One Case

Zeyang Yu, Jiangning Wang, and Lei Gao

18.1 Case Summary

Patient, male. Main cause: admitted to the hospital with redness and high fever in the right buttock for 3 days.

[Present Illness History] The patient had redness in the right buttock without obvious cause 3 days ago; the central area was harder to touch, and accompanied by a rise in body temperature, up to 39 °C. He was treated with medication at a hospital in Beijing, the symptoms did not improve significantly. He came to our hospital for further diagnosis and treatment. The outpatient department admitted him to our department with "soft tissue infection."

[Past History] Hypertension for 10 years, oral medication treatment, blood pressure control is stable; schizophrenia for 10 years, oral olanzapine treatment, the current condition is stable. No food or drug allergy history; no surgery and blood transfusion history; denied other disease history. Smoking history for 30 years, up to 60 Support/Day.

Z. Yu · J. Wang (✉) · L. Gao
Department of Orthopedics, Beijing Shijitan Hospital, Capital Medical University, Beijing, China
e-mail: xiaobo723810@126.com; wangjn@bjsjth.cn; gaolei3337@bjsjth.cn

[Admission Examination]

1. Specialist examination. A red and swollen area of about 8.0 × 8.0 cm can be seen on the skin near the anus of the patient's right buttock. It feels relatively hard, with high skin temperature. In the center of the swollen area, two white tips can be seen, and a small amount of purulent secretion can be squeezed out. The skin sensation and blood circulation are normal (Fig. 18.1).
2. Laboratory examination. ① Blood routine: WBC 10.76 × 10^9/L, neutrophils 9.4 × 10^9/L, HGB 96 g/L. ② Blood biochemistry: albumin 34.0 g/L. ③ CRP 113.97 mg/L. ④Wound bacterial culture results: saprophytic *Staphylococcus*, fecal *Streptococcus*.
3. General examination. Blood pressure 130/80 mmHg, body temperature 39.0 °C.
4. Imaging examination. Pelvic CT shows that the subcutaneous fat space of the right buttock is cloudy, with a strip-like appearance, and obvious subcutaneous edema.

[Preliminary Diagnosis] Right buttock soft tissue infection, stage 2 hypertension (high risk), schizophrenia.

[Treatment and Outcome] After admission, the patient completed relevant preoperative examinations, received symptomatic treatment such as anti-infection and swelling reduction, and underwent emergency debridement and exploration of necrotic tissue in the right buttock + inci-

J. Wang, L. Gao (eds.), *Refractory Wounds*, Experts' Perspectives on Medical Advances,
https://doi.org/10.1007/978-981-96-2067-8_18

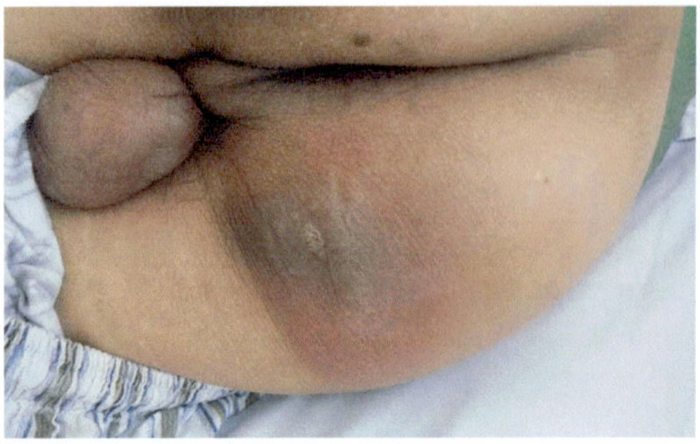

Fig. 18.1 Wound condition at admission

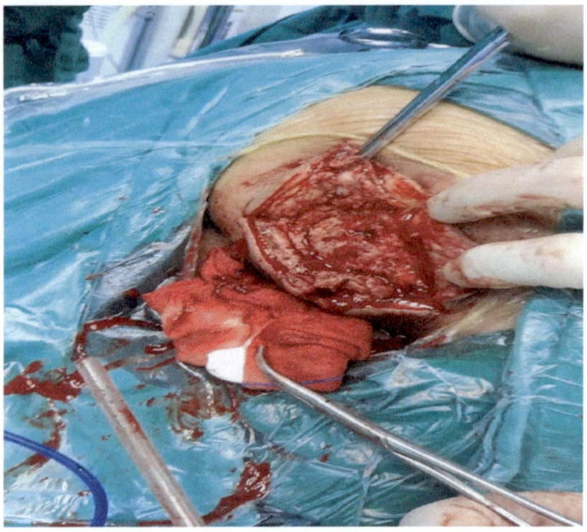

Fig. 18.2 The first debridement

sion and drainage under spinal anesthesia on the day of admission. During the operation, a cross incision was made, severe soft tissue edema and local abscess formation were observed, the abscess and local necrotic soft tissue were thoroughly removed, the wound was opened for drainage and dressing change, the body temperature returned to normal after the operation, and daily dressing change was carried out. The second debridement + flap transfer operation was performed 1 week later; regular dressing change after the operation; the wound healed well (Figs. 18.2, 18.3, and 18.4).

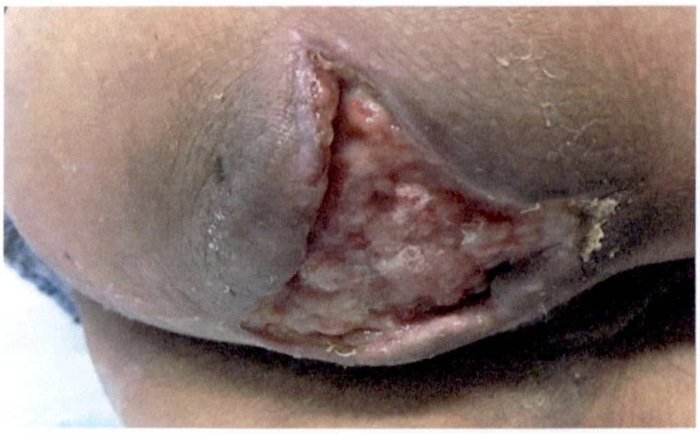

Fig. 18.3 Postoperative soft tissue edema is significantly improved compared to before, but local edema still exists

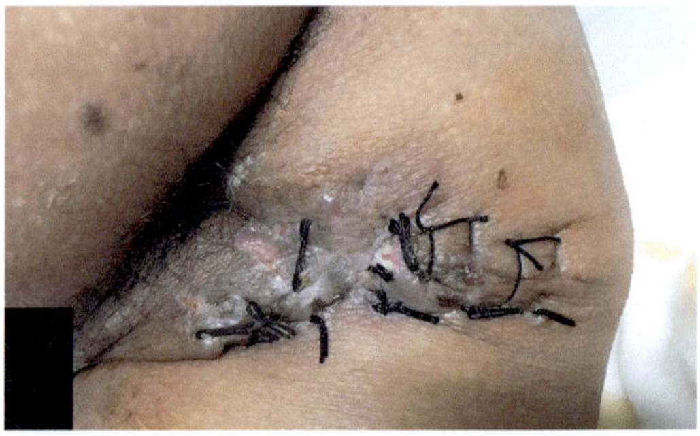

Fig. 18.4 The second debridement + 1 week after flap transfer operation

18.2 Case Analysis

Skin and soft tissue infections (SSTI) involve various pathological conditions of the skin and underlying subcutaneous tissue, fascia, or muscle, ranging from simple superficial infections to severe necrotizing infections. Successful management of severe SSTI patients requires early diagnosis, appropriate use of antimicrobial therapy, timely surgical debridement or drainage, and resuscitation when necessary.

The US Food and Drug Administration (FDA) classifies SSTIs into two major categories, namely simple and complex, for evaluating clinical trials of new antimicrobial therapies. Simple SSTIs include surface infections such as cellulitis, simple abscesses, impetigo, and furuncles, which require the use of antimicrobial drugs or surgical incision and drainage of abscesses. Complex SSTIs include deep soft tissue infections such as necrotizing infections, infectious ulcers, infectious burns, and severe abscesses, which require major surgical intervention for drainage and debridement.

This case involves an infection of the skin and subcutaneous tissue of the buttocks, requiring surgical intervention, including drainage and debridement of necrotic tissue, in addition to antimicrobial therapy.

Once the diagnosis is established, surgical debridement must be performed immediately, thoroughly removing necrotic skin, subcutaneous tissue, and fascia until normal fascia appears, and the wound is left open. A recheck is usually needed 24 h later to ensure the initial debridement was sufficient.

Initial antimicrobial therapy should cover anaerobes, *Enterobacteriaceae*, *Staphylococcus aureus*, and *Streptococcus*. Empirical treatment includes three combination schemes: ① vancomycin + cefoperazone + gentamicin + metronidazole; ② vancomycin + piperacillin/tazobactam + gentamicin; ③ vancomycin + imipenem or meropenem, for those who cannot tolerate vancomycin, linezolid or daptomycin can be used.

Bibliography

1. Auiwattanakul S, Ungpinitpong W, Yutthakasemsunt S, et al. Prevalence of pressure ulcer and nutritional factors affecting wound closure success in Thailand. Mater Sociomed. 2017;29(3):196–200.
2. Zhong W, Ahmad A, Xing MM, et al. Impact of textiles on formation and prevention of skin lesions and bedsores. Cutan Ocul Toxicol. 2008;27(1):21–8.
3. Luan XR, Li WH, Lou FL. Applied analysis of humanized nursing combined with wet healing therapy to prevent bedsore. Eur Rev Med Pharmacol. 2016;20(19):4162–6.

Case of Charcot Foot with Plantar Ulcer

19

Lei Gao and Jiangning Wang

19.1 Case Summary

Patient, female, 60 years old. Admitted to the hospital due to a sprained right foot for half a year and a plantar ulcer for over a month.

[Present Illness] The patient sprained her right foot while walking half a year ago. She immediately felt swelling and pain in her right foot. She was diagnosed with a sprained right foot at a local tertiary hospital. After symptomatic treatment such as anti-infection and swelling reduction, the swelling of her right foot eased. However, she noticed a gradual deformity in her right foot after long term walking. A month ago, she found a chicken egg-sized blister on the sole of her right foot, which burst on its own and bled continuously. She was treated at a local tertiary hospital, suspected of having Charcot foot, and was given debridement, anti-infection, and wound dressing changes. The wound did not heal. She came to our hospital for further diagnosis and treatment. The outpatient department admitted her to our department with the diagnosis of "Charcot foot." Since the onset of the disease, the patient had been clear-minded, with normal spirit, diet, bowel movements, and no weight loss.

[Past History] The patient's general health had been average. She had hypertension for 6 years and had been self-administering irbesartan tablets (1 tablet/morning) and benidipine hydrochloride tablets (1 tablet/morning), with satisfactory blood pressure control. She had diabetes for over 12 years and had been self-injecting insulin (NovoRapid injection: 11 IU in the morning, 5 IU at noon, 7 IU in the evening; Lantus, 14 IU before bed). Blood sugar control is stable; coronary heart disease, self-administered isosorbide mononitrate tablets to control the condition; had a history of surgery and drug allergy (penicillin class). Denied history of hyperlipidemia and stroke; denied history of hepatitis, tuberculosis, and close contact history; denied history of trauma and blood product transfusion; no food allergy history; vaccinations were carried out as planned.

[Admission Examination]

1. Specialist examination. The right foot was significantly swollen, the sole of the foot was raised, presenting a "rocking chair" deformity, a hard lump about 5.0 cm × 5.0 cm could be seen on the inner side of the right foot, no local varicose veins, a round wound about 3.0 cm × 3.0 cm could be seen on the sole of the foot, deep to the bone, with secretions seeping out, no local redness and swelling, toe

L. Gao · J. Wang (✉)
Department of Orthopedics, Beijing Shijitan Hospital, Capital Medical University, Beijing, China
e-mail: gaolei3337@bjsjth.cn; wangjn@bjsjth.cn

J. Wang, L. Gao (eds.), *Refractory Wounds*, Experts' Perspectives on Medical Advances,
https://doi.org/10.1007/978-981-96-2067-8_19

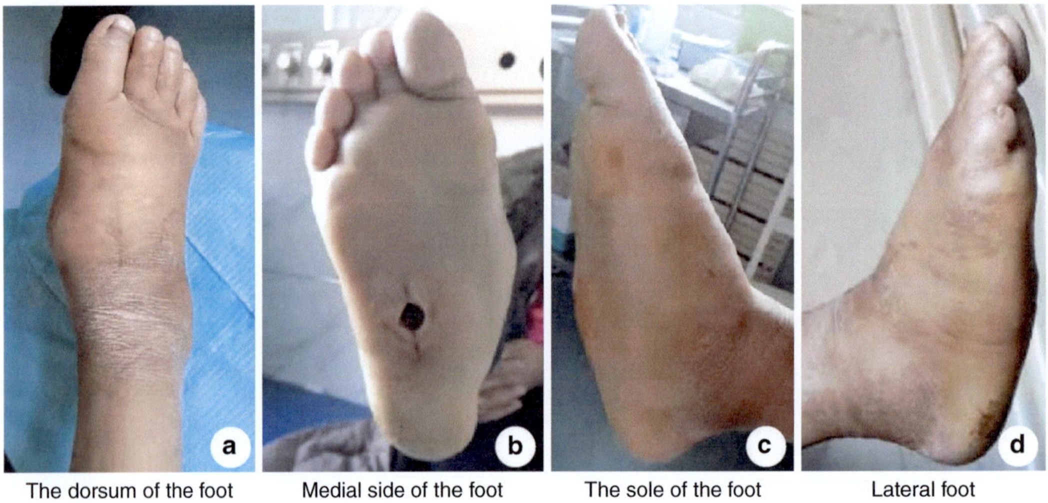

Fig. 19.1 Patient's right foot wound condition and appearance upon admission. (**a**) The dorsum of the foot. (**b**) The sole of the foot. (**c**) Medial side of the foot. (**d**) Lateral foot

flexion and extension slightly limited, peripheral blood circulation normal (Fig. 19.1).

2. Routine examination. ① Biochemical full item: alanine aminotransferase 7 U/L, aspartate aminotransferase 8 U/L, total bilirubin 7.5 μmol/L, direct bilirubin 3.4 μmol/L, indirect bilirubin 4.1 μmol/L, total protein 68.9 g/L, sodium 135 mmol/L, chloride 113 mmol/L, calcium 2.23 mmol/L, phosphorus 1.2 mmol/L, serum iron 9.8 μmol/L, serum magnesium 0.86 mmol/L, potassium 3.75 mmol/L, creatinine 54 μmol/L, uric acid 152 μmol/L, blood glucose 13. 8 mmol/L, creatine kinase 26 U/L, lactate dehydrogenase 121 U/L, globulin 30.1 g/L, albumin 38.7 g/L, alkaline phosphatase 123 U/L, blood urea nitrogen 3.58 mmol/L. ② Blood routine (venous blood): WBC 10.23×10^9/L, neutrophil percentage 80.6%, PLT 210×10^9/L, HGB 137 g/L. ③ CRP 10.14 mg/L. ④ PCT 0.02 ng/mL.
3. Imaging examination. ① Right foot X-ray examination: The alignment of the metatarsal bones and tarsal bones of the right foot is poor, the joint space is not clearly displayed, the joint surface is rough, some bones show destruction and cystic changes, suspected bone defect, peripheral soft tissue swelling; the rest of the bones are in good alignment, the joint space is not narrow (Fig. 19.2). Diagnosis: The findings of the right foot are consistent with the manifestations of diabetic foot. ② Foot CT scan: Osteoporosis in both feet, multiple bone destruction and cystic changes seen in the right foot, Soft tissue swelling in both feet, gas can be seen in the soft tissue of the right foot (Fig. 19.3). Diagnosis: Both feet show changes consistent with diabetic foot, with the right foot being more pronounced. ③ CTA examination of both lower limbs: The wall of the abdominal aorta is diffusely and unevenly thickened with multiple punctate calcified plaques, and the lumen is unevenly narrowed by about 10–20%. The walls of both iliac arteries are diffusely and unevenly thickened, and the lumen is unevenly narrowed by about 10–30%, with the left iliac artery being more pronounced. The wall of the lower segment of the right femoral artery is unevenly thickened in a ring shape, and the lumen is unevenly narrowed by about 10–30%. No obvious abnormal changes were seen in the left femoral artery, both popliteal arteries, both anterior tibial arteries, and posterior tibial arteries (Fig. 19.4). Diagnosis: Mild atherosclerosis of the abdominal aorta, both iliac arteries, and right femoral artery. ④ Lower limb venous

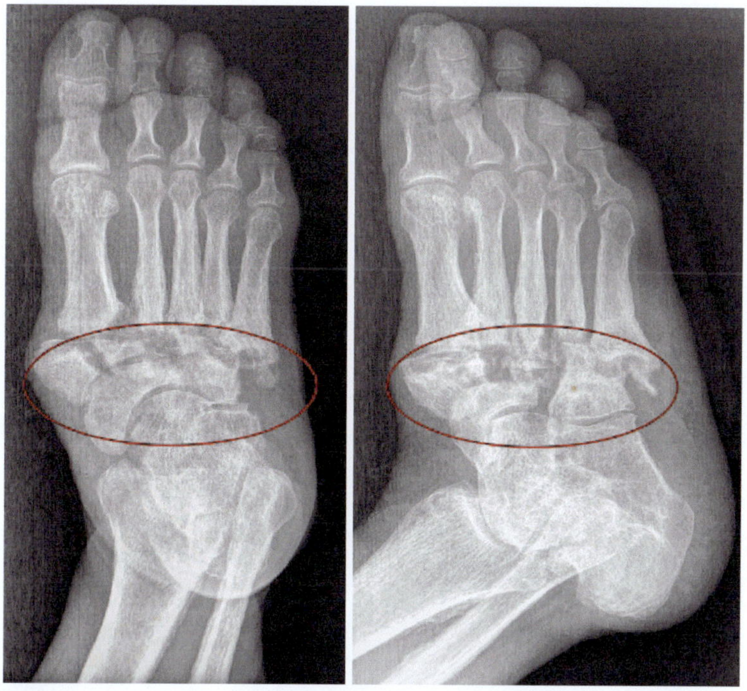

Fig. 19.2 Right foot X-ray examination

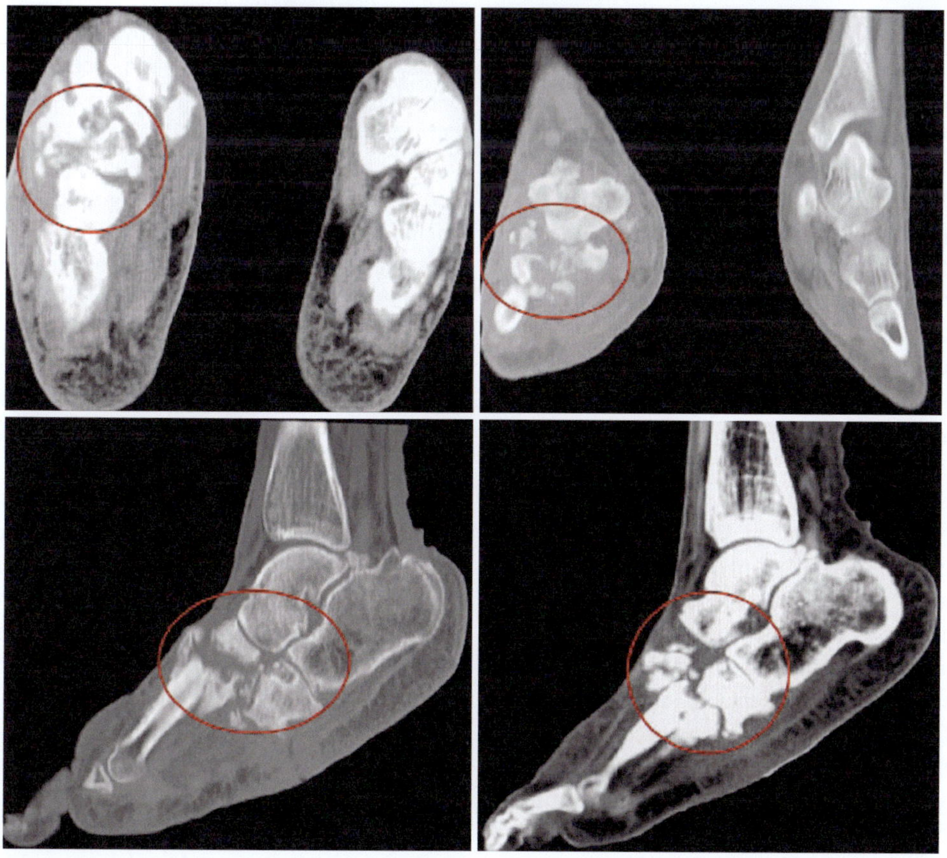

Fig. 19.3 Foot CT scan

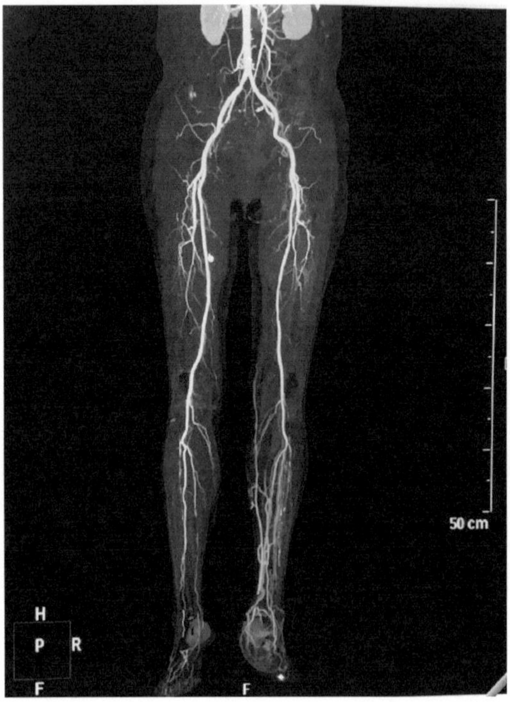

Fig. 19.4 Lower limb CTA

ultrasound: No obvious abnormalities were found in the blood vessels within the examination range. ⑤ Lower limb arterial ultrasound: Widespread hardening of the arteries in both lower limbs. ⑥ Cardiac ultrasound: The diameters of all cardiac chambers are within the normal range; the aorta and pulmonary artery are not wide. No obvious abnormalities were seen in the structure and movement of the valves. ⑦ Foot MRI examination: The soft tissue of the right foot is diffusely and significantly swollen, and a soft tissue defect can be seen on the sole of the foot; multiple tarsal bones show abnormal shape and signal, with disordered joint alignment; the cortical bone at the base of the metatarsal bones is rough and shows patchy long T1 abnormal signal, the shape of the phalanges is still acceptable, and no obvious abnormal bone signal is seen. Small patchy and round abnormal signals are seen under the joint surface of the calcaneus and talus. Liquid abnormal signal is seen in the right ankle joint and between the tarsal bones. No other obvious abnormal signals are seen (Fig. 19.5). Diagnosis: Right foot diabetic foot with Charcot joint formation, multiple tarsal bone destruction, and local tissue loss on the right foot sole.

[Preliminary Diagnosis] Type 2 diabetic foot ulcer and peripheral vascular disease, type 2 diabetic foot ulcer and peripheral neuropathy, cuboid, wedge, tarsal bone osteomyelitis (right), type 2 diabetic foot, type 2 diabetes, hypertension stage 3 (extremely high risk), coronary atherosclerotic heart disease, hyperlipidemia, anemia, hypoproteinemia, pericardial effusion, nephrotic syndrome.

[Treatment and Outcome] After admission, the patient was given wound dressing changes, symptomatic treatment such as anti-infection, swelling reduction, circulation improvement, nutritional nerve and anticoagulant drugs. Antibiotics covering *Staphylococcus* and *Streptococcus* were used. After preoperative preparation, the patient underwent right foot vascular, nerve, tendon exploration, necrotic tissue debridement, and sequestrum removal under spinal anesthesia. After the operation, under the premise of insulin control of blood sugar, continued to use anti-infection, swelling reduction, circulation improvement, nutritional nerve and anticoagulant drugs for symptomatic treatment. Postoperative wound was treated with silver ion gel dressing change (Figs. 19.6 and 19.7).

On the first day after surgery, routine blood and related infection indicators were reviewed. ① Biochemical full item: alanine aminotransferase 12 U/L, aspartate aminotransferase 15 U/L, total bilirubin 9.6 μmol/L, direct bilirubin 3.2 μmol/L, indirect bilirubin 6.4 μmol/L, total protein 69.7 g/L, sodium 136 mmol/L, chloride 109 mmol/L, calcium 2.18 mmol/L, phosphorus 1.12 mmol/L, serum iron 8.5 μmol/L, serum magnesium 0.86 mmol/L, potassium 3.98 mmol/L, creatinine 38 μmol/L, uric acid 110 μmol/L, blood glucose 10.55 mmol/L, creatine kinase 32 U/L, lactate dehydrogenase 144 U/L, globulin 32.1 g/L, albumin 37.6 g/L, alkaline phosphatase 98 U/L, blood urea nitrogen 3.45 mmol/L. ② Routine blood (venous blood):

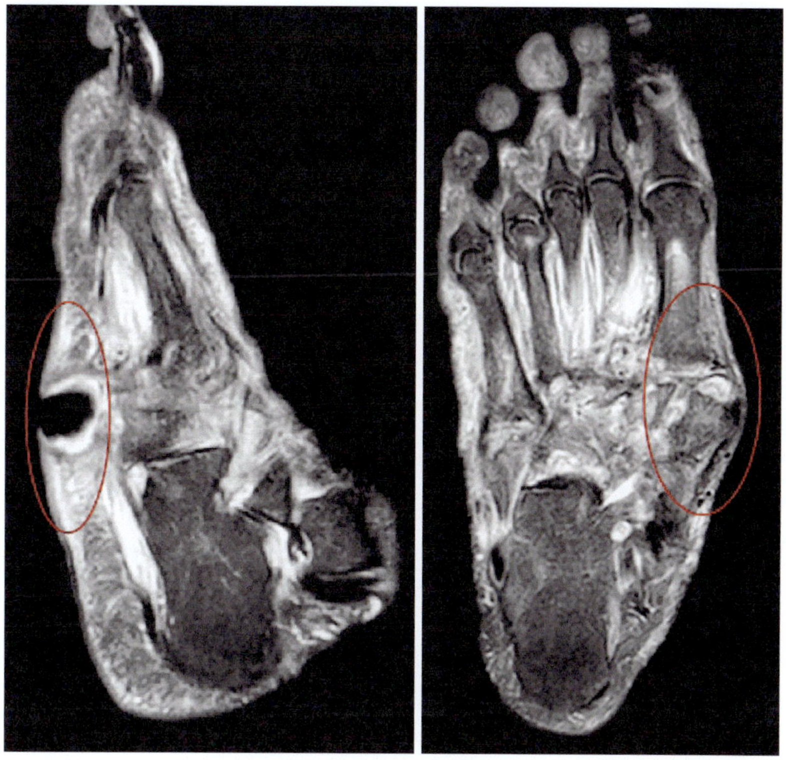

Fig. 19.5 Foot MRI

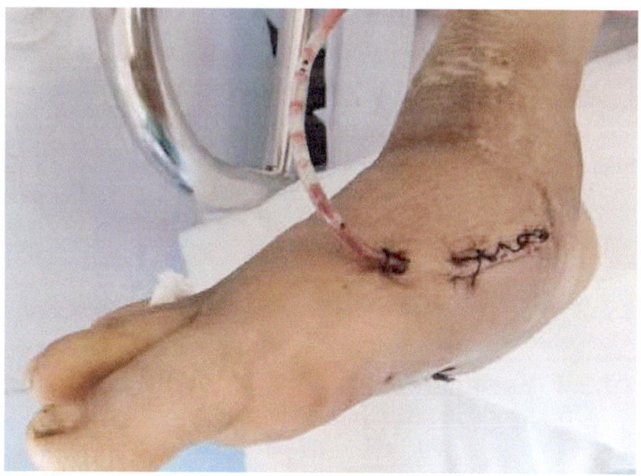

Fig. 19.6 Post-admission surgical treatment

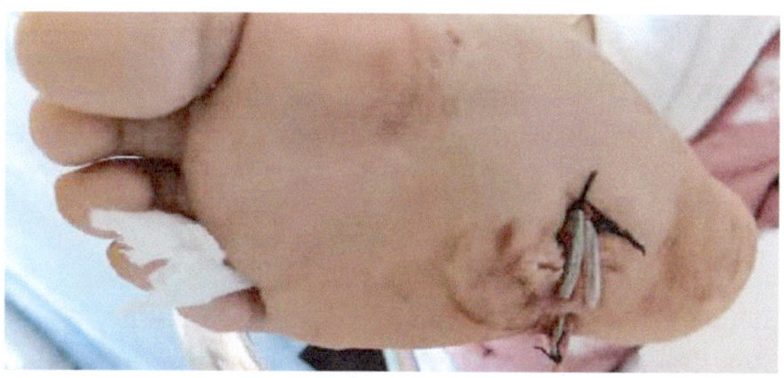

Fig. 19.7 Postoperative wound

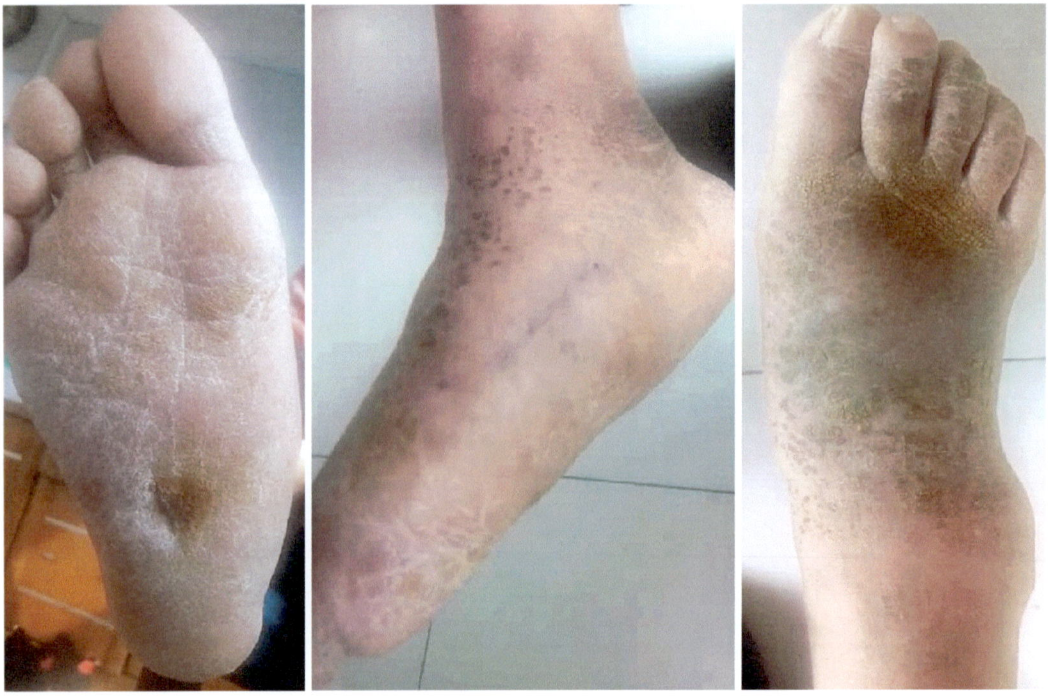

Fig. 19.8 Wound 1 month after discharge

WBC 6.25×10^9/L, neutrophil percentage 70.4%, PLT 352×10^9/L, HGB 127 g/L. ③ CRP 5.13 mg/L. ④ PCT 0.02 ng/mL. The patient was discharged 2 weeks after surgery with the wound healed, and was re-examined 1 month after discharge (Fig. 19.8).

19.2 Case Analysis

19.2.1 Surgical Treatment of Charcot Foot

Charcot foot is a special manifestation of peripheral neuropathy. Autonomic neuropathy leads to high blood flow in the foot, which increases bone resorption. Due to the involvement of multiple peripheral neuropathies, the loss of protective sensation increases the risk of acute or chronic minor injuries.

The surgical treatment of Charcot foot includes debridement of necrotic tissue and bone, thorough removal of the infection site, internal fixation bone fusion, and external fixation bone fusion. The use of internal fixation is limited to patients without evidence of infection. Patients with bone infection need staged surgery, the first stage is to eradicate the infection, and the second stage is to correct the deformity through internal fixation. Two-stage treatment usually takes a long time to achieve the purpose of eradicating infection and finally correcting deformity. The concept of Ilizarov external fixation can complete infection resection and deformity correction in one surgery. Osteoporosis is a limitation of traditional internal fixation methods, and the incidence of mechanical complications is high. Due to the combination of diabetes and various diseases, these patients have a higher risk of complications when receiving implants.

19.2.2 Use of Antimicrobial Drugs for Diabetic Foot Osteomyelitis

Patients who do not need emergency surgery can use a two-step method to treat mixed infections of soft tissue and bone: select antimicrobial drugs to treat soft tissue infections. (Use medication as necessary, then combine with bacterial culture results for medication.) Then proceed with antimicrobial therapy for ≥2 weeks, followed by bone biopsy (proceed with further treatment only if osteomyelitis is indicated).

Many antimicrobial drugs have shown efficacy in treating diabetic foot osteomyelitis, including clindamycin, various β-lactams, β-lactamase inhibitors (such as ampicillin/sulbactam), and fluoroquinolones. When prescribing antimicrobial therapy for patients with diabetic foot osteomyelitis, clinicians must consider the following issues: ① The penetration of antimicrobial drugs in bones is variable, but most categories can reach sufficient levels in infected bones. We recommend giving higher-end antimicrobial drugs within the recommended dose range, usually with a significantly longer total duration of use than for soft tissue infections. ② Rifampin (or rifampicin) may be particularly effective against biofilm-associated staphylococcal infections (usually *Staphylococcus aureus*), and must be used with caution (especially in patients taking multiple drugs or at risk of tuberculosis), especially when used in combination with another drug sensitive to the pathogen (such as fluoroquinolones). ③ Oral antimicrobial therapy for complex bone and joint infections (including diabetic foot osteomyelitis) is as effective as intravenous therapy and is safer and cheaper.

19.2.3 Design of Orthotic Devices After Closure of Charcot Foot Wounds

For patients with Charcot foot, the shoes worn after wound healing need to achieve the following functions: ① Reduce excessive pressure areas, such as the metatarsal head area and foot callus at the bony protrusion of the foot sole. ② Reduce the pressure area to evenly distribute pressure and reduce the incidence and recurrence rate of ulcers. ③ Reduce vertical pressure or shock, which is very important for patients with foot bony protrusions or abnormal bone structure. ④ Reduce shear force, which is the force generated by the foot moving forward and backward in the shoe, reducing shear force can reduce the formation of calluses. ⑤ The shoes used should adapt well to foot deformities. ⑥ Many foot deformities need to be stabilized and supported, which can relieve pain and prevent further collapse of the foot structure.

19.2.4 Conclusion

The surgical treatment of Charcot foot has traditionally been limited to debridement of infected wounds, adjustment of deformity correction, and amputation of irreparable feet. Charcot foot, due to its pathophysiological mechanism, may develop into progressive deformity, progressing to soft tissue injury or osteomyelitis. Surgeons should have the mindset of reconstructing functional feet for limb salvage treatment, while combining the design of orthotics from a biomechanical perspective to provide a guarantee for the patient's prognosis.

Bibliography

1. Raspovic KR, Wukich DK. Self-reported quality of life in patients with diabetes: a comparison of patients with and without Charcot neuroarthropathy. Foot Ankle Int. 2014;35(3):195–200.
2. Hastings MK, Johnson JE, Strube MJ, et al. Progression of foot deformity in Charcot neuropathic osteoarthropathy. J Bone Joint Surg. 2013;95(13):1206–13.
3. Rogers LC, Frykberg RG, Armstrong DG, et al. The diabetic Charcot foot syndrome: a report of the joint task force on the Charcot foot by the American diabetes association and the American podiatric medical association. Diabetes Care. 2011;34:2123–9.
4. Pinzur MS. Surgical treatment of the Charcot foot. Diabetes Metab Res Rev. 2016;32(Suppl 1):287–91.

20 Lumbar Sympathetic Ganglion Radiofrequency Ablation for the Treatment of Diabetic Peripheral Neuropathy: One Case

Tianbo Li, Jiangning Wang, and Lei Gao

20.1 Case Summary

Patient, female, 49 years old. Admitted to the hospital due to numbness, coldness, and pain in the left lower limb for 9 months.

[Present History] The patient had pain in the left lower limb accompanied by coldness and numbness 9 months before admission without any obvious cause. The symptoms did not alleviate after taking painkillers and circulation-improving drugs.

[Past History] She has a 3-year history of diabetes, regularly treated with subcutaneous insulin injections, fasting blood glucose controlled at around 8.2 mmol/L, and controlled at around 10.3 mmol/L after 2 h of meals. She was diagnosed with depression half a year ago due to emotional tension and irritability, and was treated with venlafaxine.

[Admission Examination]

1. Specialist examination. The skin temperature of the left knee and lower leg is significantly reduced (32.85 °C), the foot is sensitive to pain stimuli, with a Visual Analog Scale (VAS) score of 9, dorsalis pedis and posterior tibial pulses were not palpable, and the ankle joint and toes showed poor mobility.
2. Laboratory examination. (1) Complete blood count: WBC 6.6 × 10^9/L, neutrophil percentage 59.3%, HGB 123 g/L; (2) Blood biochemistry: albumin 39.9 g/L, fasting blood glucose 9.9 mmol/L, glycated hemoglobin 8.5%.
3. Imaging examination. The results of vascular ultrasound suggest a narrowing of the middle and lower segments of the femoral artery in the left lower limb, and angiography of the lower limb arteries shows occlusion of the bilateral internal iliac, left deep femoral artery, and left artery (Fig. 20.1).

[Treatment and Outcome] After admission, the patient was given pain relief, blood sugar control, nutritional nerve, and improved microcirculation treatments. Then, the patient underwent destruction of the left L2, L3 lumbar sympathetic ganglia under local anesthesia, under the guidance of a C-arm; percutaneous puncture was performed using a 21 G, 150 mm puncture needle, after confirming the accurate puncture position with iodixanol angiography, 80 °C radiofrequency ablation was performed (Fig. 20.2). Three minutes later, the patient reported significant pain relief, the affected foot felt hot, the skin color was red; then, 5 mL of anhydrous ethanol was injected for ablation, and the patient had no obvious discomfort after the operation.

T. Li · J. Wang (✉) · L. Gao
Department of Orthopedics, Beijing Shijitan Hospital, Capital Medical University, Beijing, China
e-mail: ltb32167@126.com; wangjn@bjsjth.cn; gaolei3337@bjsjth.cn

J. Wang, L. Gao (eds.), *Refractory Wounds*, Experts' Perspectives on Medical Advances,
https://doi.org/10.1007/978-981-96-2067-8_20

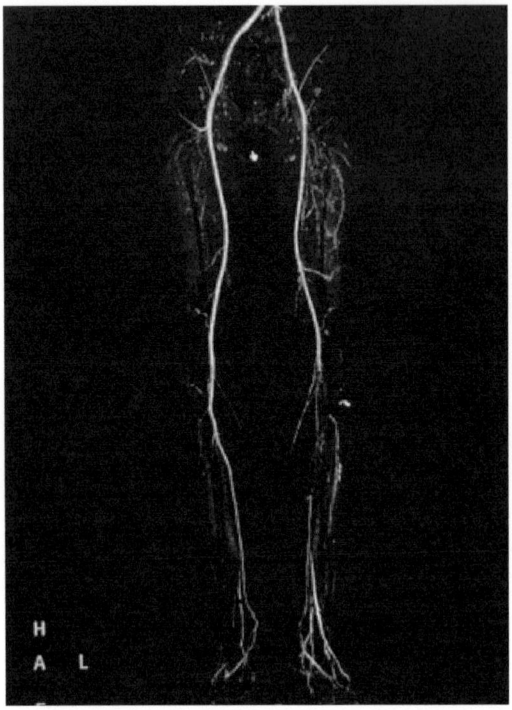

Fig. 20.1 Preoperative lower limb CTA examination

At discharge, the specialist examination showed that the skin temperature of the affected foot had risen to 36.79 °C (Figs. 20.3 and 20.4). The pain has significantly reduced, with a VAS score of 3, and the symptoms of numbness and coldness in the sole have improved. Complete blood count: WBC 5.6 × 10^9/L, neutrophil percentage 42.3%, HGB 125 g/L; blood biochemistry: albumin 41.9 g/L, fasting blood glucose 8.9 mmol/L.

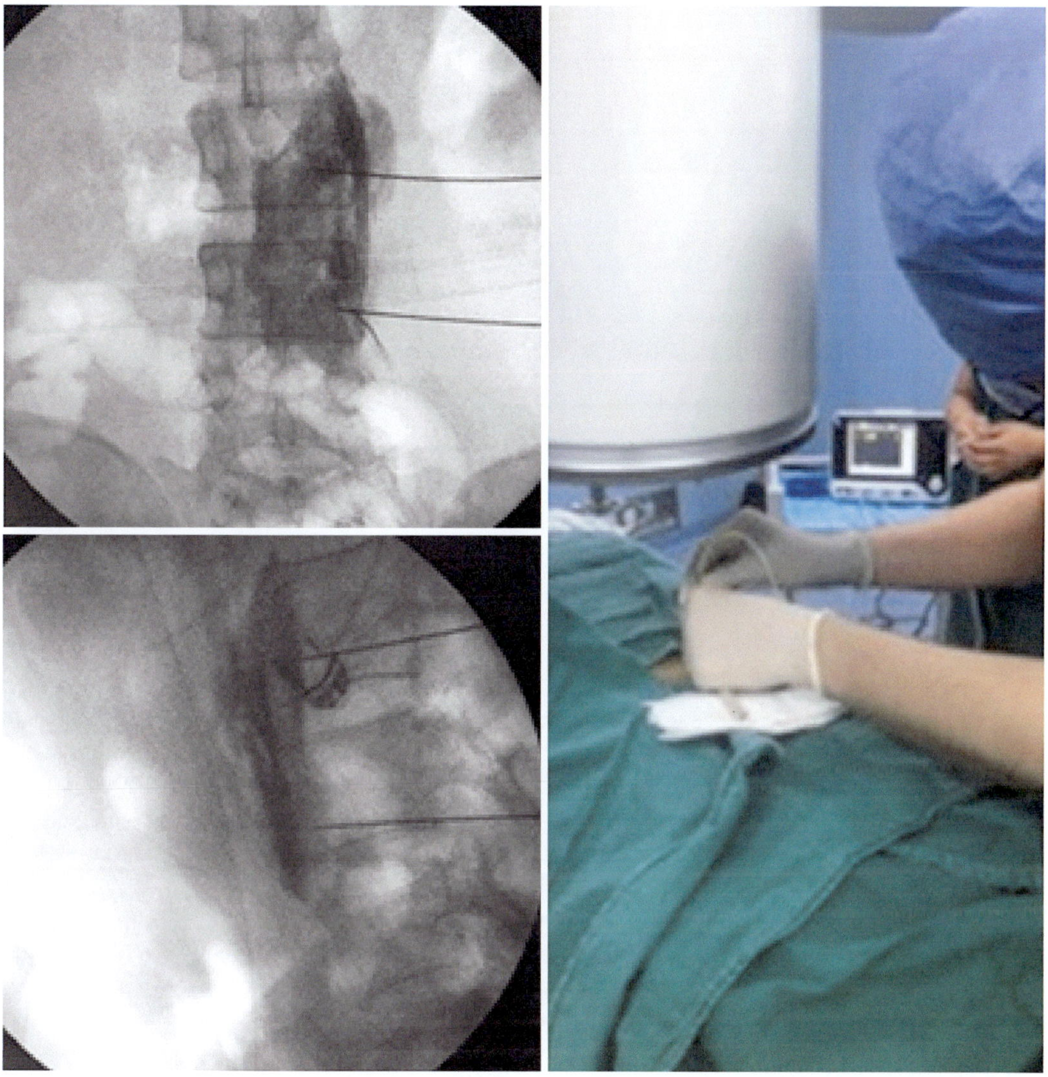

Fig. 20.2 Radiofrequency thermal ablation after satisfactory iodixanol angiography during the operation

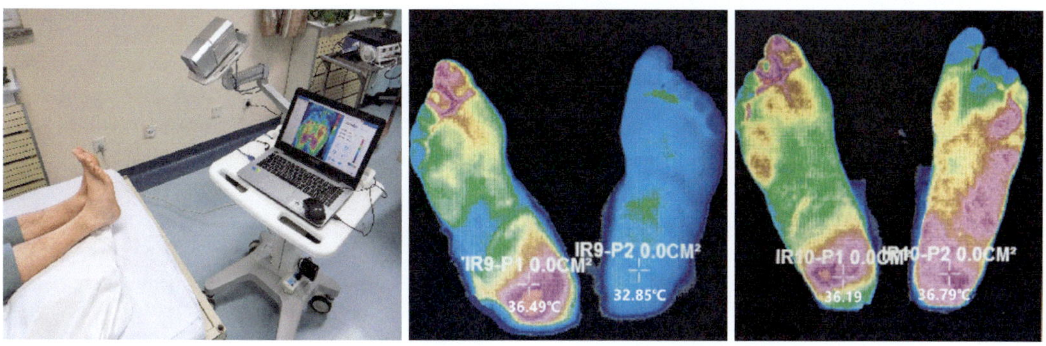

Fig. 20.3 Preoperative and postoperative infrared thermal imaging for foot skin temperature check

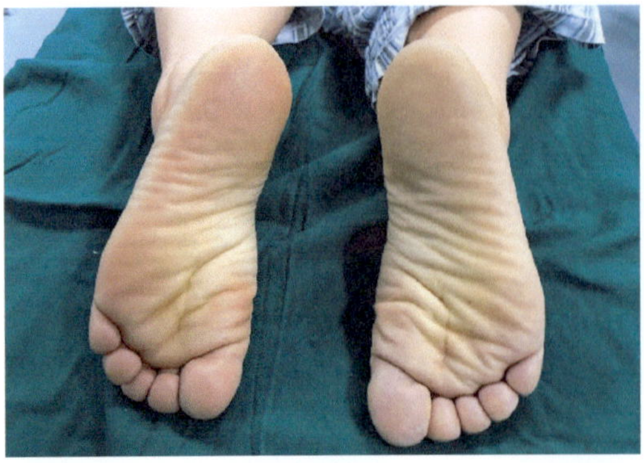

Fig. 20.4 Postoperative left foot skin color is significantly redder than the right side

20.2 Case Analysis

20.2.1 Diabetic Peripheral Neuropathy

Diabetic foot is one of the complications of diabetes, with an annual incidence of new foot lesions in diabetic patients of 3% to 7%. Diabetic foot is caused by the combined effects of diabetic neuropathy and vascular disease, and its occurrence is closely related to microvascular disease, poor blood glucose control, and infection. Diabetic foot neuropathy is a chronic complication of diabetes and is one of the important causes of disability and death in diabetic patients. It is mainly due to the microvascular disease of diabetic patients. The long-term hyperglycemic state causes the patient's foot microvessels to narrow and occlude, and the metabolism of nerve cell membranes is disordered, leading to degeneration and necrosis.

The onset of diabetic foot neuropathy is insidious and easy to be ignored by patients. Early symptoms are often sensory disturbances, presenting as symmetrical pain and sensory abnormalities. Foot neuropathy is characterized by stabbing and burning pain, and severe cases can present with insomnia and depression. Sensations are often numbness, ant crawling, and abnormal symptoms such as fever. Diabetic foot neuropathy not only affects the patient's work and life ability but also imposes a huge economic burden on the family. Therefore, timely detection and treatment of diabetic foot neuropathy and blood glucose control are key to relieving patient pain and improving quality of life.

20.2.2 Lumbar Sympathetic Ganglion Destruction Surgery

The lumbar sympathetic nerve destruction procedure is increasingly being used to treat a variety of lower limb pain disorders. Its indications include neuropathic pain, vasospastic pain, lower back and leg pain caused by chronic movement disorders, and unexplained joint and muscle pain. After the lumbar sympathetic nerve is destroyed, vasodilation and microcirculation improve, blocking the transmission of pain signals, accelerating the clearance of pain-causing substances, and thus playing a role in treating lower limb pain disorders. Due to the anatomical position of the lumbar sympathetic nerve, it is often chosen for destruction in clinical practice. The methods of lumbar sympathetic nerve destruction include surgical removal, chemical lumbar sympathetic nerve destruction, and physical destruction. The most commonly used method is chemical lumbar sympathetic nerve destruction.

Bibliography

1. Abramov R. Lumbar sympathetic treatment in the management of lower limb pain. Curr Pain Headache Rep. 2014;18(4):403.
2. Xiugao Y, Yonggao Z, Jianlong C, et al. Clinical study on the treatment of lower limb sympathetic nerve maintenance pain by lumbar sympathetic nerve destruction. Chin J Pain Med. 2014;20(6):434–6.
3. Redman DR, Robinson PN, Al-Kutoubi MA. Computerised tomography guided lumbar sympahectomy. Anaesthesia. 1986;41(1):39–41.
4. Cheng J, Daftari A, Zhou L. Sympathetic blocks provided sustained pain relief in a patient with refractory painful diabetic neuropathy. Case Rep Anesthesiol. 2012;2012:1–5.

21 Case of Type 2 Diabetes Complicated with Complex Suppurative Sweat Gland Inflammation

Lei Gao and Jiangning Wang

21.1 Case Summary

Patient, male, 37 years old. The main reason for admission was a rupture and pus discharge in the right buttock and the formation of a sinus tract for more than 2 years.

[Present Illness History] The patient had a local rupture in the right buttock without any obvious cause 2 years ago, with purulent exudate, local swelling, and pain. He intermittently sought treatment at a nearby local hospital, where he received local dressing changes, but the wound never healed. In order to seek further treatment, he came to our hospital for consultation. The out patient department admitted him with a diagnosis of "soft tissue infection."

[Past History] Type 2 diabetes for over 10 years, irregular oral administration of metformin and gliclazide for treatment, average blood sugar control. Denies history of hypertension, hyperlipidemia, coronary heart disease, and stroke; denies history of hepatitis, tuberculosis, and close contact history; denies history of surgery, trauma, and blood product transfusion; and denies history of drug and food allergies. Vaccinations were carried out as planned.

L. Gao · J. Wang (✉)
Department of Orthopedics, Beijing Shijitan Hospital, Capital Medical University, Beijing, China
e-mail: gaolei3337@bjsjth.cn; wangjn@bjsjth.cn

[Admission Examination]

1. Specialized physical examination. Right buttock shows about 15.0 cm of skin swelling, local skin temperature is high, multiple sinus tract scars can be seen, purulent exudate can be seen in the local sinus tract, touch pressure pain, soft tissue hardening (Fig. 21.1).
2. Laboratory examination. ① Blood routine: WBC 10.88 × 10^9/L, neutrophil percentage 81.9%, HGB 138 g/L. ② Blood biochemistry: albumin 40.6 g/L, serum glucose (fasting) 10.02 mmol/L, glycated hemoglobin 10.1%. ③ CRP 11.24 mg/L. ④ ESR 51 mm/h. ⑤ Deep wound bacterial culture result: *Staphylococcus epidermidis*.
3. Imaging examination. Buttock MRI: Abnormal signal in the subcutaneous soft tissue of the right buttock, considering infectious lesions and local sinus tract formation in combination with the history; multiple lymph nodes in the pelvic and bilateral inguinal regions (Figs. 21.2 and 21.3).

[Treatment and Outcome] After admission, the patient was given symptomatic supportive treatment such as anti-infection, improving circulation, nourishing nerves, reducing swelling, controlling blood sugar, correcting hypoalbuminemia, and nutritional support. After excluding surgical contraindications, the patient underwent right buttock incision, sinus tract excision, vascular nerve tendon exploration, and tissue flap

J. Wang, L. Gao (eds.), *Refractory Wounds*, Experts' Perspectives on Medical Advances,
https://doi.org/10.1007/978-981-96-2067-8_21

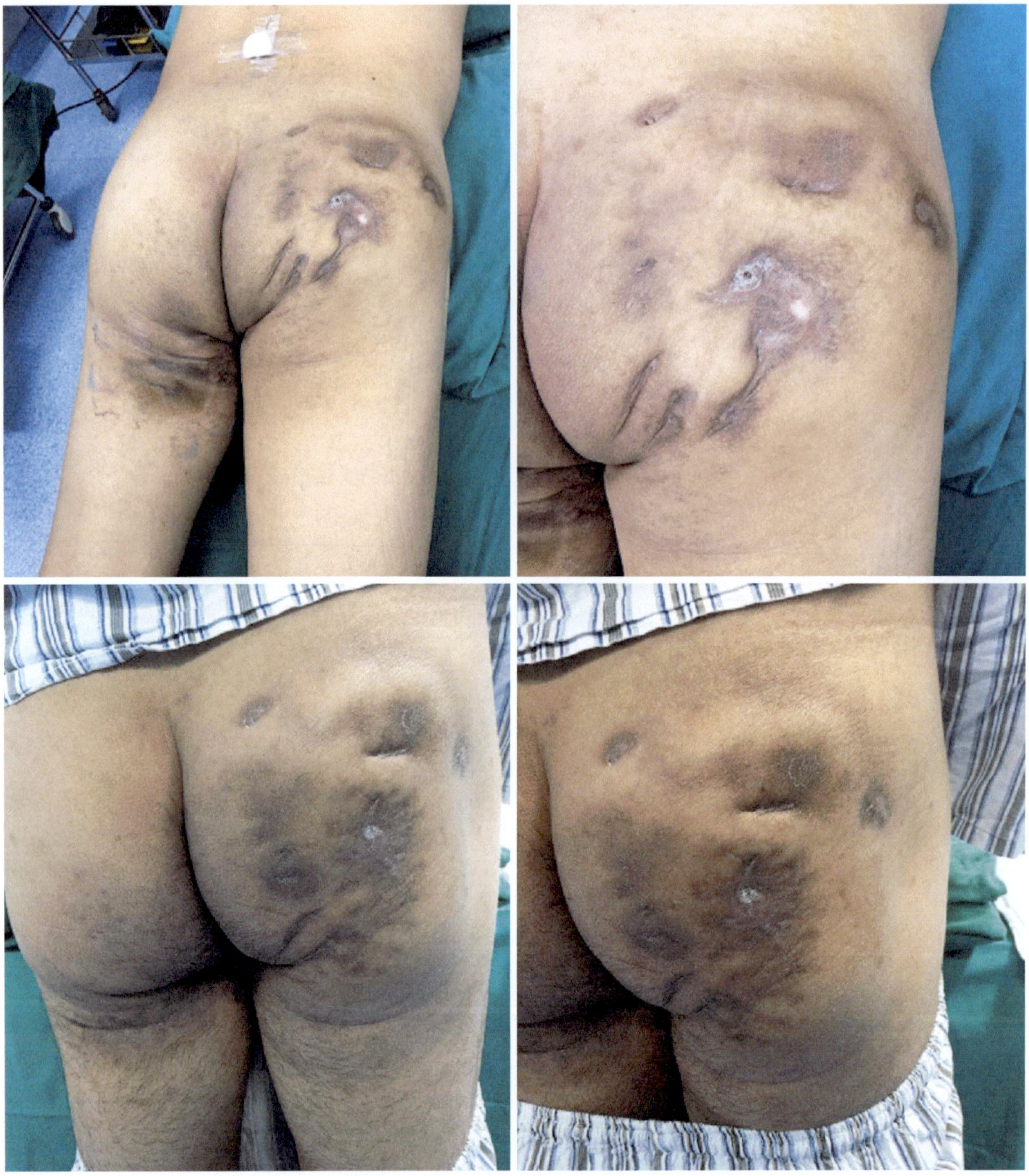

Fig. 21.1 Presentation of the right buttock upon admission

transfer under spinal anesthesia. Regular dressing changes were performed postoperatively (Fig. 21.4).

The wound on the right buttock healed well, dry and without exudate. Laboratory results at discharge: WBC 4.55 × 10^9/L, neutrophil percentage 56%, HGB 132 g/L, albumin 39.5 g/L, fasting blood glucose 6.35 mmol/L, glycated hemoglobin 7.2%, CRP 7.43 mg/L, ESR 15 mm/h (Fig. 21.5).

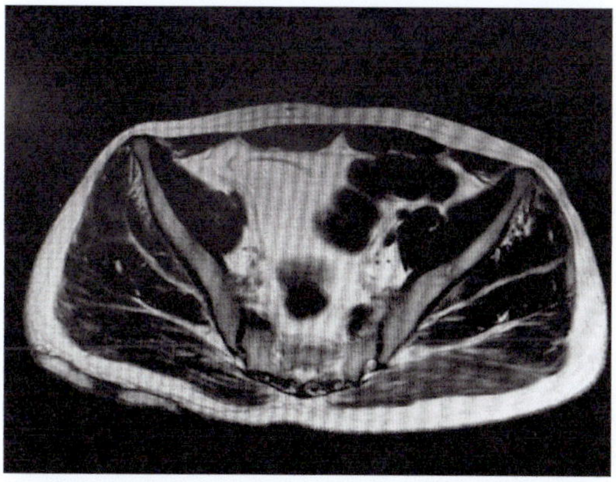

Fig. 21.2 Hip MRI

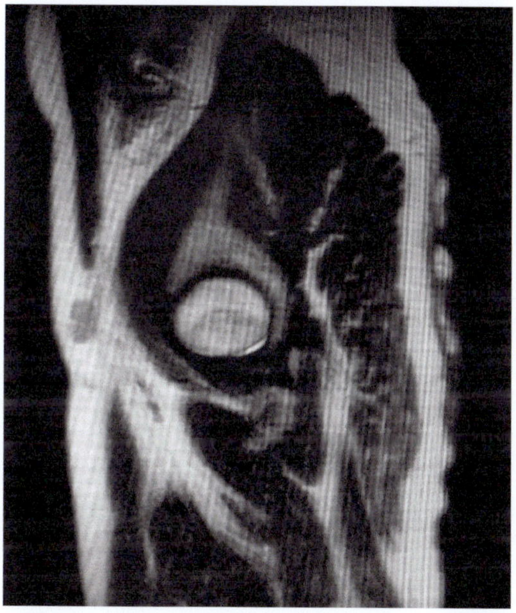

Fig. 21.3 MRI

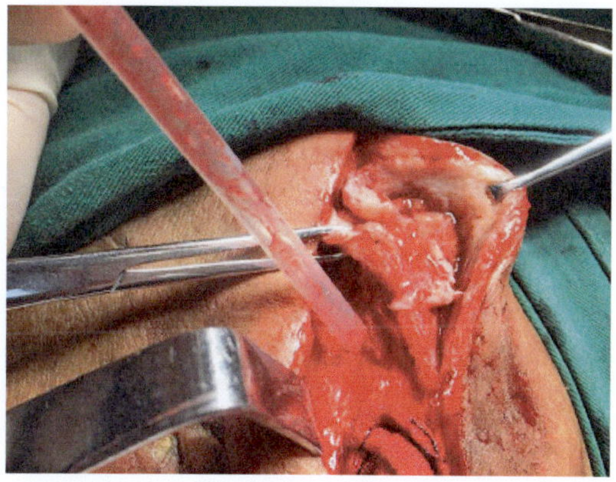

Fig. 21.4 During surgery

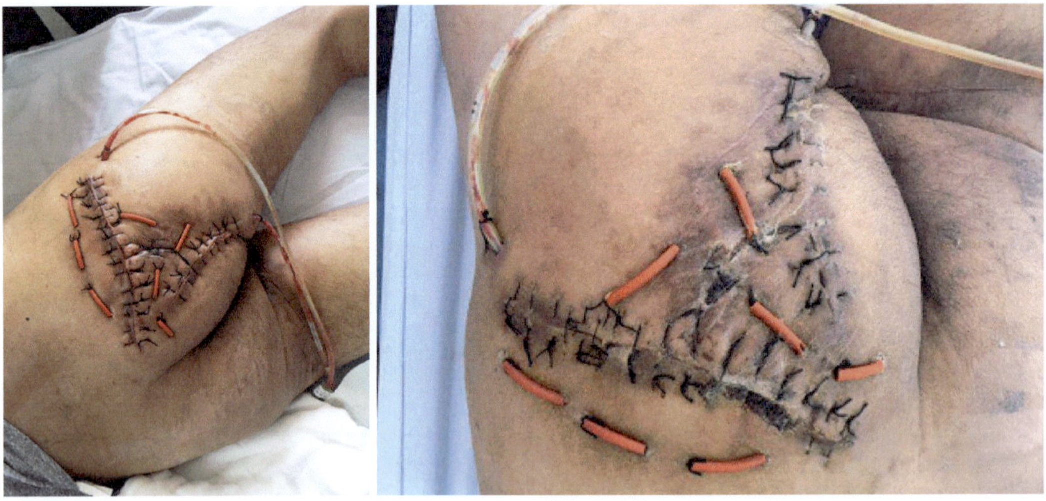

Fig. 21.5 Postoperative wound on the right buttock healed well

21.2 Case Analysis

Hidradenitis suppurativa (HS) is a chronic, recurrent, inflammatory skin disease that often occurs in areas rich in sweat glands, such as the armpits, groin (inner thigh, pubic area, scrotum, labia), buttocks, perineum, and perianal area. Other less common sites of disease include the back, neck, and behind the ears. Its incidence rate is about 1%, often starting insidiously after puberty and persisting. Late-stage lesions form extensive complex abscesses and sinus tracts after repeated purulent infections, with skin thickening and hardening, potential for malignancy, and requiring extensive surgical excision. The cause of HS is not yet fully understood. It was previously mostly believed to be caused by bacterial infection following sweat gland obstruction, but the latest research has found that its onset is mainly related to lymphocyte infiltration and hyperkeratosis of the hair follicle sebaceous gland unit. In addition, smoking, obesity, and a hot and humid living environment are all high-risk factors for HS. The clinical features include recurrent abscess formation, initially as a single hard and painful nodule, which after repeated rupture merges into patches and then forms complex labyrinthine sinuses, as well as irregular scar hyperplasia and/or contraction, severely affecting the patient's psychological, physiological, social and quality of life. Due to repeated stimulation of chronic inflammation, long-term unhealed HS may become malignant, according to Jackman's report of 125 cases of perianal suppurative hidradenitis, four cases of which turned into squamous cell carcinoma, with an incidence rate of 3.2%.

The diagnosis of HS mainly relies on medical history and clinical manifestations. Generally speaking, the diagnosis must meet one of the following two criteria: ① During the active period of the disease, there are one or more primary lesions in specific areas (such as the armpits and groin), and there have been three or more painful or purulent nodules in specific areas after puberty. ② During the quiescent period of the disease, there are no primary lesions, but there have been five or more painful or purulent nodules in specific areas after puberty. The clinical staging of HS is of great significance for diagnosis and treatment. Hurley divided this disease into three stages based on the range of lesions and the presence or absence of scars and sinuses: stage I, one or more abscesses, no sinuses or scars; stage II, one or more separate recurrent abscesses, accompanied by sinus formation; stage III, extensive interconnected sinuses and abscesses with scar formation.

Common treatments for HS include local treatment, oral antibiotics, immunosuppressants, lasers, surgery, and traditional Chinese medicine. For stages I and II patients, local treatment, oral antibiotics, lasers, and small lesion excision can be used; for stage III patients, these methods are usually ineffective, and surgical removal of all affected areas is the only cure. There are many methods for surgical treatment of HS, and different methods need to be chosen according to different conditions, such as acute or chronic phase, affected area and range, and the general condition of the patient. Small lesions in stages I and II can be locally excised and sutured; in stage III, minor surgeries such as incision and drainage can be performed during acute infection to relieve symptoms. After infection control, all lesions need to be surgically removed. To reduce the possibility of postoperative recurrence, the excision range should be as wide as possible. Parks and others suggest that the excision range should include all affected glands and all hairy skin, and the depth should reach the deep fascia. Preoperative injection of methylene blue into the sinus to mark the lesion range helps to remove the lesion at the base.

The repair of the wound after lesion excision is also crucial and is closely related to postoperative hospital stay, appearance, and functional recovery. There are many methods of repair, such as delayed healing, direct repair, suturing repair, free skin grafting, and flap or musculocutaneous flap transplantation. There are many cases of delayed healing reported abroad, and although it takes a longer time, some scholars believe that delayed healing has fewer complications, and the newly formed granulation tissue has no sweat gland components, which can reduce the risk of recurrence. However, for Asians who are prone to scarring, this method may cause severe scar hyperplasia or contraction, causing serious functional impairment to the patient, so it is not suitable. Direct suturing is only suitable for the repair of small wounds. For stage III patients, postoperative direct suturing is an important factor for the high recurrence rate of HS, because the range of lesions removed by the directly sutured wound is usually not enough.

Free skin grafts and flap transplantation are two common methods for repairing HS lesion excision wounds. Both have their pros and cons, and the method used depends on the patient's condition, the location and size of the lesion, etc. Free skin grafting is simple to operate and suitable for wounds of all sizes. Kagan believes that free skin grafting is the first choice for HS postoperative repair, because it has no requirements for the size of the wound; further, all lesions and the surrounding reddened skin can be removed, which is more thorough, so the possibility of recurrence is lower. However, HS is an infected wound, the skin graft transplanted after debridement is usually thin, and not only is the postoperative appearance not beautiful, but there may also be severe skin graft contraction and/or scar hyperplasia, seriously affecting the patient's quality of life.

Moreover, the skin graft has poor anti-infection ability, which will affect its survival if the debridement is not thorough, and often requires a longer time for dressing changes due to residual small wounds after surgery, or even reoperation, which can prolong the hospital stay. Flaps have good blood supply, stronger anti-infection ability than skin grafts, are not easy to contract, and the appearance and function recovery after repair are much better than skin grafts. The author believes that as long as the size and location of the lesion allow, flaps should be used for repair as much as possible. There are many flaps to choose from for the common HS-prone areas. For example, the repair of axillary wounds can use local flaps, V-Y advancing flaps, scapular flaps, and thoracodorsal artery perforator flaps, etc.; groin and perineal wounds can be treated with anterolateral thigh flaps or medial thigh flaps, etc.; buttock and perianal wounds can be treated with local flaps, superior gluteal, inferior gluteal, or deep femoral artery perforator flaps. In addition to flaps, musculocutaneous flaps are also highly regarded by many scholars due to their rich blood supply and strong anti-infection ability, such as latissimus dorsi musculocutaneous flaps for repairing axillary wounds, rectus abdominis musculocutaneous flaps for repairing groin wounds, and gluteus maximus musculocutaneous flaps for repairing buttock wounds. Tanaka compared the recurrence rates of musculocutaneous flaps and skin grafts and found no significant difference; however, due to the rich blood supply of musculocutaneous flaps, recurrent lesions after surgery can be cured by oral antibiotics, while recurrent lesions after skin grafting are not easy to control and may even erode the surviving skin graft. Among the common sites of HS, the axilla has the highest requirements for shape and function restoration. Direct skin grafting can cause significant local depression, pigmentation, skin graft contraction, and scar hyperplasia, and neither the shape nor the function can compare with flaps/musculocutaneous flaps. Flaps from the lateral chest and back are two common choices for repairing axillary wounds. Although the lateral chest flap has a similar texture to the axilla, both heterotopic and advancing flaps will cause varying degrees of tension on the upper arm at the apex of the axilla. Various flaps from the back (scapular flaps, latissimus dorsi musculocutaneous flaps, thoracodorsal artery perforator flaps), although they do not cause tension on the upper arm, often make the axilla appear swollen after repair, which also affects the postoperative shape and function, especially in some obese patients. To solve this problem, the method of latissimus dorsi musculocutaneous flap combined with free skin grafting was adopted, with the following advantages: ① The latissimus dorsi has a rich blood supply, which can play a role in biological clearance for possible residual infections. ② The latissimus dorsi is large in area and can repair large defects, and the donor area can be directly sutured without skin grafting. ③ The muscle is soft and has a certain thickness, and it can repair the wound after the axillary HS is removed, without making the axilla too depressed or too swollen, and the shape is beautiful. ④ Thick and medium-thick skin grafts can be used on the muscle flap, reducing the possibility of postoperative skin graft contraction, and with postoperative functional exercise, the patient's shoulder joint movement is not significantly hindered.

Bibliography

1. Jemec GB. Clinical practice. Hidradenitis suppurativa. N Engl J Med. 2012;366(2):158–64.
2. Revuz JE, Canoui-Poitrine F, Wolkenstein P, et al. Prevalence and factors associated with hidradenitis suppurativa: results from two case-control studies. J Am Acad Dermatol. 2008;59(4):596–601.
3. Yirui Z, Suwen X. Clinical summary of 32 cases of treatment for hidradenitis suppurativa. Chin J Colorectal Dis. 2001;21(5):43.
4. Nazary M, van der Zee HH, Prens EP, et al. Pathogenesis and pharmacotherapy of hidradenitis suppurativa. Eur J Pharmacol. 2011;672(1–3):1–8.
5. Yazdanyar S, Jemec GB. Hidradenitis suppurativa: a review of cause and treatment. Curr Opin Infect Dis. 2011;24(2):118–23.
6. Poli F, Wolkenstein P, Revuz J. Back and face involvement in hidradenitis suppurativa. Dermatology. 2010;221(2):137–41.
7. Syed ZU, Hamzavi IH. Atypical hidradenitis suppurativa involving the posterior neck and occiput. Arch Dermatol. 2011;147(11):1343–4.
8. Losanoff JE, Sochaki P, Khoury N, et al. Squamous cell carcinoma complicating chronic suppurative hydradenitis. Am Surg. 2011;77(11):1449–53.
9. Rambhatla PV, Lim HW, Hamzavi L. A systematic review of treatments for hidradenitis suppurativa. Arch Dermatol. 2012;148(4):439–46.
10. Zifu H, Guodong L, Yuming K, et al. Treatment of perianal suppurative hidradenitis with integrated traditional Chinese and Western medicine in 6 cases. Chin J Integr Tradit West Surg. 2012;18(5):521–2.
11. Unal C, Yirmibesoglu OA, Ozdemir J, et al. Superior and inferior gluteal artery perforator flaps in reconstruction of gluteal and perianal/perineal hidradenitis suppurativa lesions. Microsurgery. 2011;31(7):539–44.

Severe Infection Combined with Osteomyelitis in One Case

22

Shuo Wang, Jiangning Wang, and Lei Gao

22.1 Case Summary

Patient, male, 50 years old. The main reason for admission was recurrent rupture and pus discharge from the skin of the left buttock for 8 years and high fever for 10 days.

[Present Illness] The patient was diagnosed with a thoracic vertebral fracture due to trauma in 2003 and underwent thoracic surgery at a local hospital. After the surgery, the patient lost most of the sensation and movement below the navel, resulting in paralysis. Two years later, the patient underwent a procedure to remove the surgical pins. Long-term bed rest led to the development of an ulcer on the left buttock, accompanied by a small amount of fluid seepage. The patient self-treated with medication changes, but the results were not satisfactory, and the wound gradually deepened with increased seepage. Ten days ago, the patient began to experience high fever, with a maximum temperature of 39.6 °C. The local hospital treated the patient with cephalosporin drugs, and the body temperature dropped slightly. The patient came to our hospital for further treatment and was admitted with a diagnosis of "left buttock soft tissue infection."

S. Wang · J. Wang (✉) · L. Gao
Department of Orthopedics, Beijing Shijitan Hospital, Capital Medical University, Beijing, China
e-mail: shenkemao@qq.com; wangjn@bjsjth.cn; gaolei3337@bjsjth.cn

[Past Medical History] The patient has had hypertension for over 10 years and has been treated with nifedipine and captopril, with blood pressure controlled at 140/80 mmHg. The patient denies a history of diabetes, hyperlipidemia, coronary heart disease, and stroke; denies a history of hepatitis, tuberculosis, and close contact with these diseases; denies other trauma history and blood transfusion history; and denies drug and food allergies. Vaccinations have been carried out as planned.

[Admission Examination]

1. Specialist examination. Body temperature 41 °C, pulse 109 beats/min, blood pressure 80/50 mmHg, respiration 23 times/min; there is an oval wound about 3.0 cm × 3.0 cm × 4.0 cm in size on the left buttock, which is white in color, with a small amount of purulent exudate, higher skin temperature, and good blood circulation (Fig. 22.1); there is an oval skin defect about 3.0 cm × 4.0 cm in size on the left hip, which is pink in color, with normal skin temperature, and good blood circulation.
2. Routine examination. WBC 15.07 × 10^9/L, neutrophil percentage 84%, PCT 51.03 ng/mL, CRP 229.31 mg/L, myoglobin 165.8 ng/mL, troponin 0.11 ng/mL.
3. Imaging examination. Pelvic CT: Left ischial branch osteomyelitis and soft tissue infection (Fig. 22.2).

J. Wang, L. Gao (eds.), *Refractory Wounds*, Experts' Perspectives on Medical Advances,
https://doi.org/10.1007/978-981-96-2067-8_22

[Preliminary Diagnosis] Left buttock soft tissue infection, thoracic spinal cord injury, incomplete paralysis, stage 2 hypertension (very high risk).

[Treatment and Outcome] After admission, the patient was given symptomatic treatment such as anti-infection, swelling reduction, circulation improvement, and anticoagulant drugs. After the use of antibacterial drugs, the body temperature dropped to 38 °C on the fourth day, and on the fifth day, necrotic tissue removal and necrotic bone removal surgeries were performed under local anesthesia combined with intravenous enhanced anesthesia. An 18-gauge Benos drainage tube was placed, the wound was regularly changed after surgery, and the wound healed well (Figs. 22.3 and 22.4). On the ninth day after surgery, the drainage tube was removed (Figs. 22.5 and 22.6), and the inflammatory indicators were rechecked: CRP 50.3 mg/L, WBC 8.05×10^9/L, neutrophil percentage 72.6%, PCT 0.33 ng/mL.

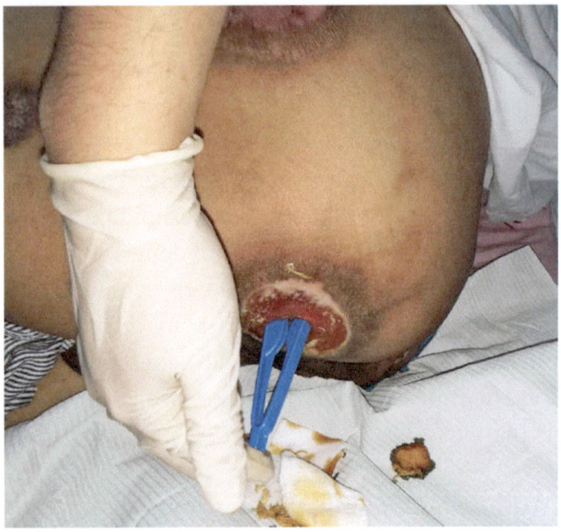

Fig. 22.1 Patient's left buttock upon admission

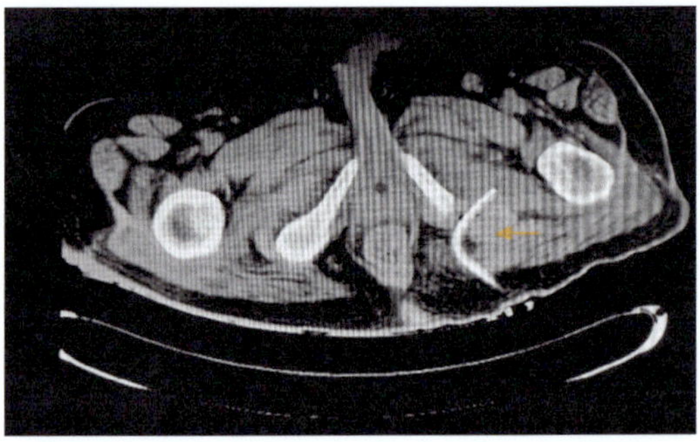

Fig. 22.3 Postoperative pelvic CT

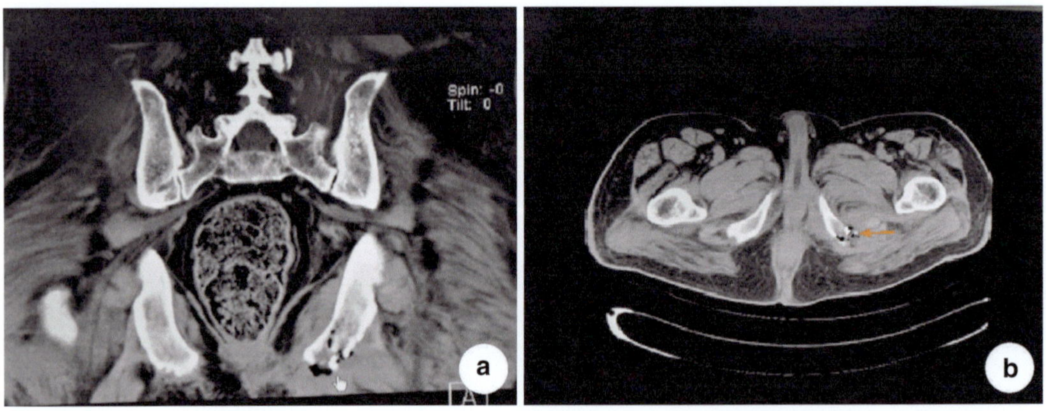

Coronal plane   Cross section

Fig. 22.2 CT shows destruction of the left ischial branch bone. (**a**) Coronal plane; (**b**) Cross section

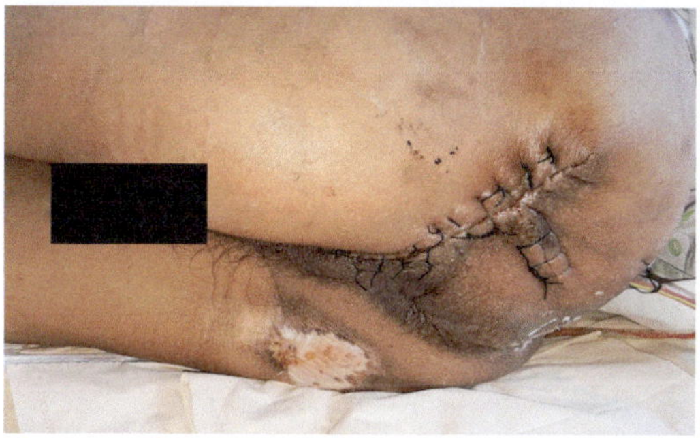

Fig. 22.4 Postoperative wound

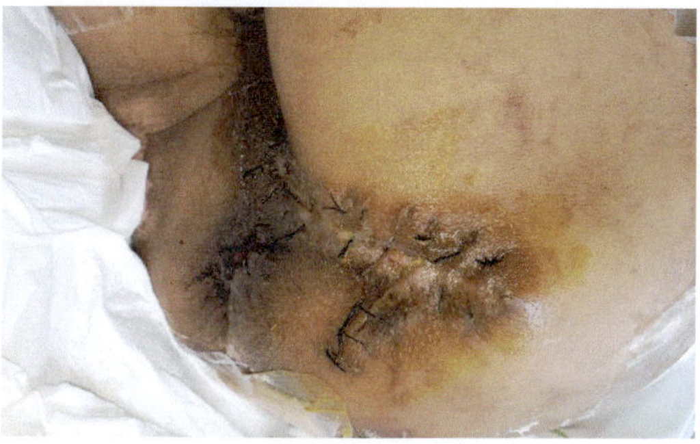

Fig. 22.5 Postoperative wound drainage tube removal

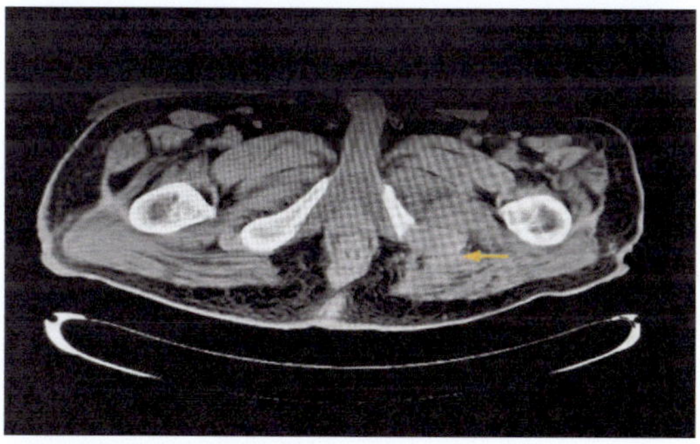

Fig. 22.6 Pelvic CT after tube removal

22.2 Case Analysis

Soft tissue infections are common in long-term bedridden patients, which can cause multiple ulcers, long-lasting non-healing necrosis, and exudation. The wound can reach deep into the bone and even penetrate organs such as the rectum. In severe infections, high fever and septic shock can occur, requiring bacterial culture and appropriate antibacterial drug treatment. This case was admitted to the hospital with a soft tissue infection. After symptomatic use of antibacterial drugs according to the wound condition, the inflammatory indicators decreased, the body temperature decreased, and after completing the relevant examinations, the diagnosis of osteomyelitis was confirmed. A one-stage surgery was performed to thoroughly debride, remove necrotic tissue, and close the wound. The patient's inflammatory indicators gradually returned to normal, and the body temperature also returned to normal.

For patients with soft tissue infections, in addition to symptomatic medication changes, it is also necessary to conduct drug sensitivity culture, carry out anti-infection treatment, and it is essential to improve CT or MRI to clarify the range and depth of the wound, and to confirm whether there is osteomyelitis, so as to thoroughly remove necrotic tissue during surgery.

Bibliography

1. Qingyu H, Naihang G, Deheng S. Bacteriological investigation and drug resistance analysis of patients with chronic wound infection. China Mod Med J. 2018;20(11):7–10.
2. Yanrong Y, Min L, Liting Z, et al. Analysis of pathogen colonization and infection in different types of wounds. Med Anim Control. 2019;35(1):98–100.
3. Guoqi W, Peifu T. Progress in the treatment of chronic wounds. J PLA Med Sch. 2018;39(5):444–6.
4. Guisheng X. Distribution and drug resistance analysis of pathogens in skin and soft tissue infections. China Disinfect J. 2018;35(7):53–6.
5. Bouvet C, Gjoni S, Zenelaj B, et al. *Staphylococcus aureus* soft tissue infection may increase the risk of subsequent staphylococcal soft tissue infections. Int J Infect Dis. 2017;60:44–8.
6. Jiangning W, Gengjia T, Zhaofan X, et al. Comprehensive treatment of pressure sores. Beijing: People's Health Publishing House; 2018.
7. Jiangning W, Lei G, Tiangui C, et al. Professor Wang Jiangning's team's detailed explanation of comprehensive diagnosis and treatment of diabetic foot cases. Beijing: Science and Technology Literature Publishing House; 2018.

23 ECMO Local Perfusion Free Flap Repair of Diabetic Foot Wound One Case

Lei Gao and Jiangning Wang

23.1 Case Summary

Patient, male, 46 years old. Admitted to our department due to recurrent rupture of the right foot for 24 years, with increased exudation and odor for 1 week.

[Medical History] Twenty-four years before the patient's admission, the right foot was fractured due to an open wound, causing the second and third metatarsal fractures. The patient underwent debridement and fracture fixation surgery in our hospital. The wound did not completely heal after the surgery, and the patient changed the dressing at home. One week ago, the rupture increased with more exudation and a strong odor, so the patient came to our hospital for further diagnosis and treatment. During the course of the disease, the patient's mental state and sleep were not good; there was no significant increase or decrease in body temperature.

[Past History] The patient's general health condition is average, with diabetes for 15 years, irregular use of hypoglycemic drugs, and poor blood sugar control. The patient denies having hypertension, hyperlipidemia, coronary heart disease, and stroke history; denies hepatitis, tuberculosis history, and close contact history. In 2012, the patient underwent percutaneous screw fixation surgery for a right femoral neck fracture, and the screw was later removed; in 2019, the patient had gastric bleeding and received 800 mL of blood transfusion, with no adverse reactions to the transfusion. The patient denies a history of trauma and drug and food allergies and has been vaccinated as scheduled.

[Admission Examination]

1. Specialized physical examination. An 8.0 cm × 3.0 cm wound can be seen at the first metatarsal of the right foot, with gray-black necrotic fascia tissue accompanied by gray-black exudate, strong odor, obvious redness and swelling of the surrounding skin, and tenderness. The pain, temperature, and touch functions of the right foot are reduced, and the pulsation of the dorsalis pedis artery and the posterior tibial artery is weakened (Fig. 23.1).
2. Laboratory examination. ① Blood routine: WBC 12.73 × 10^9/L, neutrophil percentage 82%. ② Blood biochemistry: albumin 34.3 g/L, Glu 24.22 mmol/L. ③ CRP 121.81 mg/L. ④ PCT 0.11 ng/mL. ⑤ ESR 80 mm/h.
3. Imaging examination. MRI: Uneven swelling of the soft tissue of the right foot; STIR shows diffuse net-like and strip-like slightly high signals; the skin edge of the medial side of the foot is ruptured; the first metatarsal and phalanges show diffuse abnormal signals; T2WI

L. Gao · J. Wang (✉)
Department of Orthopedics, Beijing Shijitan Hospital, Capital Medical University, Beijing, China
e-mail: gaolei3337@bjsjth.cn; wangjn@bjsjth.cn

J. Wang, L. Gao (eds.), *Refractory Wounds*, Experts' Perspectives on Medical Advances,
https://doi.org/10.1007/978-981-96-2067-8_23

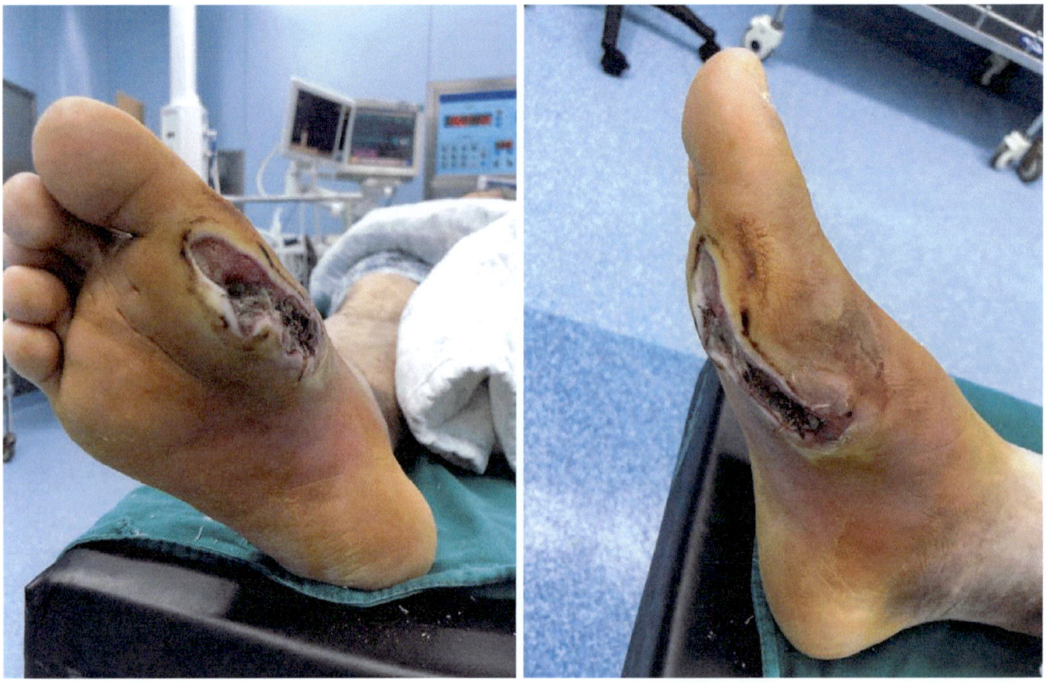

Fig. 23.1 Foot wound

fat suppression sequence shows slightly high signals; a small amount of effusion is seen in the first metatarsophalangeal joint. Linear slightly long T1 abnormal signals are seen at the distal end of the second metatarsal and the base of the third metatarsal, no abnormal signals are seen in the T2WI fat suppression sequence; the remaining multiple bone marrow cavities show uneven slightly long T2. Abnormal signal, no clear signal reduction seen in T1WI. A small amount of liquid abnormal signal is seen in the right ankle joint cavity (Fig. 23.2). No abnormalities were found in the lower limb arterial color Doppler ultrasound.

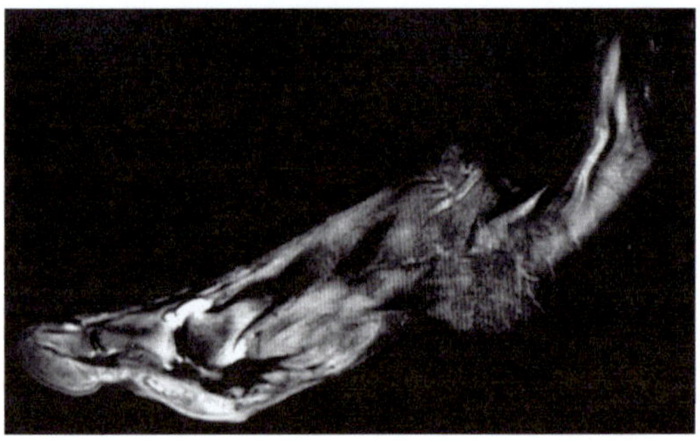

Fig. 23.2 Right foot MRI

[Treatment and Outcome] After the patient was admitted to the hospital, relevant examinations were completed, surgical indications were confirmed, emergency debridement surgery was performed, and postoperative control of blood sugar, anti-infection, swelling reduction, and nutritional nerve treatments were given (Fig. 23.3). The wound was dressed daily, and debridement surgery was performed twice (Fig. 23.4). After thoroughly removing the infected bone and soft tissue, a free flap graft was performed to cover the exposed bone and tendon wound (Figs. 23.5 and 23.6). At the same time, extracorporeal membrane oxygenation (ECMO) technology was used to perfuse the flap after surgery, establishing collateral circulation in the flap (Fig. 23.7). Eventually, the flap survived (Fig. 23.8).

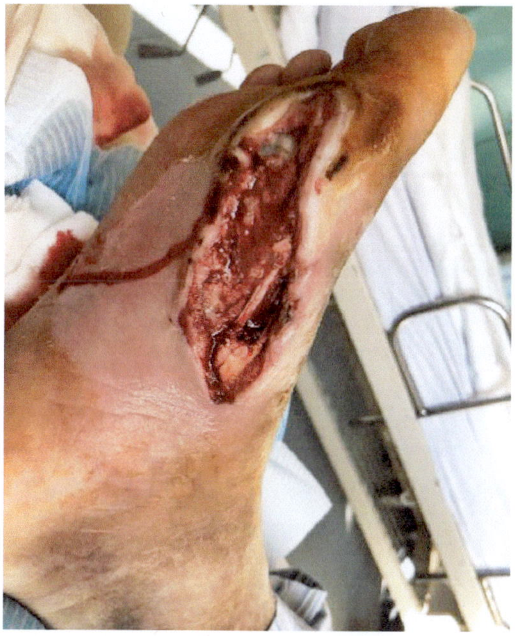

Fig. 23.3 Debridement surgery after admission

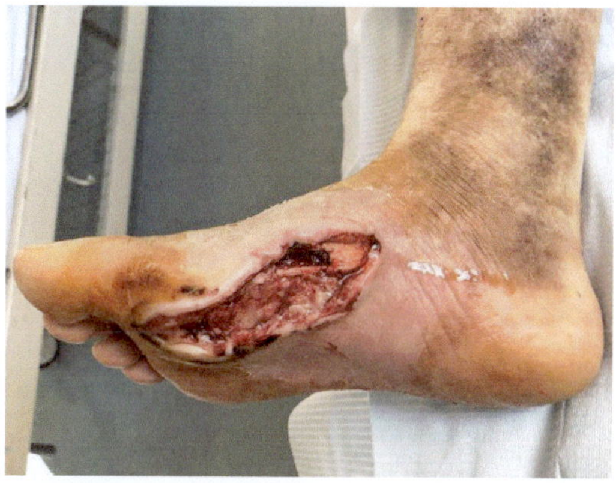

Fig. 23.4 Twice debridement to thoroughly remove necrotic bone tissue

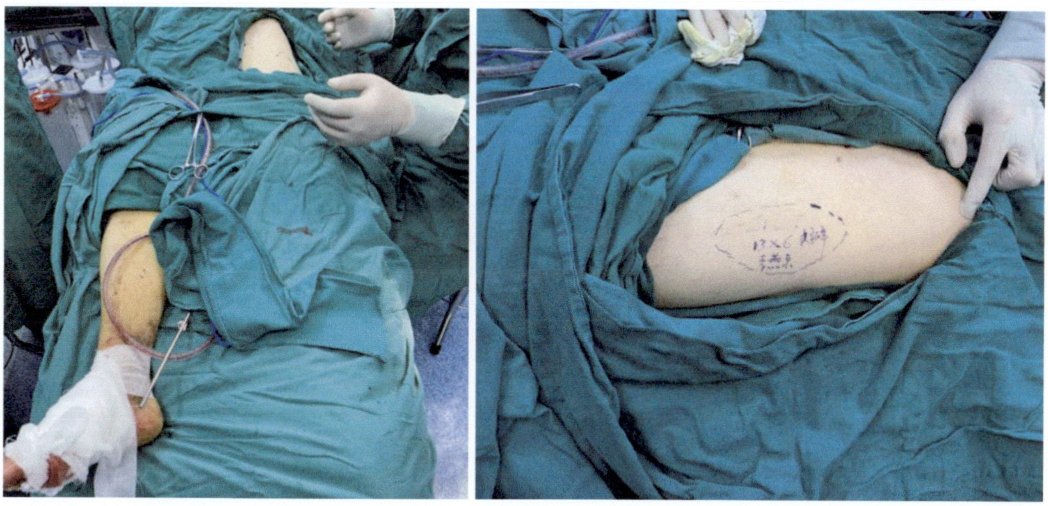

Fig. 23.5 Anterolateral thigh free flap used for foot wound repair

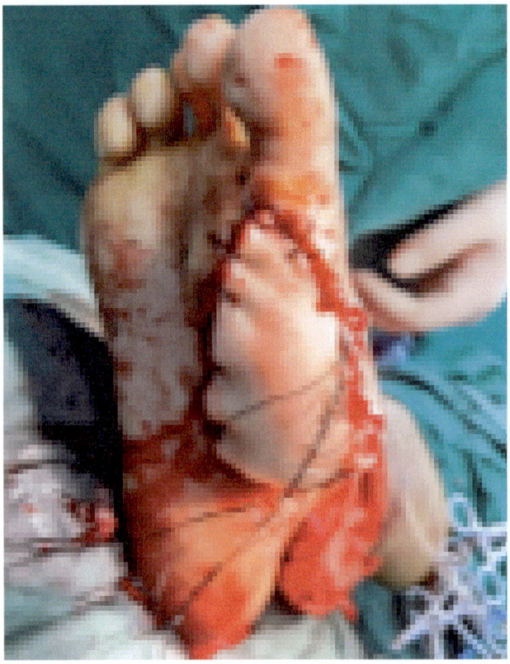

Fig. 23.6 Free flap graft surgery to cover the exposed bone and tendon wound

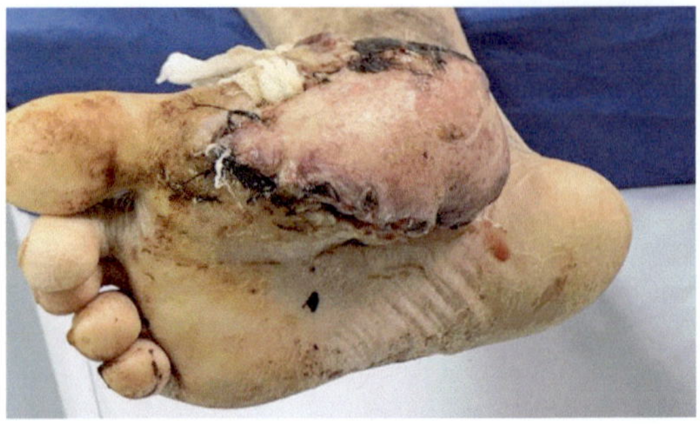

Fig. 23.8 Flap survival

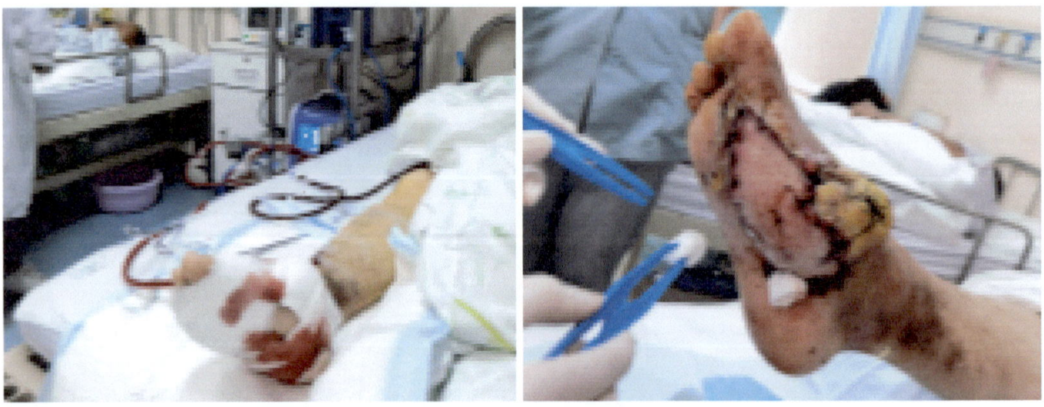

Fig. 23.7 Postoperative ECMO perfusion of the flap to establish collateral circulation in the flap

23.2 Case Analysis

23.2.1 The Limitations of Using Free Flaps Alone to Repair Diabetic Foot Wounds

Diabetic foot is one of the long-term complications of diabetes and one of the complications with the highest amputation and mortality rates. One important reason for these severe conditions is vascular disease, where the lumen of the diseased vessels narrows and blocks, obstructing blood flow, resulting in insufficient or even no supply of nutrients to the nerves and soft tissues of the lower limbs. This leads to nerve disease, easy damage to soft tissues that cannot heal, and symptoms such as soft tissue infection.

Orthopedics and microsurgery often repair diabetic foot wounds with flaps. In some cases with better vascular physiological conditions, the use of local free flaps to repair exposed bone wounds has been proven effective. However, due to severe vascular disease in the late stage of diabetic foot, it is impossible to find a vascularized flap to transfer, and no suitable vessels can be found at the distal end of the foot, making it impossible to implement a vascularized flap.

23.2.2 ECMO Local Perfusion Flap Technique

After the vascularized flap is separated from the distal end, it is connected to the large artery with good physiological conditions in the lower limb and the distal vein through the Extracorporeal Membrane Oxygenation (ECMO) power pump for pressurization, ensuring the blood supply of the flap and the survival rate of the flap. After the flap survives, it is implanted in the diabetic foot wound without disconnecting the autologous blood supply. Using the principle of capillary reconstruction, the pedicle is severed after 21 days, ensuring the survival of the flap, further solving the problem of low flap survival rate due to limb blood circulation disorders, or even inability to survive, thereby improving the flap survival rate.

23.2.3 Flap Perfusion and Arterialized Venous Flap

Venous flaps are flaps whose main blood supply enters and exits through the venous system. Compared to traditional arterial flaps, venous flaps have their own advantages, including easy design, no need for deep dissection, no sacrifice of the main blood vessels of the flap supply area, unrestricted position of the flap supply area, and fewer complications in the flap supply area. Based on the direction of blood flow in the vessels entering and leaving the flap, three types of venous flaps have been proposed. Type I: single pedicle venous flap; type II: double pedicle venous flap; type III: arterialized venous flap, which is perfused after the proximal artery and the proximal vein of the flap are anastomosed, and flows out from the distal vein. This case uses ECMO technology to foster free flaps. When the collateral circulation is established, the flap is then cut off, and the final flap survives. There is a risk of failure, and the chosen one is an arterial flap, such as the selected anterolateral thigh flap, then the dissection range is larger, damaging the main blood vessels of the flap supply area. Therefore, in order to simplify the operation procedure and be more conducive to flap survival, later research chose venous flaps, imitating the principle of type III venous flaps. The arterial end of the extracorporeal perfusion system is connected to the vein of the flap, and the autologous venous blood is drawn out for oxygenation, and then used to perfuse the vein of the venous flap. The theoretical basis for arterialized venous perfusion is: after the vein is arterialized, the main route of early blood flow in the tissue is the arterial blood flow into the small veins, and then backflow to the small veins that cause backflow through the inter-venous communication branches; after venous diversion, the microveins can replace the role of capillaries. It is currently believed that arterialized veins can effectively dilate venous vessels through blood pressure, close or make venous valves ineffective, blood flows through the ischemic area for circulation, and then opens the microvenous shunt, effectively providing blood supply for the surrounding tissues. As the vascularization of the ischemic tissue is completed, the blood flow gradually becomes physiological blood circulation, thereby effectively ensuring tissue survival.

23.2.4 Conclusion

Due to the severe vascular disease in the late stage of diabetic foot, it is impossible to find a vascular flap that can be transferred, and free flaps cannot be found at the distal end of the foot. Therefore, vascular flaps cannot be implemented. If the joint bone is exposed and cannot be repaired by skin grafting, it can only be repaired by transferring flaps or free flaps. Some patients face the risk of amputation, but due to limb blood circulation disorders, the survival rate of the flap is low or even unable to survive. Therefore, we want to separate the vascular flap from the distal end, and connect it with the large artery and distal vein with good physiological conditions in the lower limb through the arteriovenous pump pressure, to ensure the blood supply of the flap and ensure the survival rate of the flap. After the flap survives, it is grafted onto the wound of the diabetic foot without interrupting the autologous blood supply, further solving the low survival rate of the flap caused by limb blood circulation disorders, or even the inability to survive, thereby improving the survival rate of the flap.

Bibliography

1. Lechleitner M, Abrahamian H, Francesconi C, et al. Diabetic neuropathy and diabetic foot syndrome (update 2019). Wien Klin Wochenschr. 2019;131(Suppl 1):141–50.
2. Jiangning W, Lei G. New progress in the treatment of chronic wounds of diabetic foot. Chin J Repair Reconstr Surg. 2018;32(7):832–7.
3. Alexandrescu VA, Brochier S, Limgba A, et al. Healing of diabetic neuroischemic foot wounds with vs without wound-targeted revascularization: preliminary observations from an 8-year prospective Dual-Center Registry. J Endovasc Ther. 2020;27(1):20–30.
4. Khin NY, Dijkstra ML, Huckson M, et al. Hypertensive extracorporeal limb perfusion for critical limb ischemia. J Vasc Surg. 2013;58(5):1244–53.
5. Lei W, Xin N, Yefeng Y, etc. Use of Vascular Ning to treat lower limb crush injury crush syndrome model pigs under extracorporeal circulation perfusion system. Chin Tissue Eng Res. 2019;23(11):1723–9.
6. Lei Y, Lei G, Lei W, etc. Pressurized perfusion under extracorporeal circulation system improves lower limb blood circulation in model pigs. China Tissue Eng Res. 2018;22(4):553–7.
7. Lei G, Jiangning W, Yefeng Y. 2019 interpretation of the "international diabetes foot working group diabetes foot prevention and treatment guidelines". Chin J Repair Reconstr Surg. 2020;34(1):16–20.
8. Lane RJ, Phillips M, McMillan D, et al. Hypertensive extracorporeal limb perfusion (HELP): a new technique for managing critical lower limb ischemia. J Vasc Surg. 2008;48(5):1156–65.

ECMO Technology for the Treatment of Lower Limb Ischemia in Diabetic Foot: One Case

24

Lei Gao and Jiangning Wang

24.1 Case Summary

Patient, male, 60 years old. The main reason for admission was the nonhealing ulceration of the fifth toe of the right foot for more than 10 days.

[Present Illness History] The patient's right foot's fifth toe ulcerated more than 10 days before admission, which was not taken seriously. Later, the wound gradually enlarged, with increased exudation and pain. The patient came to our hospital for further diagnosis and treatment. Since the onset of the disease, the patient's bowel movements, spirit, and appetite have been okay, with no significant increase in body temperature and no weight loss.

[Past History] Generally healthy, diabetes for 30 years, blood sugar control is okay, self-injection of Novolin 30 R insulin 16 IU before breakfast and dinner. Denies hypertension, hyperlipidemia, and coronary heart disease. Has a history of stroke, diagnosed as cerebral infarction in a local hospital in July 2019, did not undergo surgical treatment, and had a good effect after conservative treatment. Denies history of hepatitis, tuberculosis, and close contact history; denies surgical history, trauma history, blood product transfusion history; denies drug and food allergy history. Vaccination history is as planned.

L. Gao · J. Wang (✉)
Department of Orthopedics, Beijing Shijitan Hospital, Capital Medical University, Beijing, China
e-mail: gaolei3337@bjsjth.cn; wangjn@bjsjth.cn

[Admission Examination]

1. Specialized physical examination. A 1.0 cm × 1.0 cm wound can be seen between the fourth and fifth toes of the right foot, accompanied by pale yellow serous exudation. The wound edge to the surrounding area of the fifth metatarsophalangeal joint is obviously red and swollen, with tenderness. The posterior tibial and dorsal foot arteries are not palpable, the peripheral blood circulation is poor, and the pain, temperature, and tactile sensation of the affected foot are reduced (Fig. 24.1).
2. Laboratory examination. ① Complete blood count: WBC 13.73×10^9/L, neutrophil percentage 85%. ② Blood biochemistry: albumin 34.3 g/L, Glu 14.22 mmol/L. ③ CRP 80.81 mg/L. ④ PCT 0.21 ng/mL. ⑤ ESR 80 mm/h.

[Treatment and Outcome] After the patient was admitted to the hospital; relevant examinations were completed; surgical indications were clarified; debridement and suturing surgery was performed; postoperative control of blood sugar, anti-infection, swelling reduction, nutritional nerve treatment, and ECMO technology perfusion of the affected limb (Fig. 24.2); the wound was dressed daily and healed smoothly (Fig. 24.3).

J. Wang, L. Gao (eds.), *Refractory Wounds*, Experts' Perspectives on Medical Advances,
https://doi.org/10.1007/978-981-96-2067-8_24

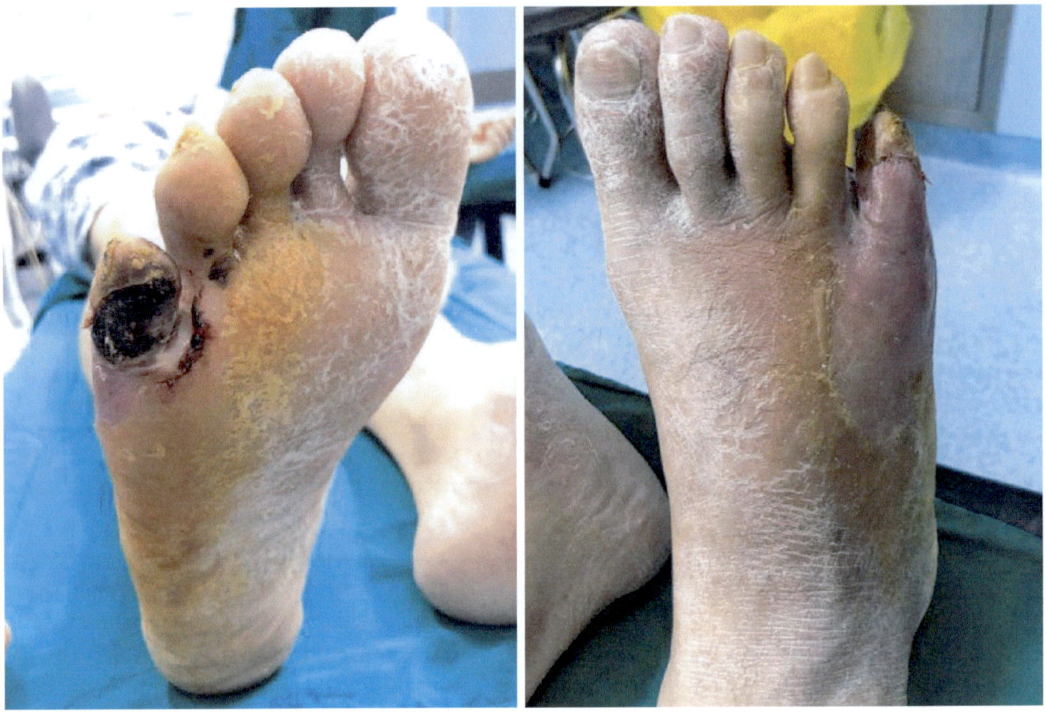

Fig. 24.1 Right foot wound

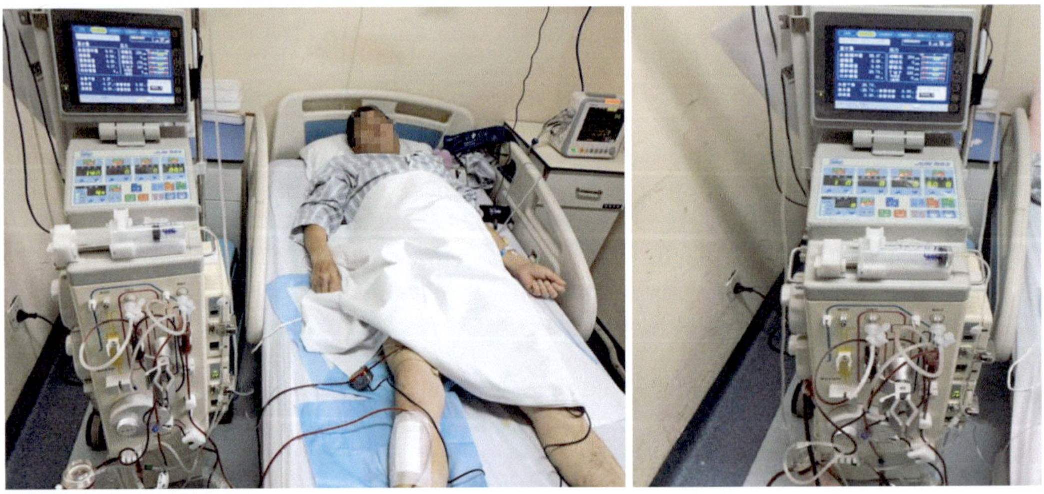

Fig. 24.2 ECMO extracorporeal membrane oxygenation technology perfusion treatment of diabetic foot disease

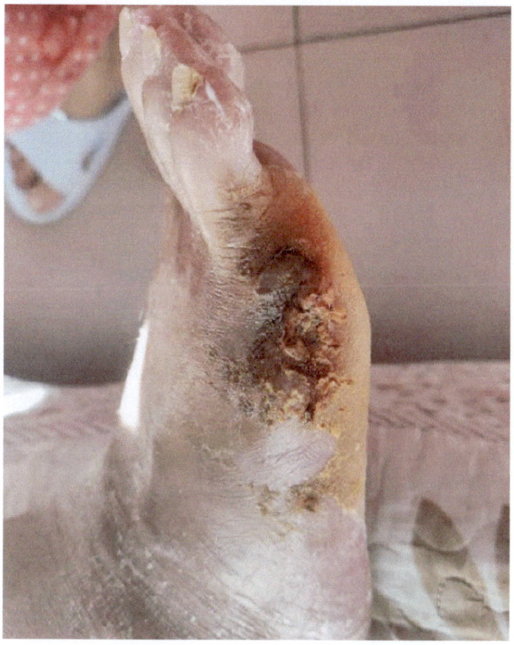

Fig. 24.3 Wound healing

24.2 Case Analysis

24.2.1 Theoretical Basis of ECMO Treatment for Diabetic Foot

The theoretical basis of this technology is feasible. In the early stage, we confirmed in the study of the extracorporeal simulation of the physiological environment system that this method can effectively preserve the severed limb for a long time; saves more time in rescuing patients with severe hemorrhagic shock, severe multiple organ damage, and other systemic trauma, and myocardial infarction combined with severed limbs. It also removes a large amount of toxins produced by ischemia and compression of the severed limb, as well as harmful substances such as myoglobin, potassium, phosphorus, magnesium ions, and acidic products released in large quantities with muscle necrosis, before the severed limb is replanted into the human body. This reduces the entry of harmful substances into the body through the restored blood circulation after replantation, alleviates the systemic response of the body after trauma, reduces the degree of kidney damage caused by the large amount of myoglobin released after muscle tissue necrosis being filtered through the renal tubules, and deposits in the renal tubules under acidosis and acidic urine conditions, avoids acute renal failure, thereby greatly reducing the mortality rate after limb replantation and increasing the success rate of limb replantation.

24.2.2 Improvement of ECMO Technology

As this technology is applied in clinical practice, we have found the following disadvantages: ① If the extracorporeal circulation power system uses the roller pump in the extracorporeal circulation machine, it will cause mechanical damage to the red blood cells in the circulating blood, reducing the effective red blood cell content in the blood and lowering the blood's oxygen-carrying capacity. ② If the centrifugal pump is chosen as the power system in the ECMO technology for lung replacement therapy, although it avoids mechanical damage to red blood cells, it is expensive, increases the proportion of medical insurance payments, and the machine is large, which is not convenient for clinical operations. ③ ECMO oxygenates the human venous blood and then perfuses it into the arteries, so arterial cannulation is required. Arterial cannulation is prone to thrombosis, which can easily cause blockage of the membrane lung and circulation tubing.

Therefore, we have improved this technology. First, we improved the perfusion oxygenation system, using the centrifugal pump as the power pump, choosing lower-cost membrane lung materials to make the oxygenation device, thereby reducing the price of consumables; in addition, the oxygenated venous blood is re-perfused into the vein, performing lower limb venous perfusion, making the foot's distal vascular vein arterialization, and using the venous network pathway established by the superficial vein and deep vein for tissue blood supply, thereby improving the foot's blood supply to promote wound healing, and it has been clinically practiced and achieved good results.

24.2.3 Theoretical Basis of Venous Arterialization Perfusion

After venous arterialization, the main pathway of early tissue blood flow is that after arterial blood flows into the small veins, it flows back to the small veins that have a reflux effect through the inter-venous communication branches; after venous diversion, micro-veins can replace the role of capillaries. It is currently believed that venous arterialization can effectively dilate venous vessels through blood pressure, close or make venous valves ineffective, blood flows through the ischemic area for circulation, and then opens the micro-venous shunt, effectively providing blood supply for the surrounding tissues. As the vascularization of the ischemic tissue is completed, the blood flow gradually becomes physiological blood flow circulation, thereby effectively ensuring tissue survival.

24.2.4 Conclusion

ECMO has very high clinical application value and social benefits. By improving the blood supply of ischemic extremities, shortening the wound healing time, effectively reducing the amputation rate of diabetic foot patients, and saving medical costs, it reduces the national medical insurance payment amount and reduces the economic burden on families and society.

Bibliography

1. Lei W, Xin N, Yefeng Y, et al. Application of Vascularin in the treatment of lower limb crush injury and crush syndrome model pigs under extracorporeal circulation perfusion system. Chin J Tissue Eng Res. 2019;23(11):1723–9.
2. Lei Y, Lei G, Lei W, et al. Pressurized perfusion under extracorporeal circulation system improves lower limb blood circulation in model pigs. Chin J Tissue Eng Res. 2018;22(4):553–7.
3. Tengfei L, Jiangning W, Lei G, et al. The effect of distal ischemic perfusion method on preserving amputated limbs in an extracorporeal system simulating the physiological environment in vivo. Chin J Repair Reconstr Surg. 2016;30(1):91–4.
4. Junlong B, Jiangning W. Progress in the treatment of thromboangiitis obliterans. J Pract Med. 2015;31(10):1563–5.
5. Shaochun Z, Xinyuan Q, Youwei Z, et al. The effect of Vascularin on the ischemia/reperfusion injury model of the extracorporeal system simulating the physiological environment in vivo. Chin J Tissue Eng Res. 2014;18(36):5825–9.
6. Yin YF, Si XL, Wang JN, et al. Crossover replantation of carpometacarpal after traumatic amputation. Plast Reconstr Surg. 2013;131(3):468e–70e.
7. Wang JN, Tong ZH, Zhang TH, et al. Salvage of amputated upper extremities with temporary ectopic implantation followed by replantation at a second stage. J Reconstr Microsurg. 2006;22(1):15–20.

25 A Case of Type 2 Diabetic Foot Gangrene with Large Area Skin Defect

Lihua Liu, Jiangning Wang, and Lei Gao

25.1 Case Summary

Patient, female, 65 years old. Main reason for admission was the right lower leg and foot ulceration for 5 months and the right foot fell off 1 month ago.

[Present Illness] The patient started experiencing numbness in the right foot and lower leg without any apparent cause a year ago, which worsened with activity. The local hospital diagnosed it as "type 2 diabetes and type 2 diabetic peripheral neuropathy." The patient refused to take medication, instead controlling their diet and increasing exercise to regulate blood sugar. Five months ago, the patient accidentally discovered a rupture on the sole of the right foot. After self-treating and changing the dressing for over half a month without improvement, the wound gradually enlarged to involve the middle and rear foot, accompanied by purulent secretions and exudate. The local hospital diagnosed it as "type 2 diabetic foot gangrene," and treated it with anti-infection measures, wound cleaning, and dressing changes. After the wound was somewhat controlled, the patient went home and continued to change the dressing themselves. The ulcer gradually expanded to the lower leg, and a month ago, most of the skin on the right foot and lower leg fell off on its own. The affected limb was swollen, with wound exudate and purulent secretions. The patient was transferred to our hospital for further treatment. Since falling ill, the patient's spirits have been low, with poor appetite and sleep, and weight changes have not been monitored.

[Past History] The patient has a history of hypertension for 1 year, currently taking nifedipine controlled-release tablets 5 mg/d for blood pressure control, blood pressure has not been monitored. The patient has a history of type 2 diabetes for over 7 years, without regular blood sugar monitoring and medication. Five months ago, during a medical examination, diabetic nephropathy was discovered, and the patient is currently self-administering uremia-clearing granules for treatment. The patient denies a history of hyperlipidemia, coronary heart disease, stroke, hepatitis, tuberculosis, and close contact with tuberculosis; denies a history of trauma, denies a family history, denies a history of food or drug allergies.

[Admission Examination]

1. Specialist examination. Most of the right foot is missing, the right lower leg and remaining foot are significantly swollen, the skin and subcutaneous tissue of the middle and lower parts of the right lower leg and distal part are missing, the wound is dirty, some bone tissue is exposed, there is a lot of necrotic tissue and secretions on the wound, and granulation tis-

L. Liu · J. Wang (✉) · L. Gao
Department of Orthopedics, Beijing Shijitan Hospital, Capital Medical University, Beijing, China
e-mail: llhzyxq@163.com; wangjn@bjsjth.cn; gaolei3337@bjsjth.cn

J. Wang, L. Gao (eds.), *Refractory Wounds*, Experts' Perspectives on Medical Advances,
https://doi.org/10.1007/978-981-96-2067-8_25

sue of varying degrees is growing (Fig. 25.1). The knee joint's active and passive movements are normal, arterial pulsation can be felt, but it is weak.

2. Laboratory examination. ① Blood routine: WBC 5.42 × 10^9/L, neutrophil percentage 78%, RBC 52.96 × 10^{12}/L, HGB 87 g/L, hematocrit 282, PLT 273 × 10^9/L. ② Urine routine: Urinary occult blood (+ +), urinary protein (+ +). ③ Blood biochemistry: albumin 25.8 g/L, blood glucose 6.83 mmol/L. ④ CRP 19.71 mg/L. ⑤ ESR 117 mm/h. ⑥ PCT 0.02 ng/mL. ⑦ D-dimer 387 ng/mL. ⑧ Glycated hemoglobin (HBA1c) 5.3%. ⑨ BNP 25015.00 pg/mL. ⑩ Wound bacterial culture: *Pseudomonas aeruginosa*.
3. Imaging examination. The imaging examination of the lower leg and foot suggests that the right foot has a distal bone defect, the talus is tilted, no obvious bone destruction is seen, and the surrounding soft tissue is swollen (Fig. 25.2). Lower limb arterial ultrasound: bilateral lower limb arterial sclerosis. Lower limb venous ultrasound: no obstruction was seen in the deep and superficial veins of the lower limbs. Bilateral lower limb CTA: different degrees of calcified plaques on the walls of the abdominal aorta, bilateral common iliac arteries, internal and external iliac arteries, femoral arteries, anterior and posterior tibial arteries, and peroneal arteries. The middle and lower sections of the left lower leg are significantly narrowed, and there are signs of arteriovenous shunting in the right lower leg (Fig. 25.3).

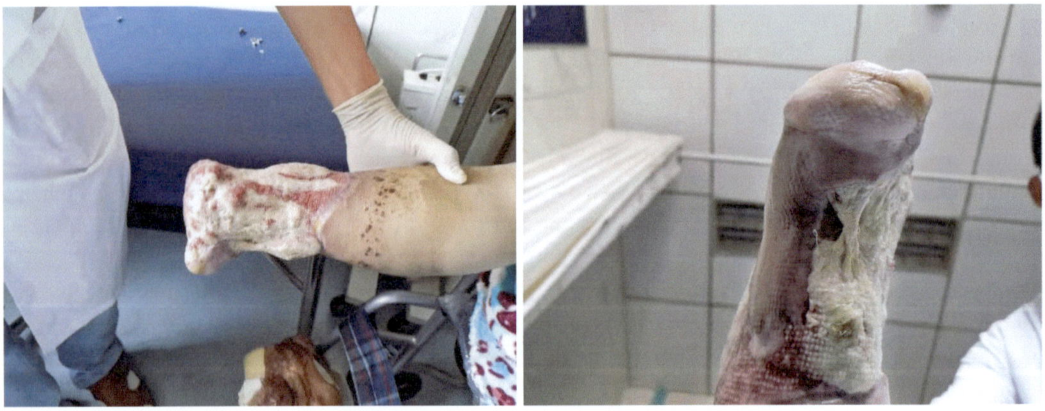

Fig. 25.1 The wound on the patient's right lower leg and foot upon admission

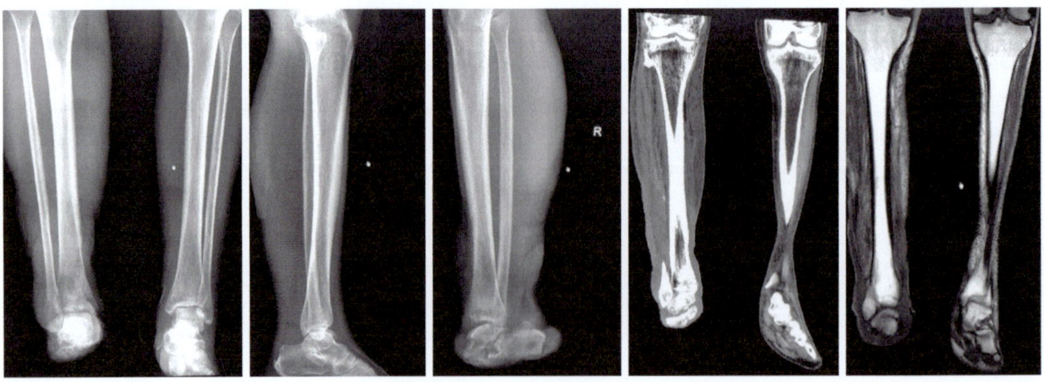

Fig. 25.2 Imaging examination of the lower leg and foot

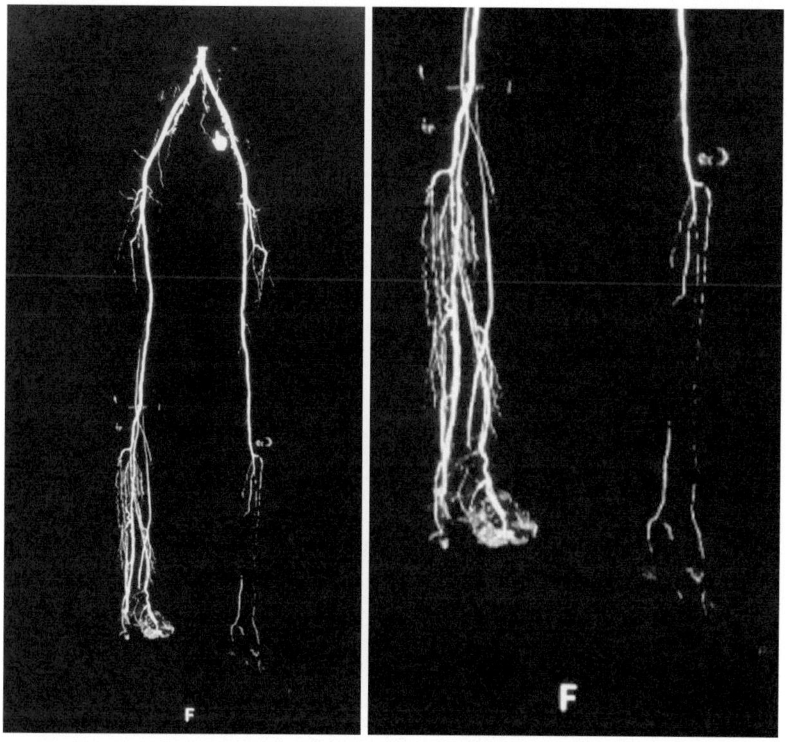

Fig. 25.3 Bilateral lower limb arterial angiography

[Preliminary Diagnosis] Type 2 diabetic foot ulcer, right foot defect, right lower leg and foot skin defect, right lower leg and residual foot soft tissue infection, type 2 diabetic peripheral neuropathy, type 2 diabetic peripheral vascular disease, type 2 diabetic foot, type 2 diabetes, diabetic nephropathy, hypertension, hypoproteinemia.

[Treatment and Outcome]

1. After admission, the patient's blood pressure and blood sugar were monitored, and insulin medication was adjusted, strengthened nutritional support, while providing symptomatic treatment with anti-infection, swelling reduction, circulation improvement, and neurotrophic drugs. The swelling of the affected limb has reduced and the patient's physical condition has improved.
2. After perfecting the preoperative preparation, the first debridement of necrotic tissue in the right lower leg and foot was performed under nerve block anesthesia on the fourth day after admission. After the debridement, the necrotic tissue and secretions on the wound surface significantly reduced, and a small amount of granulation tissue grew (Fig. 25.4).
3. Seven days after the debridement, the right lower leg and foot necrotic tissue debridement and negative pressure drainage were performed again under nerve block anesthesia. After the debridement, the swelling of the affected limb significantly reduced, the granulation tissue on the wound surface grew well, and wound surface coverage treatment was planned (Fig. 25.5).
4. The right lower leg and residual foot were grafted with autologous skin in stages, and negative pressure drainage was used as an auxiliary treatment (Figs. 25.6, 25.7, 25.8, and 25.9). The autologous skin was sourced from the inner thigh skin on both sides.
5. The wound was completely covered with autologous skin; the patient's physical condition significantly improved and was transferred to rehabilitative treatment (Figs. 25.10 and 25.11).

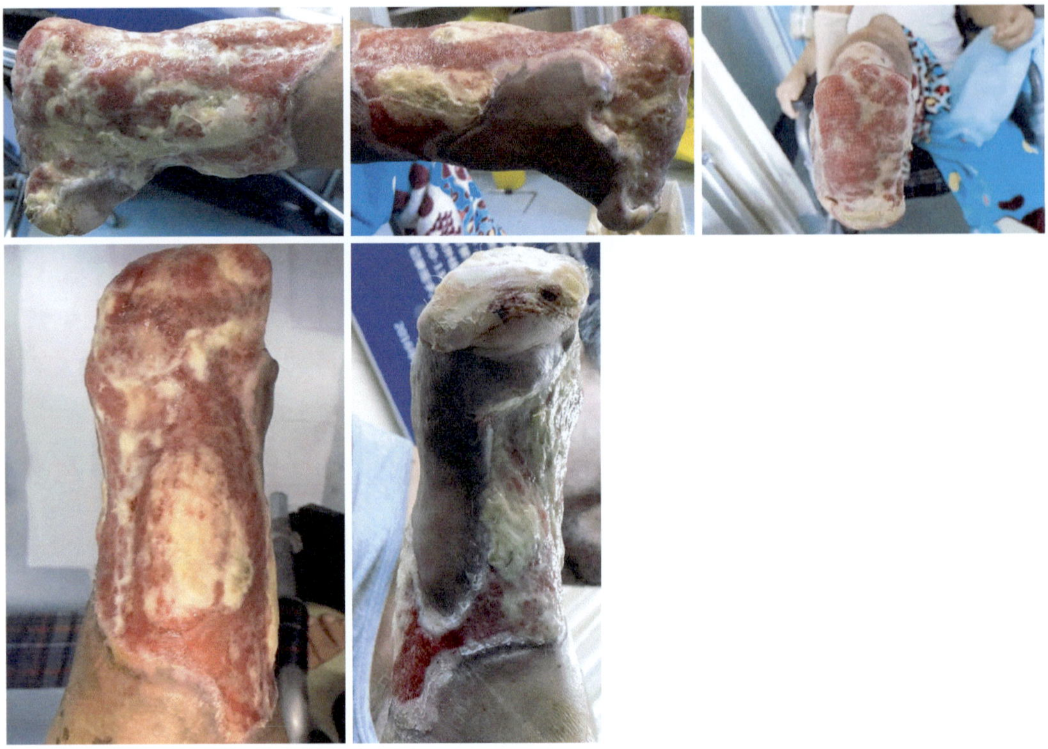

Fig. 25.4 Seven days after the first debridement

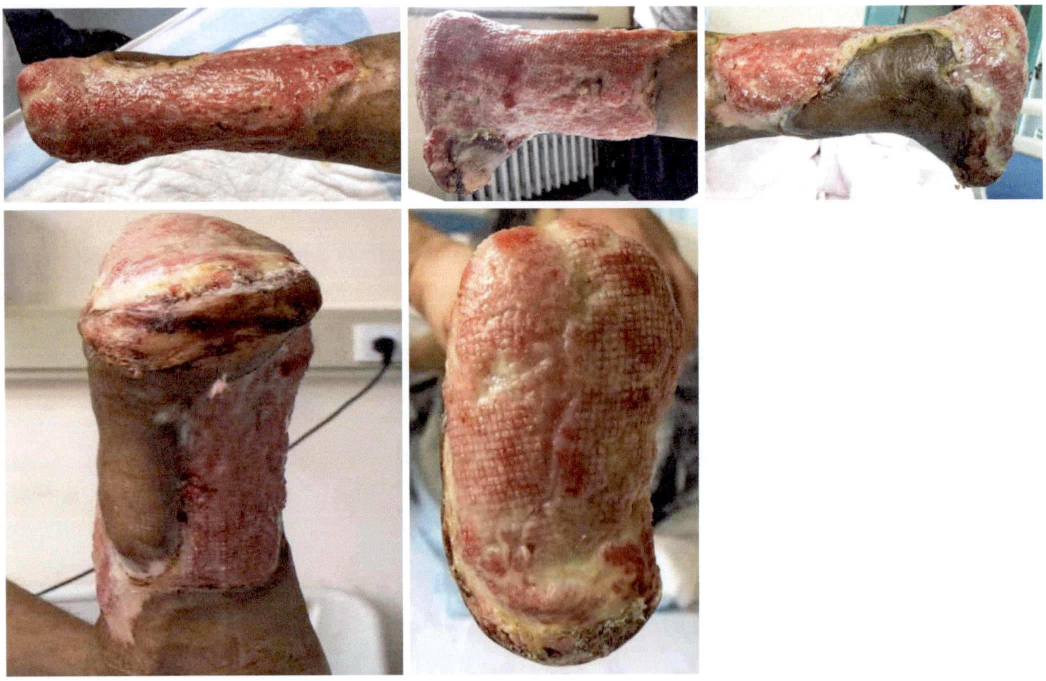

Fig. 25.5 Ten days after the second debridement and negative pressure drainage

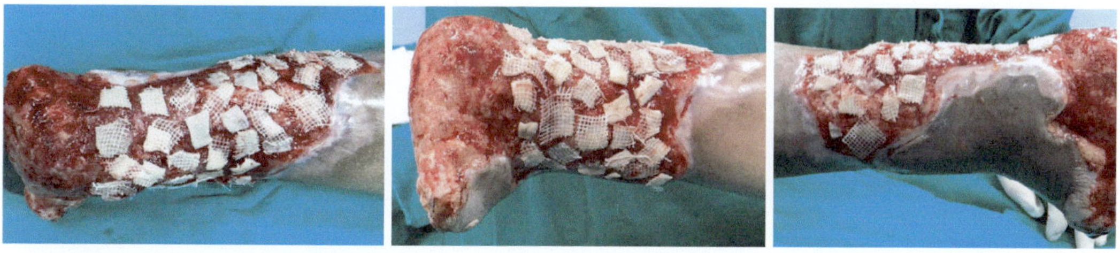

Fig. 25.6 During the first skin grafting

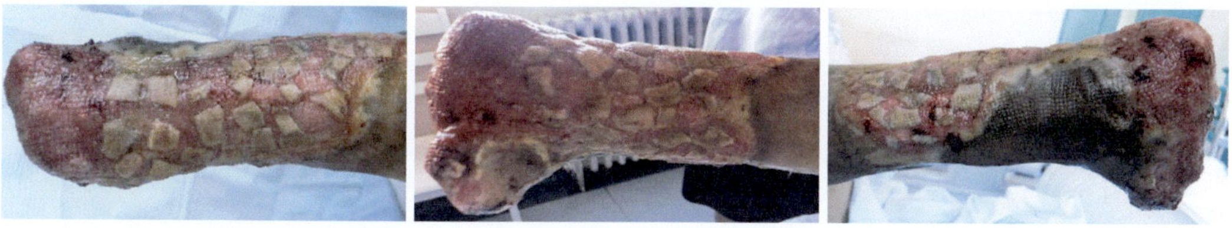

Fig. 25.7 Ten days after the first skin grafting

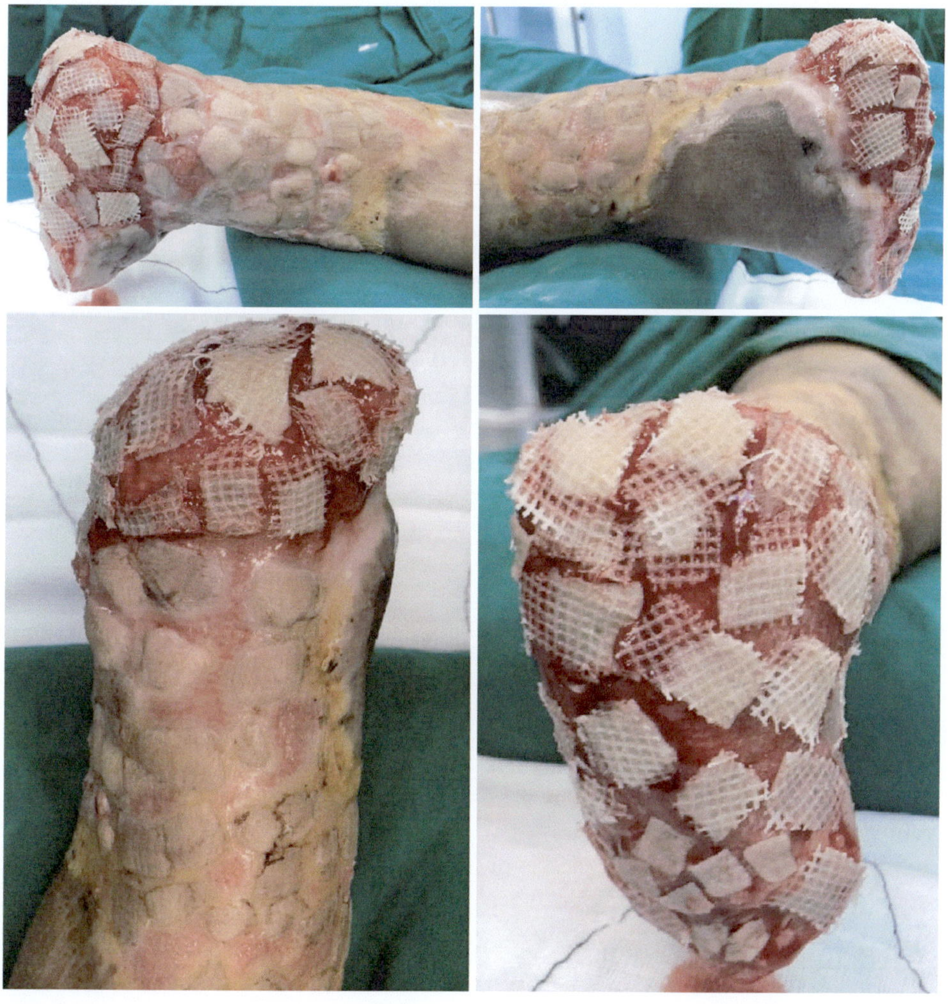

Fig. 25.8 During the second autologous skin grafting after wound cleaning and dressing change

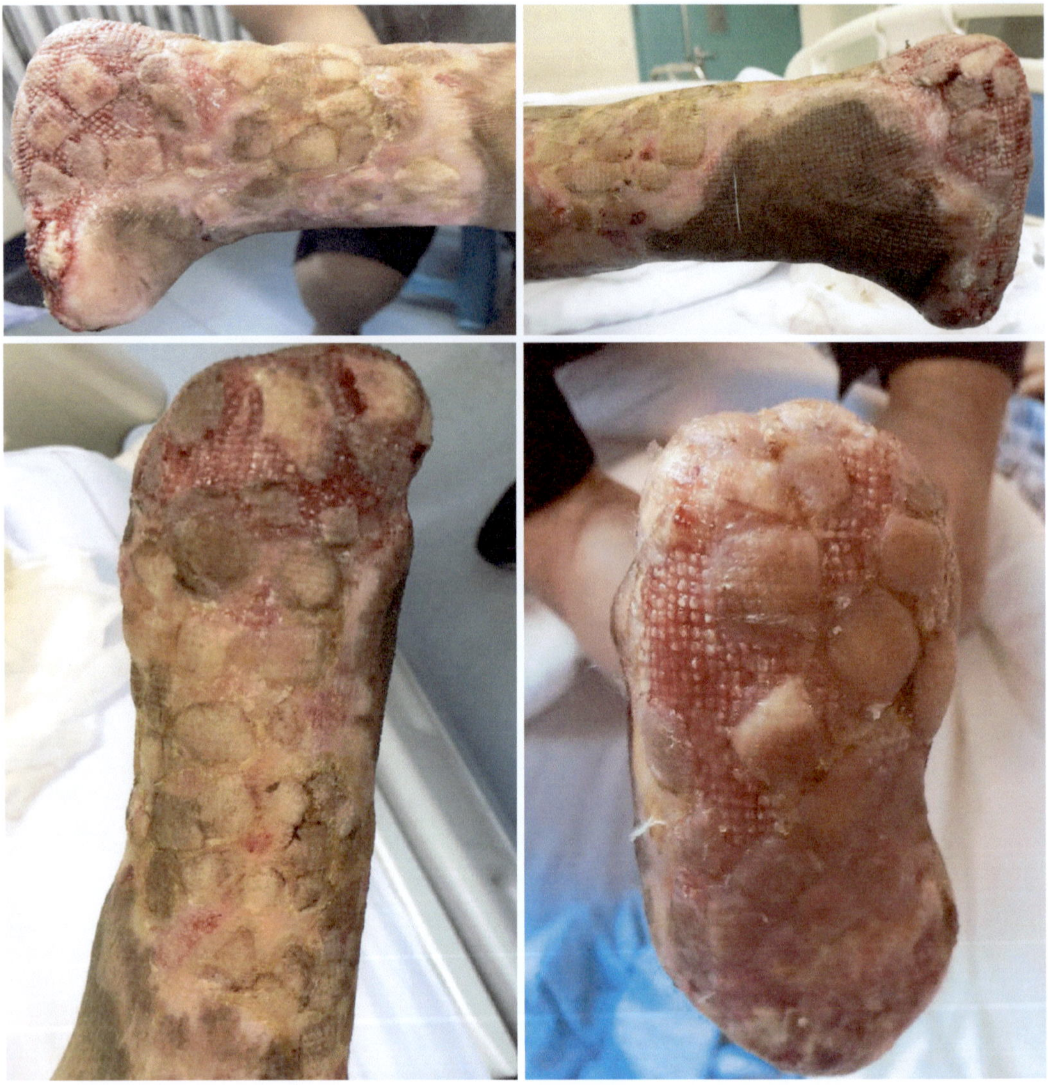

Fig. 25.9 Day 10 after the second skin grafting

The skin is the largest organ of the human body, protecting various tissues and organs from various external stimuli, and is a very important natural barrier of the human body. Smaller wounds can heal themselves or close through stretching, while larger skin defects require free skin grafting, skin flap transplantation, etc.

Free skin grafting cuts different thicknesses of autologous skin and transplants it to another place to re-establish blood circulation for repair. According to the thickness of the skin graft, it can be divided into thin skin grafts (blade thick skin grafts), medium-thick skin grafts, full-thickness skin grafts, and full-thickness skin grafts containing subdermal vascular network.

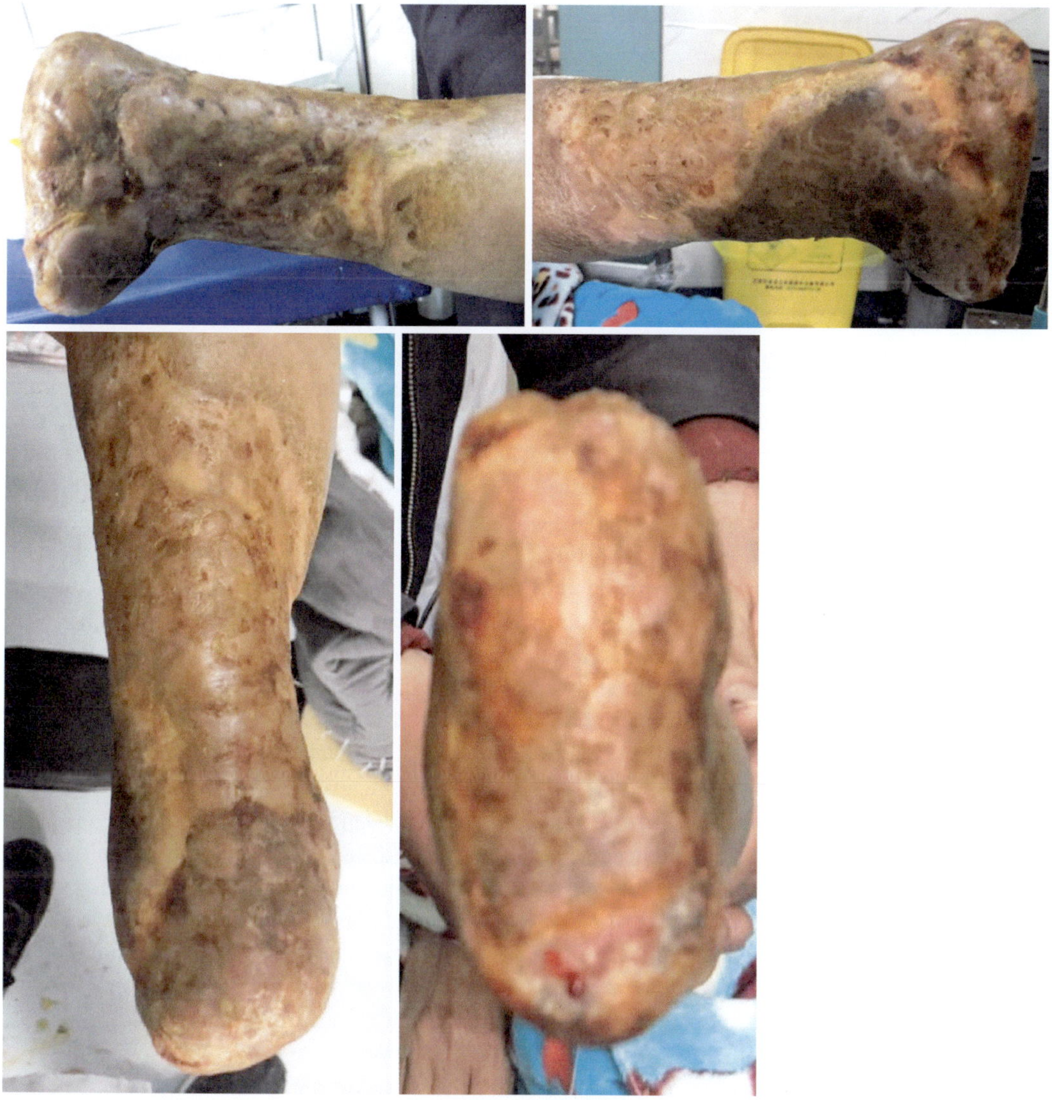

Fig. 25.10 Good skin healing 2 months after the second skin grafting

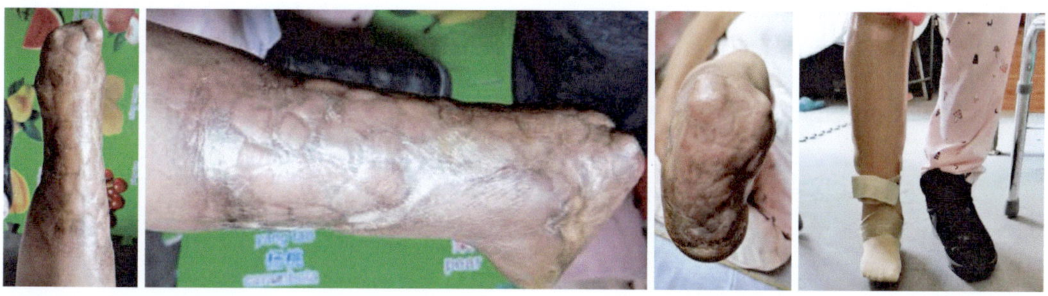

Fig. 25.11 Good skin healing 1 year after the second skin grafting, walking on the ground with the assistance of a full-contact plaster support

25.2 Case Analysis

The average thickness of the thin skin graft is 0.3 mm, histologically containing the epidermal layer of the skin and a small amount of the papillary layer of the dermis. It is suitable for large skin defects and infected granulation wounds, helping early wound healing. The advantage of thin skin grafts is that they are easy to grow, have strong resistance, and can survive and grow even in poor conditions or mildly infected granulation wounds. On the other hand, the donor area recovers quickly, and can fully heal within 7–10 days after skin grafting, leaving no significant scars; if necessary, it can be re-harvested multiple times. The disadvantage is that due to scar hyperplasia under the skin graft, the skin graft often shrinks after healing, sometimes shrinking by 40%, and the skin graft has deeper pigmentation. Functionally, the skin graft often cannot achieve the purpose of restoring function due to shrinkage, especially near the joints, limiting its application. In addition, thin skin grafts cannot withstand pressure and friction, and are prone to ulcers. The average thickness of the medium-thick skin graft is 0.3–0.6 mm, containing part of the epidermis and dermis (thin medium-thick skin graft), or up to three-quarters of the full thickness of the skin (thick medium-thick skin graft). Because the skin graft contains more elastic tissue, it has the characteristics of full-thickness skin, less shrinkage, soft, and wear-resistant. The donor area can heal itself, so it is widely used clinically and is suitable for parts with higher functional and appearance requirements, such as repairing skin defects on the face or joints, or the wounds left after scar or tumor removal. If there is exposure of tendons or bone surfaces, it is necessary to cover them with nearby soft tissues before grafting. Full-thickness skin grafts have the best grafting effect, containing all of the epidermis and dermis, but without attached adipose tissue. After grafting, the shrinkage is small, soft and elastic, resistant to pressure and wear, and the color is similar to normal skin, but it is difficult to grow, and infected wounds are not easy to survive. The donor area cannot heal itself and must be sutured, and the amount of skin taken is limited. It is generally used for defects in the skin of facial organs, such as ectropion of the eyelid, defects of the ala of the nose, etc.; repairing wounds on the palms and soles. Skin grafts containing the subdermal vascular network have higher requirements for the conditions of the recipient wound area. Hemostasis must be perfect, and immobilization must be firm. If the skin graft survives completely, the function is the best. Skin flaps are formed by skin and its attached subcutaneous fat tissue supplied by blood. Skin flaps include any type of skin flap: local flaps/nearby flaps (advancement flaps/gliding flaps, rotation flaps, transposition flaps including Z-plasty), adjacent flaps, distant flaps (direct flaps, direct carrier flaps); axial flaps: general axial flaps, island flaps, musculocutaneous flaps, free flaps (also known as anastomotic vascular flaps), compound tissue transplants with vascular pedicles, tubular skin flaps (skin tubes) and fasciocutaneous flaps. Skin flaps are suitable for repairing wounds with exposed bones, joints, tendons, important organs, large blood vessels, and nerve trunks.

Allograft skin transplantation cannot be completely autologous, and generally shows an immune rejection reaction after about 3 weeks. Therefore, it needs to be combined with autologous particulate skin transplantation, using allograft skin as a carrier to promote wound recovery.

Diabetic Foot Orthopedic Shoes: Three Cases

26

Hailiang Zheng, Lei Gao, and Jiangning Wang

26.1 Case Summary

Foot load reduction is a key part of the treatment of diabetic foot, and it is very important for the prevention of diabetic foot recurrence. Diabetic foot prevention should be a full-cycle management, not only to prevent the disease but also to prevent the patient from relapsing after surgery. Customized orthopedic shoes have a significant effect on patient recurrence, attracting attention in the industry, and there are also related reports abroad. Our department has carried out related work and achieved certain results.

This article selects the design and use of orthopedic shoes after the surgical cure of diabetic foot treated by our department in recent years, which has played a good role in protecting the skin of the patient's foot, in order to inspire others.

26.1.1 Case 1: Study on Orthopedic Shoes for Patients After Midfoot Amputation

Patient, male, 59 years old. Right foot ulcer infection for more than 1 year, infection worsened with part of the skin turning black and dry for more than 3 months.

[Present Illness History] When the patient was first admitted, the toes of the left foot were missing, the skin was cracked and dry, and the skin temperature was slightly lower than that of the left thigh; the arch of the right foot disappeared, it was everted, the lateral side and toenails turned black, the second and the fourth toe on both sides is turning black, as is the belly of the fourth toe. All toes have poor sensation and motor function. The fifth toe is missing, and there is significant swelling on the lateral side of the foot dorsum. On the lateral side of the first metatarsophalangeal joint of the right foot, there is a 3 cm × 3 cm wound, with a small amount of yellow secretion on the surface. It does not bleed when touched, and there is no tenderness around the wound. Large areas of black skin and scabs can be seen on the lateral side of the foot dorsum and the heel, with some of the blackened scabs falling off to reveal the subcutaneous tissue. There is a small amount of exudate from the wound, mild tenderness in the heel, cracked and dry skin on the foot dorsum, and the skin temperature is lower than that of the skin on the lower leg. Peripheral blood circulation is poor (Fig. 26.1). The right ankle joint has poor motor function, but the knee and hip joints are still functional. The diagnosis is "Type 2 diabetic foot, foot soft tissue infection."

[Treatment and Outcome] In November 2015, the patient underwent debridement and Vacuum

H. Zheng · L. Gao · J. Wang (✉)
Department of Orthopedics, Beijing Shijitan Hospital, Capital Medical University, Beijing, China
e-mail: 5799231@qq.com; gaolei3337@bjsjth.cn; wangjn@bjsjth.cn

J. Wang, L. Gao (eds.), *Refractory Wounds*, Experts' Perspectives on Medical Advances,
https://doi.org/10.1007/978-981-96-2067-8_26

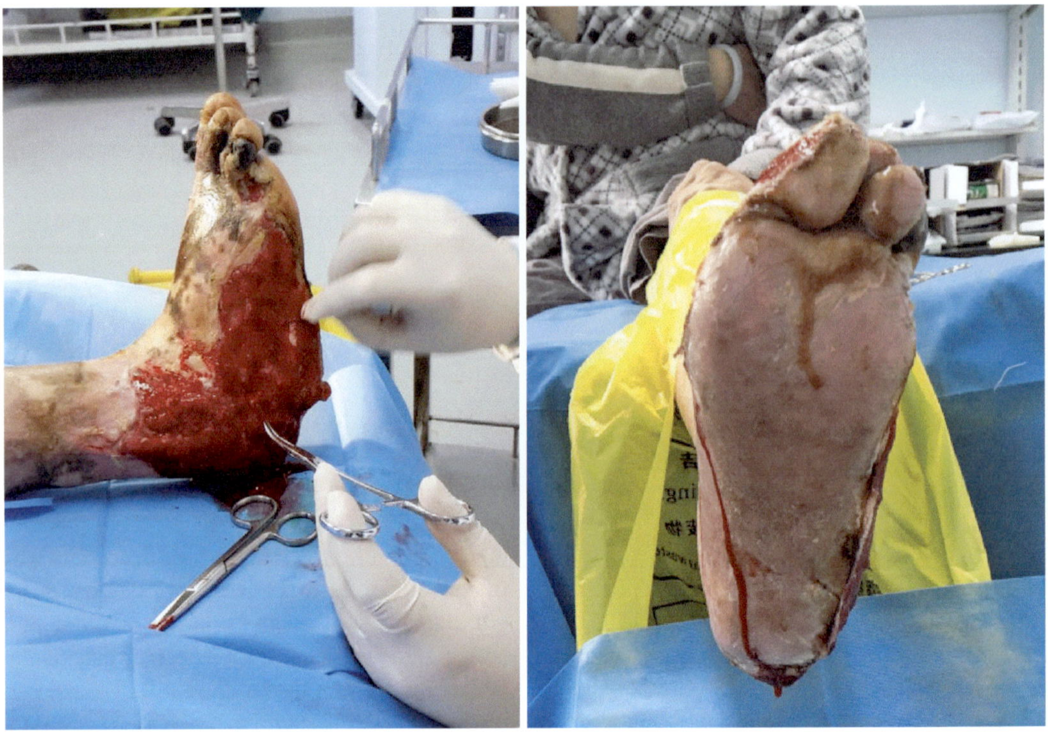

Fig. 26.1 Patient changing dressings upon admission

Sealing Drainage (VSD) suction surgery on the right foot, neurovascular exploration, and artificial skin grafting, and was then discharged.

On January 27, 2016, the patient was readmitted with a diagnosis of "diabetic foot, gangrene of the 2nd to 4th toes of the right foot, soft tissue infection of the foot, and osteomyelitis of the left foot." On the day of admission, the patient underwent amputation of the second to fourth toe bones of the right foot, debridement of the left foot metatarsal, exploration of the blood vessels, nerves, and tendons of both feet, and Vacuum-Assisted Closure (VAC) suction surgery on the right foot, and was then discharged. On February 3, the patient was admitted for the third time and underwent emergency debridement of the left lower limb, incision and decompression, and vascular nerve exploration surgery under local anesthesia and reinforcement. On March 9, the patient underwent debridement of both lower limbs, removal of necrotic bone from the left foot, and vascular nerve exploration surgery under lumbar anesthesia. Skin grafting was performed using skin taken from the right thigh, and VSD suction surgery was performed.

On March 15, the patient underwent removal of VSD from both lower limbs, exploration of the wound on the right foot, debridement of the left lower limb, and vascular nerve tendon exploration surgery under local anesthesia. On March 25, the patient underwent removal of VSD from the right lower limb, debridement of the wounds on both lower limbs, and vascular nerve tendon exploration surgery. On May 20, the patient underwent debridement of both feet, neurovascular tendon exploration, skin grafting from the left foot, and VSD suction surgery on the left foot under lumbar anesthesia. On May 27, the patient underwent debridement of the left foot and VSD removal surgery under local anesthesia. On June 22, the patient underwent debridement of both feet, neurovascular tendon exploration, skin grafting from the left foot, and VSD suction surgery on the left foot under local anesthesia. On July 5, the patient underwent debridement of the left foot, VSD removal, debridement of the right

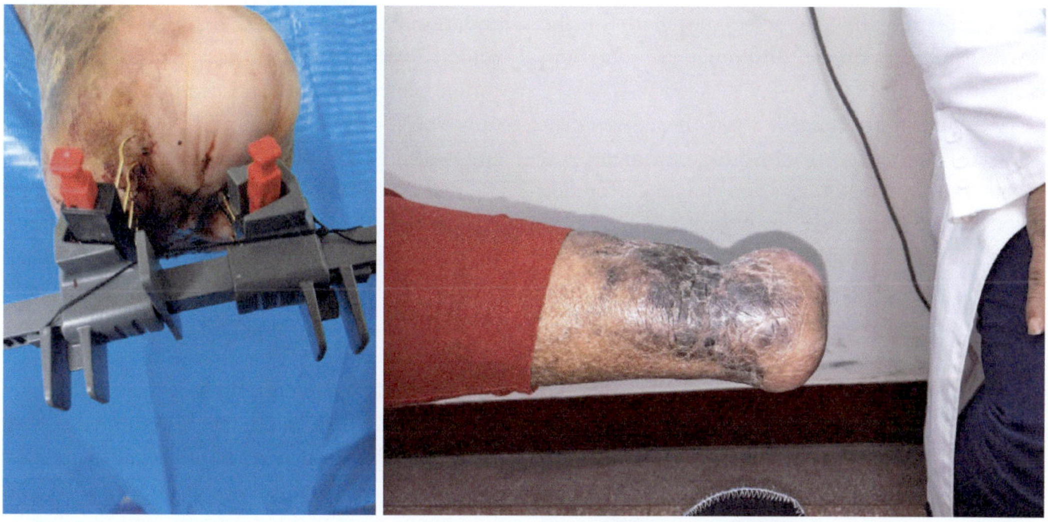

Fig. 26.2 Using a closure device to promote wound healing

foot, and VSD suction surgery under local anesthesia. On July 11, the patient underwent removal of VSD from the right foot and neurovascular tendon exploration surgery under local anesthesia, and was given anti-infection and pain relief treatment after the surgery.

On July 5, 2017, the patient underwent debridement of necrotic tissue from the left residual foot under nerve block anesthesia + Vascular nerve tendon exploration surgery + Platelet-rich fibrin membrane repair surgery + VSD suction surgery, postoperative anti-infection, and swelling treatment. On July 14, under local anesthesia, necrotic tissue debridement of the left foot + VSD removal + vascular tendon exploration surgery were performed.

On March 28, 2018, to further promote wound healing, necrotic tissue debridement of the left foot + vascular nerve tendon exploration surgery + closure device installation surgery were performed under local anesthesia. Postoperative anti-infection treatment and wound dressing changes were given. On April 2, due to the long fixation time of the closure device and reduced wound tension, necrotic tissue debridement of the left foot + vascular nerve tendon exploration surgery + closure device removal surgery was performed under local anesthesia. During the surgery, a skin traction closure device was used to close the wound (Fig. 26.2). A transitional ankle orthosis was made during the hospital stay for walking (Fig. 26.3). Because the patient's talus had osteomyelitis and was surgically removed, the calcaneus was directly connected to the tibia

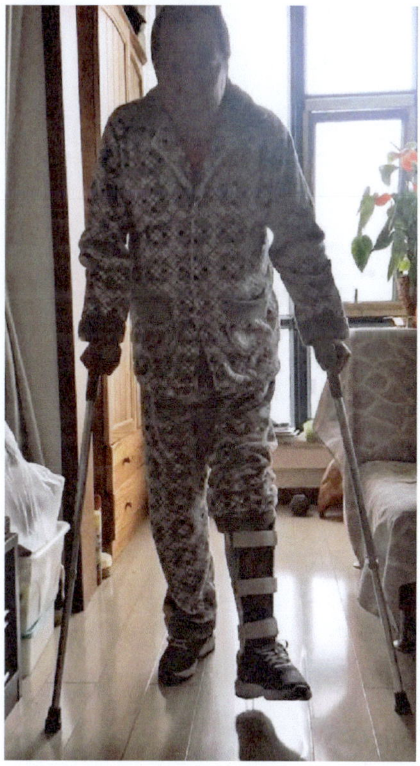

Fig. 26.3 Wearing a therapeutic foot brace

and fibula, resulting in unequal length of the lower limbs, with a difference of 2.6 cm (Fig. 26.4).

After the injury healed, a prosthesis was customized (Fig. 26.5). Because the calcaneus was retained, although there was a height difference between the two legs, it was not enough to accommodate the footplate of the prosthesis. The compromise solution adopted was: the accommodation chamber of the prosthesis was directly welded to the footplate, and the elastic energy storage plate at the heel position was removed. A rubber prosthetic foot was made for shoe wearing and walking. Walking requires crutch support. The patient complained that wearing the prosthesis was time-consuming and laborious, walking was laborious, and it was easy to smell when sweating in hot weather. He asked us if we could solve it with orthopedic shoes.

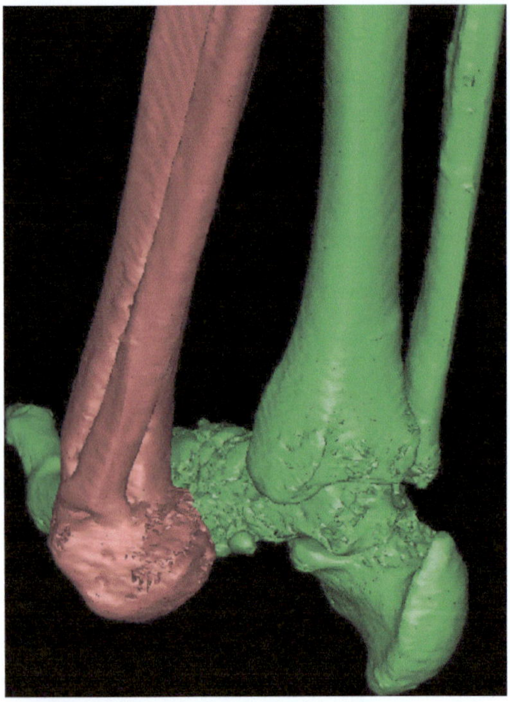

Fig. 26.4 Three-dimensional image of the patient's foot skeleton (without talus)

[Orthotic Design] A CT scan of the patient's foot was performed and a three-dimensional (3D) reconstruction was made, resulting in two design proposals. Proposal one: no filling in the shoe toe. The left foot's residual limb is designed as a cup-shaped shoe pad for support, and the shoe is designed as a horseshoe shape (Fig. 26.6). Proposal two: filling in the shoe toe. A high-top orthotic shoe is custom-made using the ankle orthosis worn by the patient, with a custom-fit soft pressure-relieving shoe pad for the right foot (Fig. 26.7).

[Wearing Effect] The patient wore shoes from both proposals (Fig. 26.8). The design of the horseshoe-shaped shoe made the patient feel difficult to find balance, while the orthotic shoe was better for walking and balance. However, the patient felt pressure pain at the residual limb. After raising the cup-shaped orthotic shoe pad, the patient felt good when the residual limb did not touch the sole of the foot. The patient could walk without crutches when wearing the shoe pad customized by my team with the prosthesis, which was the best effect.

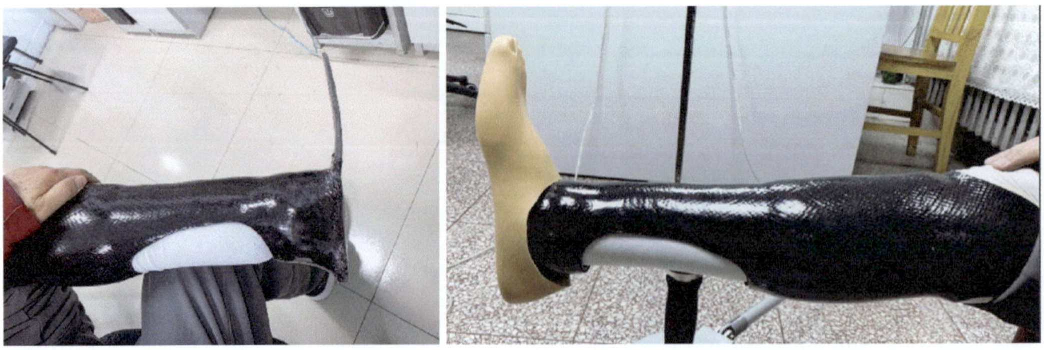

Fig. 26.5 Customized and fitted prosthesis

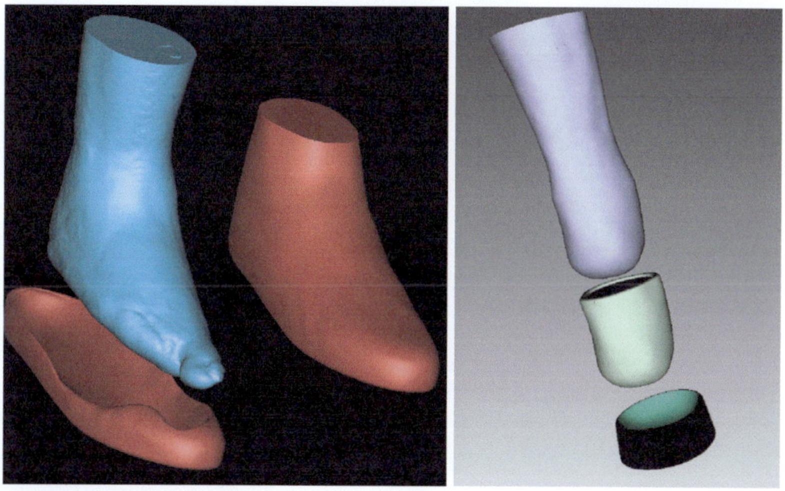

Fig. 26.6 Exploded view of the shoe toe without filling, the left foot is mirrored to the right foot and filled in the shoe toe

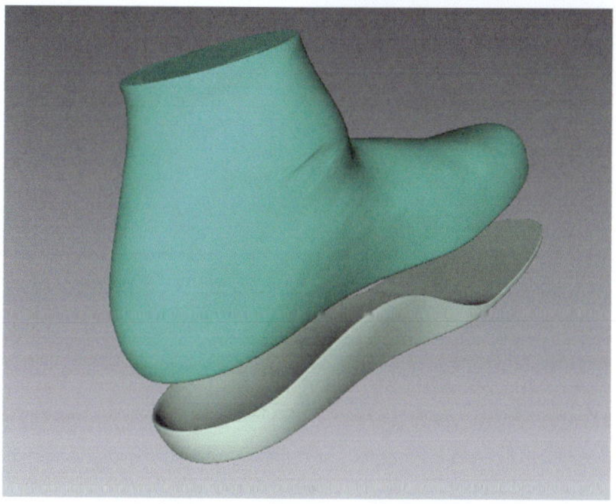

Fig. 26.7 Exploded view of the shoe toe with filling

26.1.2 Case 2: Design of Orthotic Shoes for Patients After Calcaneal Pad Removal Surgery

The patient is a male and 70 years old.

[Present Illness History] The patient developed 2 skin tears on the right heel 2 months ago. The patient had a skin crack on the foot, which was not treated. A week later, chills and high fever appeared. The patient self-administered fluid therapy. After the symptoms eased, the wound secretion increased, and the necrotic area around the wound enlarged. The patient sought treatment at the local hospital's endocrinology department, where they received symptomatic treatments such as anti-infection, circulation improvement, and dressing changes. However, the symptoms did not improve. The patient was then transferred to the vascular intervention department for treatment, including dressing changes, circulation improvement, debridement, VSD suction, and lower limb angiography balloon dilation. The treatment was not satisfactory, and the necrotic area of the wound enlarged. Three days ago, the purulent secretion from the wound increased. Today, the patient came to our hospital for further treatment. The outpatient department admitted the patient with "diabetic foot gangrene." Since the onset of the disease, the patient's diet, sleep, and bowel movements have been normal, but the weight has decreased by 5 kg.

[Diagnosis] Type 2 diabetic foot gangrene (right), type 2 diabetic peripheral vascular disease, lower extremity atherosclerotic occlusive disease, type 2 diabetic peripheral neuropathy, type 2 diabetic retinopathy, grade 3 hypertension (extremely high risk), coronary atherosclerotic heart disease, post-coronary stent implantation status, heart function grade II (NYHA classification), post-cholecystectomy.

[Treatment course] After the patient was admitted to the hospital, all examinations were completed. On March 14, 2017, the patient underwent right foot debridement + neurovascular tendon exploration + fat grafting + skin closure under nerve block anesthesia. On March 27, the patient underwent right foot necrotic tissue removal + neurovascular tendon explora-

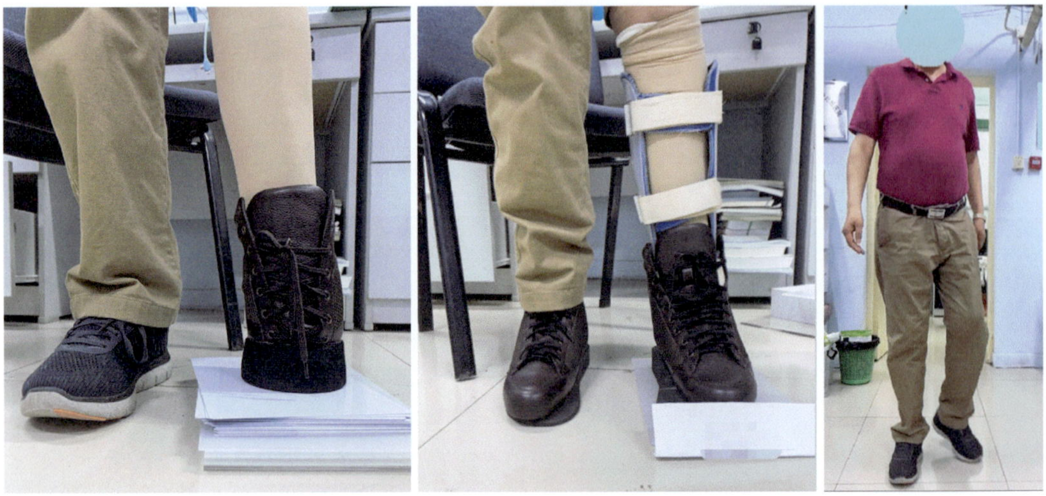

Fig. 26.8 Actual situation when worn

tion + skin closure removal under spinal anesthesia. On April 6, the patient underwent right foot necrotic tissue removal + neurovascular tendon exploration under spinal anesthesia. On April 13, the patient underwent right foot necrotic tissue removal + skin grafting + VSD suction + neurovascular tendon exploration under nerve block anesthesia. After the operation, symptomatic treatments such as anti-infection, swelling reduction, and pain relief were given, and the dressing was changed regularly.

[Orthotic design] After treatment, the patient's foot healed with no exudate (Fig. 26.9). However, because the heel healed through skin grafting and the patient could not walk, the patient could not get out of bed for a long time, and we began to consider making orthopedic shoes. Through 3D modeling, we obtained Fig. 26.10. Through reverse engineering, we designed the shoe last and orthotic insole (Fig. 26.11), and reasonably dispersed the pressure on multiple parts of the patient's heel in the design.

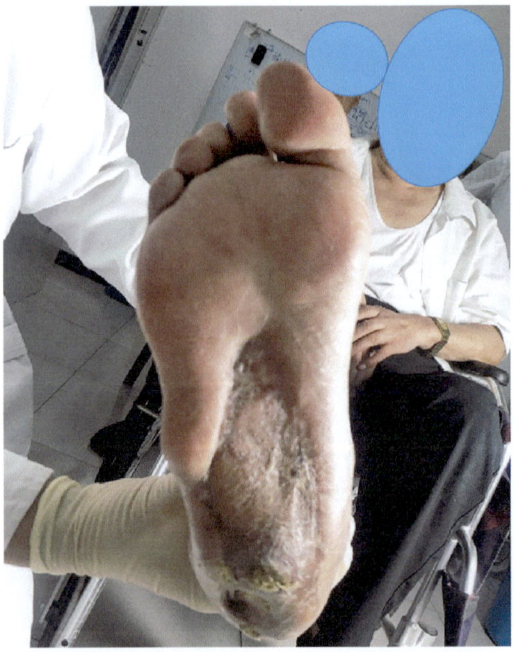

Fig. 26.9 The condition of the patient's foot at the end of treatment

[Wearing effect] The patient can walk with the help of crutches in the early stage of wearing shoes (Fig. 26.12). One month later, the patient can walk in the park on his own.

26.1.3 Case 3: Design of Orthopedic Shoes for Patients with Severe Foot Infections and Diabetic Foot

[Present Illness History] The patient had a high fever for 3 days without any cause 40 days ago. The bottom of the first metatarsal bone of the left foot was red and swollen. A 0.5-cm piece of glass was found to have pierced the skin. Two days after it was removed, purulent exudate appeared from the wound, the foot was significantly swollen, the skin turned black, and the skin temperature was high. After simple debridement at the local county hospital, the patient was transferred to a tertiary hospital for orthopedic treatment. The orthopedic department performed two debridement surgeries for infection after left foot trauma + VSD suction surgery. After the surgery,

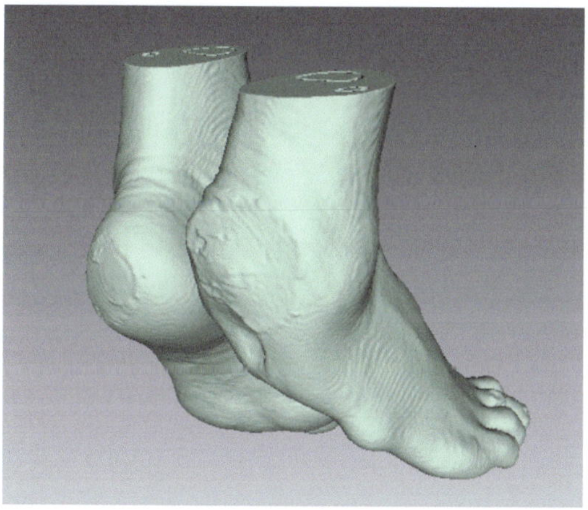

Fig. 26.10 Establishment of the patient's foot biological entity model

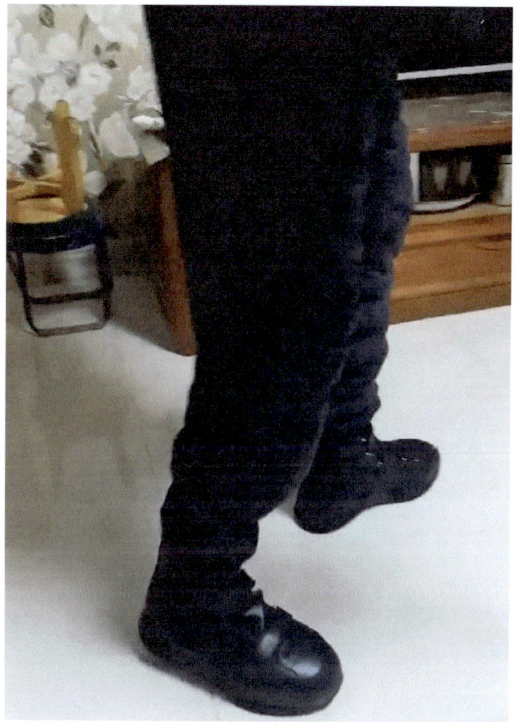

Fig. 26.12 Actual effect of the patient wearing orthopedic shoes

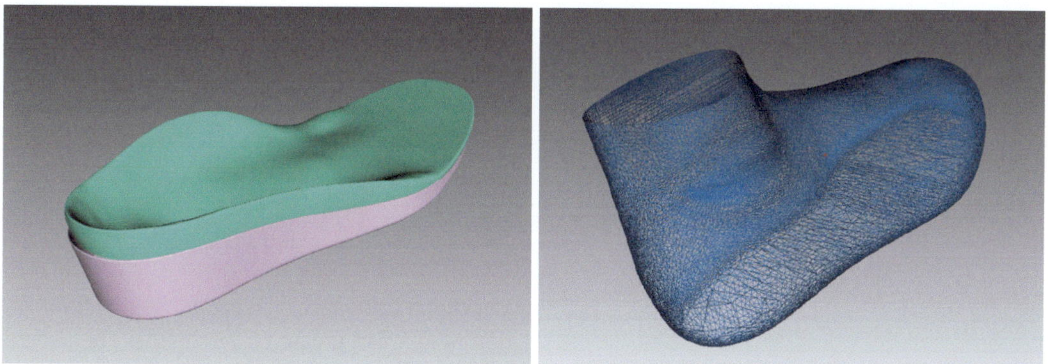

Fig. 26.11 Design of orthopedic insoles and shoe lasts

VSD and gentamicin were continuously irrigated and drained, and anti-infection and symptomatic treatment were given. Because skin grafting was needed, the patient was transferred to the plastic surgery department. On November 10, 2015, the patient underwent another debridement + VSD suction surgery for the left foot wound. After the surgery, anti-infection treatment was given, but the wound infection worsened, expanded to the heel, and then high fever occurred. The VSD was removed and symptomatic treatment was given. On November 27, the patient underwent another debridement + VSD treatment for the left foot wound, but the effect was still not good, the wound infection worsened, there was a lot of necrotic tissue in the wound, and the wound gradually enlarged. In order to seek further treatment, the patient came to our hospital for treatment. Our department admitted the patient as an emergency case with "left foot soft tissue infection" (Fig. 26.13). Before admission, the patient had a high fever, but no nausea or vomiting.

[Treatment and Outcome] After admission, all necessary examinations were actively completed.

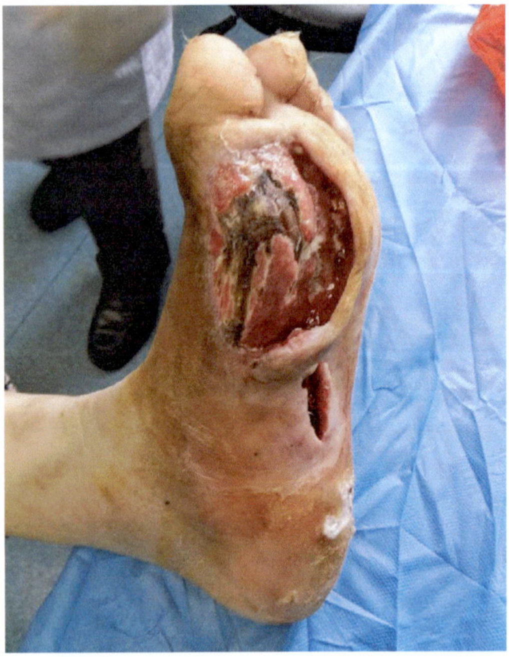

Fig. 26.13 Patient's foot at the time of hospital admission

On December 2, emergency spinal anesthesia was performed for incision and drainage of the infected tissue in the left foot. On December 18, spinal anesthesia was performed to remove necrotic tissue from the left foot and install a closure device. On December 30, spinal anesthesia was performed to remove necrotic tissue from the left foot and install a skin expander. On January 18, 2016, spinal anesthesia was performed for debridement and flap transfer of the left foot + left thigh. Skin grafting + Left foot grafting. The patient recovered well after surgery, symptomatic anti-infection, swelling reduction, and pain relief treatments were given. The patient was hospitalized for 51 days.

At discharge, the patient's mental state and sleep were good, appetite was normal, bowel movements were normal, and there were no discomfort complaints. Physical examination: body temperature 36.1 °C, pulse 78 times/min, respiration 18 times/min, blood pressure 126/83 mmHg. The dressing on the patient's left foot wound was dry, the gauze was well wrapped, the lower leg was slightly swollen, the skin color was normal, the ankle and knee joint movements were not obviously abnormal, the dressing change revealed that the wound on the bottom of the left foot was well fixed, the transplanted flap had good blood circulation, the wound was well sutured, the rest of the wound was dry with a small amount of exudate and a small amount of granulation. Ankle joint movement was normal, toe movement was poor, blood circulation was good, and the skin sensation of the affected limb was better than before (Fig. 26.14).

[Orthotic Design] After the MDT treatment in our department, the patient's affected foot healed well. The patient underwent foot pressure testing and foot contour mapping (Fig. 26.15), showing that the first metatarsal head was the area with greater pressure, the foot arch was high, and the foot was pronated. The main work of the orthotic shoe for this patient is to relieve pressure on the first metatarsal head.

After a full scan of the patient, a 3D visualization model was created (Fig. 26.16). The patient had no obvious arterial sclerosis, no bone hyperplasia or osteoporosis in the foot, and the tube

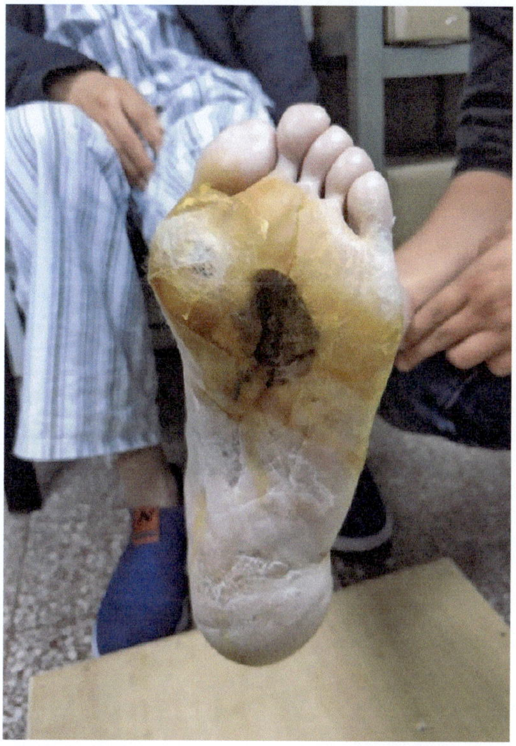

Fig. 26.14 Patient's foot at the time of consultation

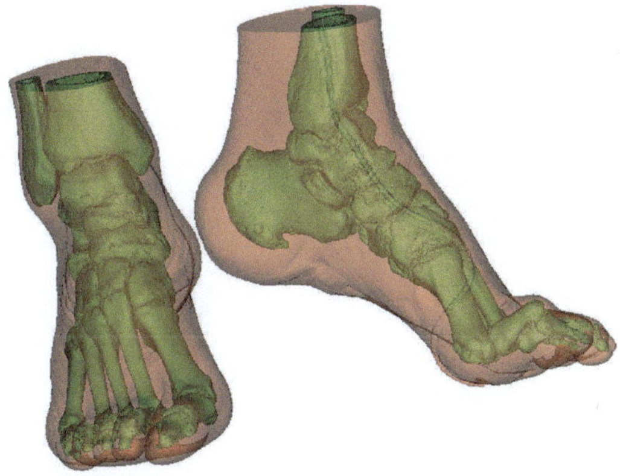

Fig. 26.16 Patient's foot 3D modeling

Fig. 26.15 Foot examination. (**a**) Plantar pressure imprint, (**b**) Contour line map

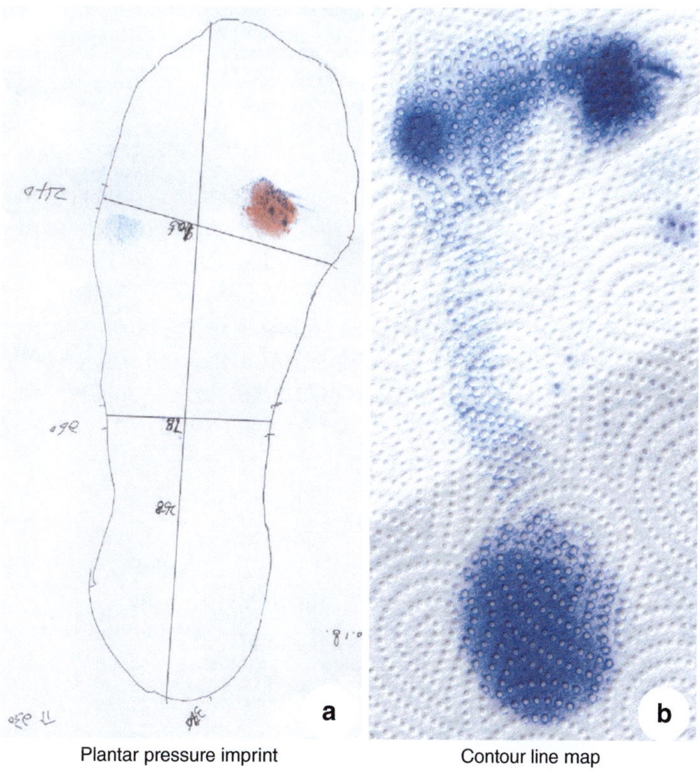

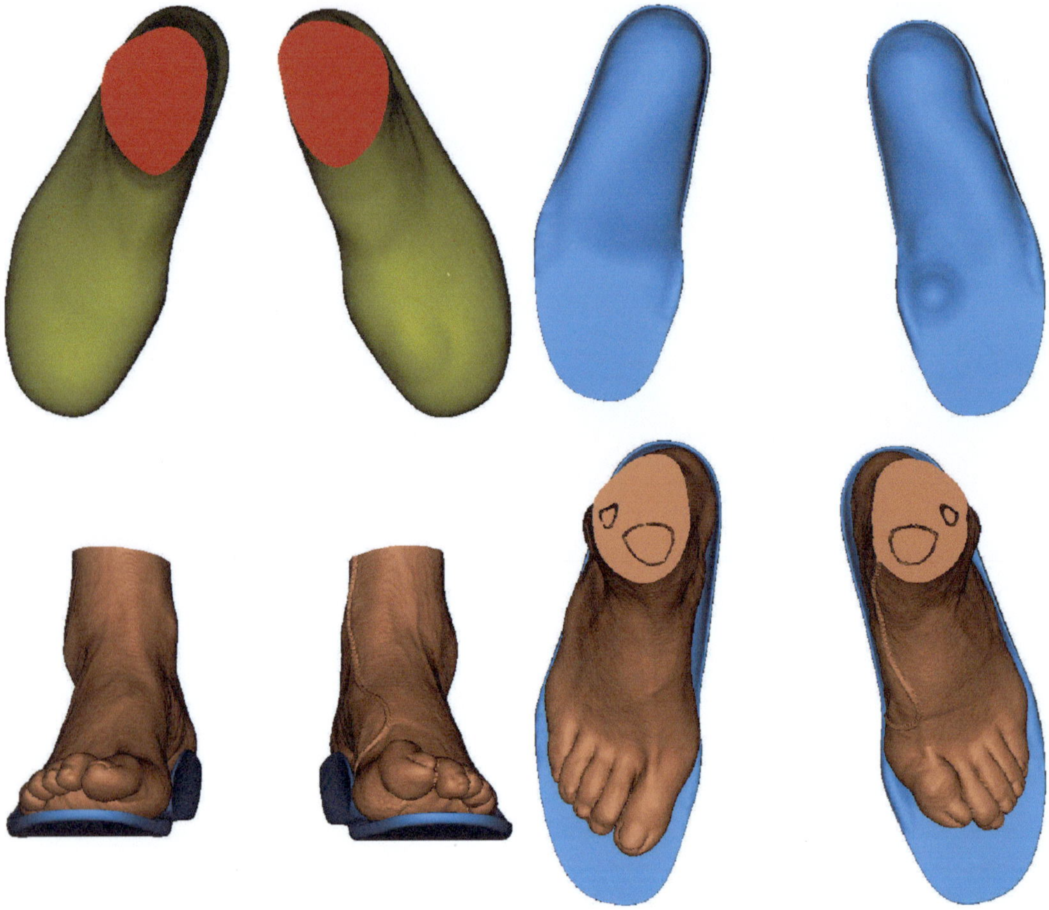

Fig. 26.17 Orthopedic shoe design

shown in the figure is a pressure perfusion catheter.

The design of the patient's orthopedic shoes and insoles can be seen in Fig. 26.17, the upper left part is the shoe last designed according to the patient's foot 3D model, and the right part is the insole and the patient's foot 3D visualization. In addition, from Fig. 26.17, it can be seen that the precisely designed orthopedic insole fits well with the patient's foot.

[Wearing effect] The patient's orthopedic shoes and actual wearing effect are shown in Fig. 26.18.

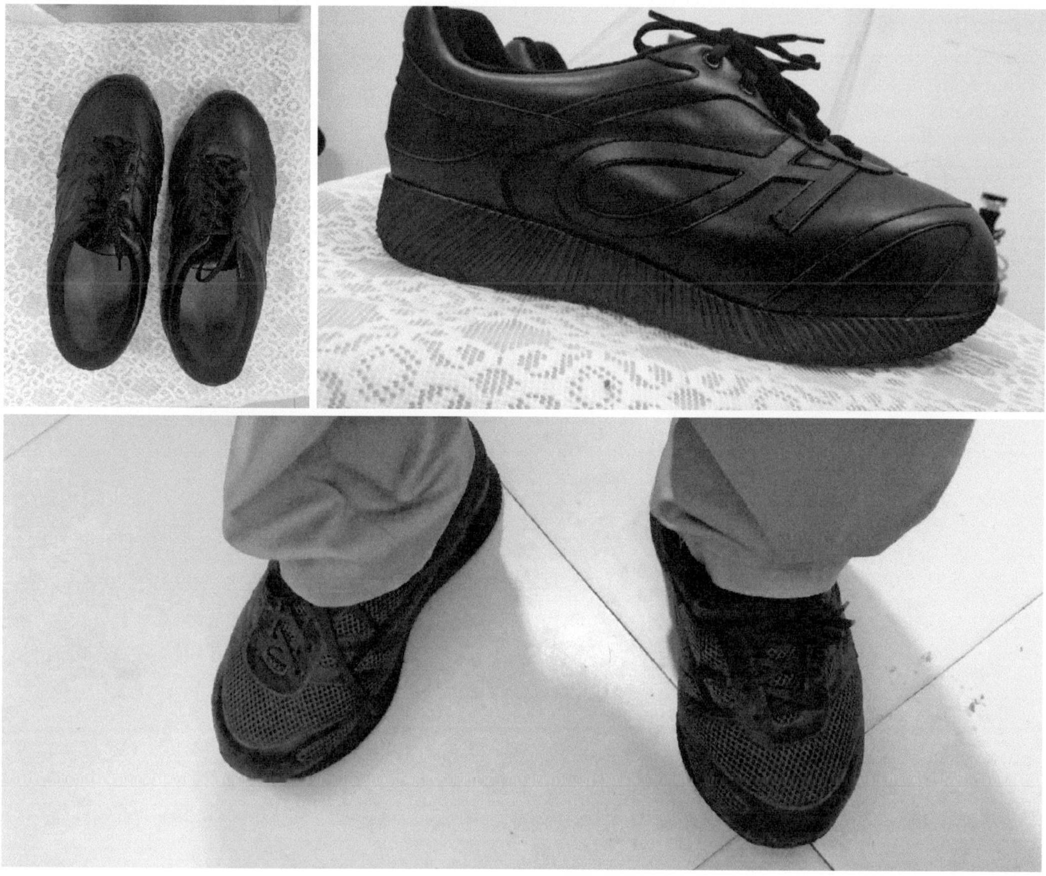

Fig. 26.18 Patient's actual wearing effect

26.2 Case Analysis

The limb preservation surgery plan for Case 1 allows the patient to retain more bones and muscle tissue, making the patient more satisfied with the surgery results. However, this plan poses a great challenge to the design of prosthetics and orthopedic shoes, requiring orthotists to be creative, fully utilize the biomechanical characteristics of the residual limb, and design customized orthopedic footwear to meet the patient's needs.

Case 2 is based on the patient's medical history and skeletal biomechanical characteristics to reasonably design orthopedic footwear, which can realize the patient's desire to walk on the ground and improve the quality of life.

Case 3 is a case where the thigh skin is used as a donor to perform skin grafting on the ulcer of the first metatarsophalangeal joint, promoting wound healing. After the success of the surgery, it is necessary to strengthen the decompression and protection of the wound, prevent skin keratinization, and avoid increasing the risk of the patient's ulcer recurrence.

Bibliography

1. Jiangning W, Lei G. New progress in the treatment of chronic wounds of diabetic foot. Chin J Repair Reconstr Surg. 2018;32(07):832–7.
2. Pendsey S. Management of modern diabetic foot. Translated by Wang Jiangning. Beijing: People's Medical Publishing House; 2017. p. 161–70.
3. Armstrong DG, Boulton AJM, Bus SA. Diabetic foot ulcers and their recurrence. N Engl J Med. 2017;376(24):2367–75.
4. Zheng Hailiang. Orthotic device functional reconstruction 1 case. Wang Jiangning, Gao Lei, Tiangui C, et al. Professor Wang Jiangning's team's comprehensive diagnosis and treatment of diabetic foot cases. Beijing: Science and Technology Literature Publishing House, 2018.
5. Lei G, Shuo W, Lei W, et al. Application of skin traction closure device in the repair of diabetic foot wounds. Chin J Repair Reconstr Surg. 2018;32(05):591–5.

Appendix A: The Cellular Mechanisms of Diabetic Foot and Diabetic Cutaneous Syndrome and the Potential of Stem Cell Regenerative Therapy

Michael Roseamann, Jiangning Wang, and Hans-Günther Machens

Author Introduction

(Germany) Michael Rosemann, Deputy Director of the Institute of Radiation Biology, Helmholtz Center for Health and Environmental Research, Munich, Germany, Project Group Leader; Associate Professor, Technical University of Munich, Mentor (Medical School Project, Doctoral Program in Medical Life Science and Technology).

Wang Jiangning, Head of Orthopedics, Chief Physician, Professor, Doctoral Supervisor at Beijing Shijitan Hospital, Capital Medical University. An internationally renowned orthopedic expert, he enjoys special government allowances from the State Council.

(Germany) Hans-Günther Machens, Director of Plastic Surgery and Hand Surgery, Professor of Plastic Surgery, Isar Right Bank Hospital, Technical University of Munich (Lifetime Professor).

Pathophysiology of Diabetic Foot Ulceration and Diabetic Cutaneous Syndrome

Diabetic foot ulcerations (ICD-11 code BD54) at its later stage affects a variety of tissues and cells, making it difficult to project the causality of it back to a single cellular origin. For a future targeted therapy aiming to stop the progression and revert the pathogenesis of diabetic foot ulcers, however, identification of the target cells that are the most vulnerable during the pathogenic process and are the starting point of this progressive condition is essential.

Because the early stage of diabetic foot ulcers resembles the diabetic skin lesions (loss of dermal thickness, pink wound bed, dermopathy without slough), a common etiology can be expected for both. Diabetic cutaneous syndrome and diabetic skin lesions (ICD-11 code EB90.0), however, most frequently affects the shin, i.e., the skin that overlays the tibia. In contrast to diabetic foot ulcers, this part of the lower leg is not prone to unrecognized micro-injuries as are suspected to occur at the bottom of feet by localized foreign bodies in shoes. Later stages of diabetic foot ulcers share many features with pressure ulcers (bed sores, ICD-11 code EH90), in which external micro-injuries by foreign bodies can be excluded, but persistent disturbances of the blood circulation in the connective tissue due to repeated or enduring external pressure are likely involved. In the later condition, a localized loss of sensation might go in parallel with the progression of the skin ulceration, although both are not necessarily causally linked. It is more likely that they develop independently from each other, but share a common causation (Fig. A.1).

Peripheral polyneuropathy (ICD-11 code 8C03.0) frequently occurs together with diabetic foot ulcers, and loss of sensation is often reported by the patient before the first symptoms of skin

M. Roseamann · H.-G. Machens (✉)
Plastic Surgery and Hand Surgery, Technical University of Munich, Munich, Germany
e-mail: Hans-Guenther.Machens@mri.tum.de

J. Wang
Department of Orthopedics, Beijing Shijitan Hospital, Capital Medical University, Beijing, China
e-mail: wangjn@bjsjth.cn

J. Wang, L. Gao (eds.), *Refractory Wounds*, Experts' Perspectives on Medical Advances,
https://doi.org/10.1007/978-981-96-2067-8

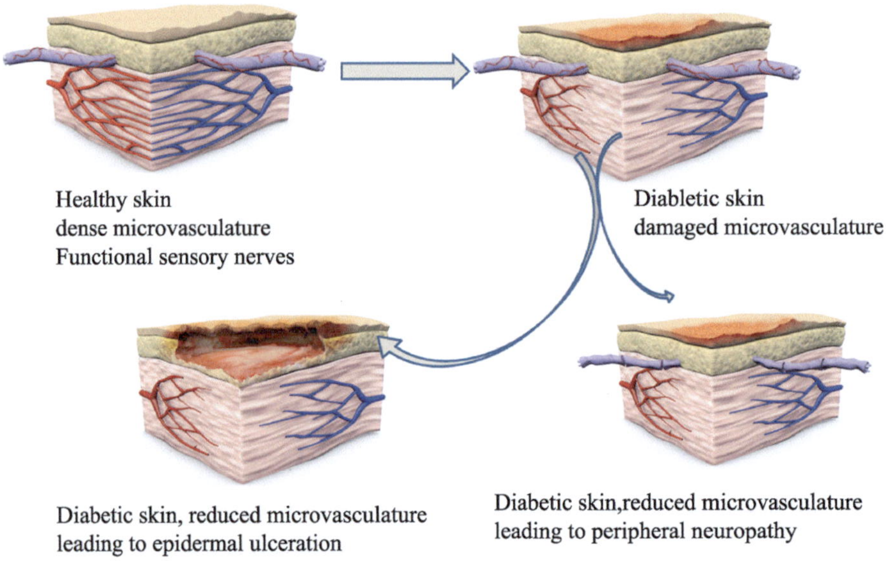

Fig. A.1 Anatomical structure damaged in T2D cutaneous syndrome

lesions are diagnosed. Although it is tempting from this temporal sequence, also a causal relationship, there are several reasons to challenge this. Among the large number of polyneuropathies that can be caused by various exogenous, heritable or acquired factors, only diabetic polyneuropathy has been linked to skin ulcerations or diabetic foot. The loss of mechanical sensation is typical for a variety of cutaneous sensory disorder, such as inflammatory polyneuropathy, toxic neuropathies (for instance Beriberi), sensory loss after spinal cord injury, or conferred by inherited conditions, but a link to skin ulceration or chronic wound healing complications has only been reported in diabetic patients. It is therefore more reasonable to consider diabetic polyneuropathy as a condition that is not essential for the pathogenesis of diabetic foot ulcers, but most likely depends on the same underlying physiological disturbance. Considering that neurons, both sensory as well as motor neurons, are highly energy dependent, they will be immediately affected in their function by a long-lasting depletion of nutrients and oxygen, as could result from a microvascular impairment. System microvascular impairment has a manifestation in several tissues of diabetic patients, such as the kidney, the heart, and the eye. The peripheral circulatory complications in type 2 diabetes (ICD-10 code E11.5) are perhaps the most prevalent long term health impairments resulting from hyperglycemia. In the affected organs, they can cause kidney failure, stroke, ischemic infarct, macular edema (ICD-11 code 9B71.02), and other diabetic retinopathies (ICD-11 code 9B71.0).

Because blood circulation is essential not only for the supply of oxygen and nutrients, but equally important for the distribution of various immune cells that fight wound infection, legs and feet affected by vasculopathies can be affected by chronic wound healing complications. The lower part of the extremities are more affected by diabetic cutaneous syndrome and wound healing complications that lead to diabetic foot ulceration, because the physiologic situation of the blood circulation unavoidably causes a higher (hydrostatic) blood pressure in the legs and feet. It is known that in healthy individuals, the systolic blood pressure at the ankle is between 10% and 50% higher than the blood pressure measured at the arm arteries (ABPI, ankle-to-brachial blood pressure index).

This higher arterial blood pressure is under healthy conditions compensated by an increased strength or thickness of the smooth muscle cells (SMCs) that mechanically stabilize the arteries.

In diabetic patients, however, SMCs frequently show dystrophic calcification, causing media sclerosis also called arteriosclerosis. When SMCs lose their elasticity and durability, they can no longer stabilize the endothelial cells of the arteries, leading to a leakage of blood products from these vessels into the skin. The damaged arteries which can no longer resist the blood pressure degenerate to avoid further hemorrhage.

Physiology of Wound Healing and the Role of Mesenchymal Stem Cells

SMCs which support the large arteries and pericytes which surround the arterioles and sinusoids are both derived from mesenchymal stem cells (MSCs).

MSCs are multipotent, tissue resident, adult stem cells which have a life-long capacity to regenerate connective tissue, bone marrow stroma, bone, and adipose tissue. They are most frequently found in highly vascularized tissue. MSCs are also an important factor during normal, scare-free wound healing (Fig. A.2).

At the early (inflammatory) phase of wound closure, MSCs secret immunomodulatory cytokines, which regulate the activity of macrophages. With the onset of the resorptive and the regenerative, MSCs may give rise to the fibroblasts which deposit contractive collagen which can reduce the wound area. In the remodeling phase, MSCs are again crucial to provide SMCs and pericytes to support the newly formed blood vessels.

And there are even some indications that MSCs are also capable to differentiate into Schwann-cells, i.e., those cells which produce the myelin sheet around peripheral neurons. Schwann cells are essential for neuronal regeneration and provide a myelin tube that directs axonal regrowth. MSCs also secrete exosomes which promote Schwann-cell mediated neuronal regeneration.

Impaired Function of MSCs Linked to Diabetic Wound Complications

Mesenchymal stem cells represent a small number of cells in connective tissue, which maintain a regenerative potential throughout life of an organism. They have a self-renewing potential, meaning that by asymmetric cell division at least one of the daughter cells retains the stem cell potential. By certain cellular defense systems (macro-autophagy, DNA repair, expression of detoxifying enzymes, and efflux pumps) they also have a dedicated pro-survival capacity against acute forms of cellular stress. After chronic forms of cellular stress, however, MSCs

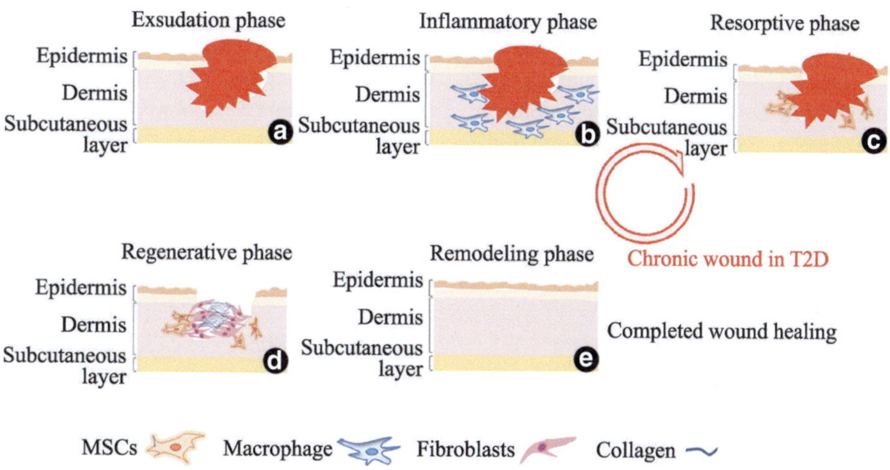

Fig. A.2 Phase of successful wound-healing and its defect in T2D cutaneous syndrome

gradually lose their stem cell capacity. We have reported that ionizing radiation can cause MSCs to spontaneously differentiate into adipocytes, and that MSCs derived from in utero low-dose irradiated mice have a higher tendency to become senescent. Proliferating stress in vitro causes a reduced capacity to recognize and repair endogenous and radiation-induced or reactive oxygen species (ROS)-induced DNA damages. MSCs are also vulnerable to oxidative stress, which causes an increase in senescence and DNA double strand breaks. Redox imbalance is a common feature affecting many cells in diabetic patients. This is related to systemic inflammation, oxidative stress, and accelerated cellular aging.

Apart from persistent oxidative stress in diabetic MSCs, the generation of advanced glycation end products (AGE) is a well-known stressor during hyperglycemia. AGE affect intra- and extracellular proteins by adding glycogen residues, thereby causing miss-folding or aggregation of proteins. It has been shown that pericytes, i.e., MSC-derived cells which are in close proximity to the vascular endothelium of small arteries, are severely damaged by AGEs, which cause a hyperosmotic intracellular pressure and can lead to cellular burst.

Equally toxic to MSCs are carbonylated proteins or lipids. Carbonylation occurs to biomolecules by the attack of reactive oxygen species. Since carbonylated proteins and lipids become dysfunctional, they can accumulate in the affected cells. Carbonylated phospholipids cause membrane dysfunction, which can affect not only the plasma-membrane, but also the ER and the mitochondrial membrane. Healthy cells induce macro-autophagy, which can catabolize carbonylated lipids and utilize the fatty acids for ATP production.

Cell-Based Therapy for Wound Healing Complications

Wound healing complications not only appear in diabetic foot or diabetic cutaneous syndrome, but are also a challenge after mechanical trauma affecting larger areas of the body surface, after thermal or after radiation burns or after surgery for malignant tumors. Adjuvant administration of autologous MSCs (together with wound dressings using organic matrices) have been demonstrated to be beneficial for faster, more complete, and scar-free wound healing.

Interestingly, an inherited skin disorder (epidermolysis bullosa, ICD-11 code EC32), which is characterized by a severe disorder of collagen VII in the epidermal basement membrane, can be successfully treated by topical administration of bone marrow derived stromal cells, which are essentially identical to MSCs. This indicates that in non-systemic, but localized skin or wound healing disorders, autologous or allogenic (in case of germline disorders) MSC therapy can have a clinical benefit.

In type 2 diabetes, however, prolonged hyperglycemia has potentially damaged MSCs anywhere in the body. Autologous engraftment to the site of skin ulceration is therefore only of limited efficiency. In a diabetic mouse model of wound healing, it has been shown that transplantation of MSCs from a diabetic donor to a diabetic recipient has little benefit, whereas MSCs derived from a healthy mouse significantly improved wound healing in a hyperglycemic mouse.

In T2D patients with skin ulcerations or diabetic foot, current treatments include anabolic steroids, negative pressure wound therapy, phototherapy, support surfaces, reconstructive surgery, ultrasound, topical phenytoin, and pressure relieving devices. There is little or no evidence to support or refute the benefits of most of these treatments compared to each other and placebo. Therapies using biologicals (such as human cells, stem cells, or growth factors) have a high potential to alleviate the disease close to its origin.

Autophagy

The role of autophagy in MSCs during normal and impaired wound healing has already been investigated by others and the involvement of the mTOR pathway and HIF-1α signaling has been found to be impaired in diabetic MSCs. We have in our study also found evidence for a significant reduction of diabetic MSCs to perform autophagy after ROS stress. In MSCs from diabetic donors, autophagy could either not be induced, or was persistently alleviated. MSCs from healthy donors, in contrast, responded to radiation-induced oxidative stress with an upregulation of autophagy (Fig. A.3).

The lack of autophagy in diabetic MSCs was also associated with an increased deposition of lipid droplets in their cytoplasm, an indicator of accumulating lipid carbonylation (Fig. A.4).

We therefore hypothesized that for a successful adjuvant MSC therapy in diabetic wounds or diabetic foot disease, the autophagy defect was to be repaired, either using modern molecular methods, pro-autophagic drugs, or caloric restriction (starvation).

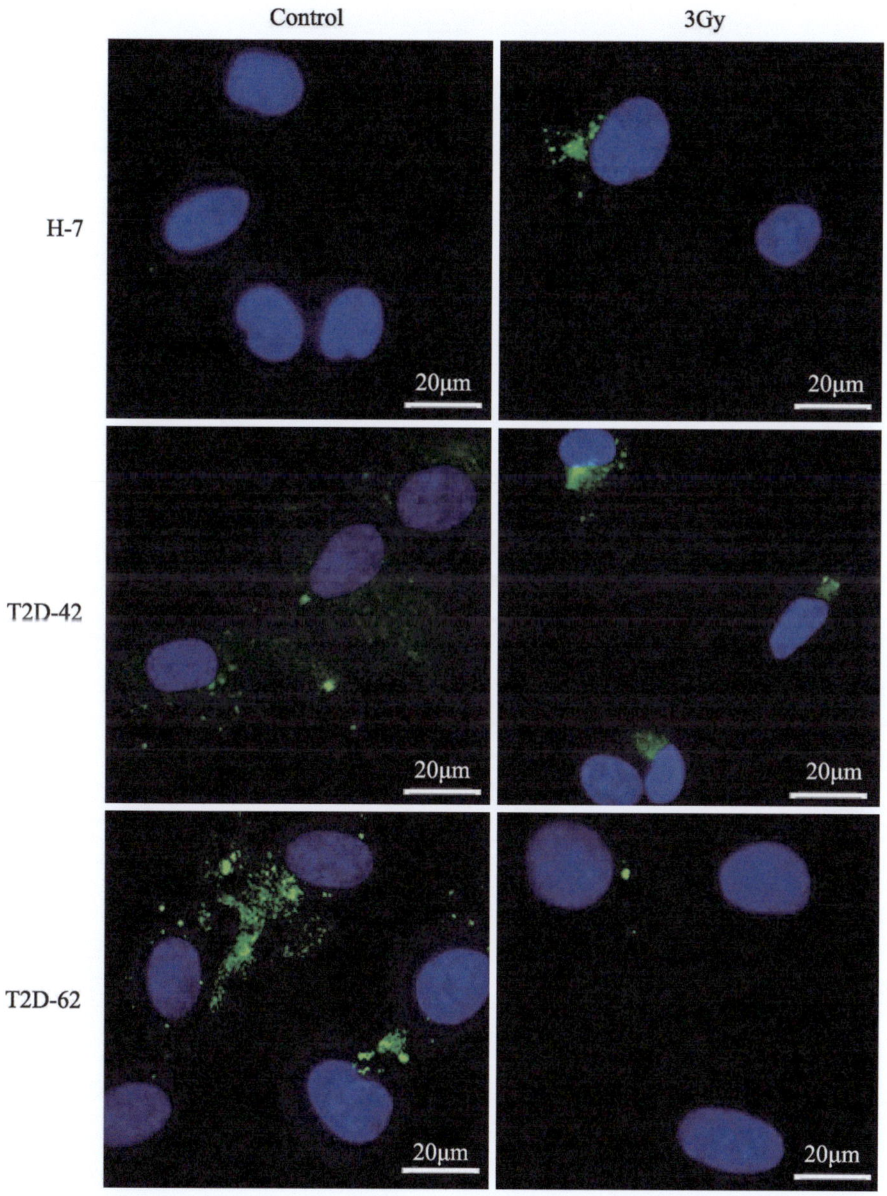

Fig. A.3 Representative immunofluorescence of LC3B in human bone marrow mesenchymal stem cells after exposure to 3 Gy radiation. Blue spots are Hoechst 33342 DNA staining, green spots are LC3B staining. H-7 represents mesenchymal stem cells from healthy donors. T2D-42 and T2D-62 represent mesenchymal stem cells donated by patients with type 2 diabetes. Cells with green spots represent autophagosomes. Fluorescence microscopy observes LC3B spots in cells

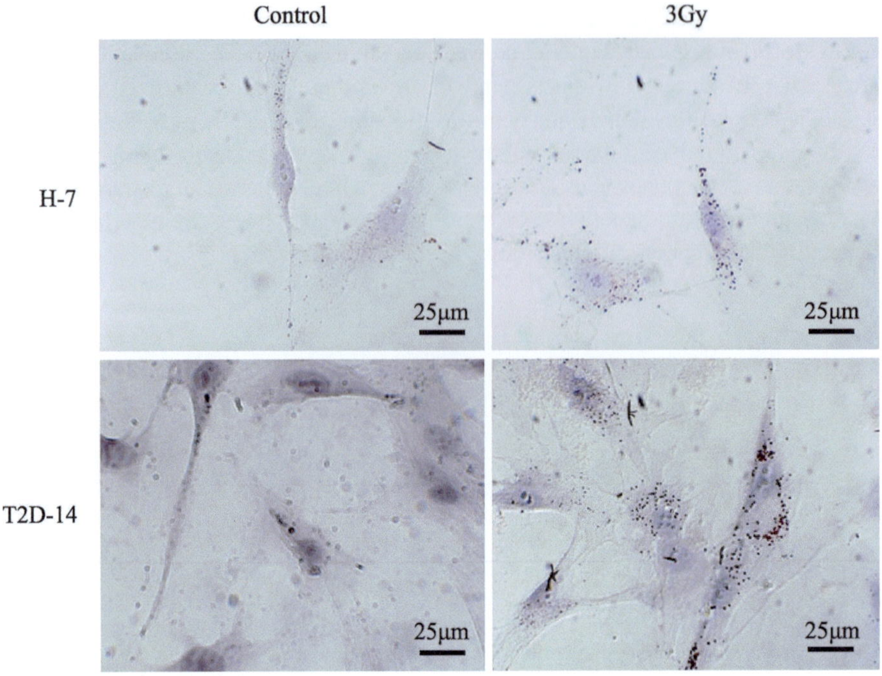

Fig. A.4 Representative image of Oil Red staining of human bone marrow mesenchymal stem cells after 3 Gy radiation. Oil Red staining shows significant lipid droplets on human bone marrow mesenchymal stem cells, displaying lipid droplets of different sizes. Hematoxylin stains the cell nucleus blue. H-7 is a healthy donor, T2D-14 is a type 2 diabetes donor

Appendix B: Clinical Guidelines for the Treatment of Diabetic Foot Wounds with Extracorporeal Circulation Perfusion Free Flap

Lei Gao and Jiangning Wang

Currently, the global prevalence of diabetes is 366 million (ages 20~70), and this number will rise to 552 million by 2030. Globally, 70% of diabetic patients undergo amputations, and the number of diabetic patients undergoing lower limb amputations exceeds one million each year. A foot ulcer complication, such as a chronic non-healing wound infection or peripheral artery disease (PAD), often leads to lower limb amputation, with one diabetic patient losing a limb every 20 seconds. The main principle of current diabetic foot treatment is to control blood sugar levels, improve local blood circulation, and nourish peripheral nerves, supplemented locally by closed negative pressure drainage technology and various dressings. Despite this, 84% of diabetic foot patients still face the choice of amputation.

In response to the severe consequences caused by diabetic foot, Professor Wang Jiangning's team took the lead in implementing the MDT diagnosis and treatment model in the department in China. The team is mainly composed of orthopedic doctors, but each has their own expertise (the team can perform vascular interventional surgery, orthopedic reconstruction surgery, flap repair surgery, etc.), forming a multidisciplinary comprehensive treatment model for diabetic foot. The comprehensive surgical treatment of diabetic foot starts from chronic wounds, including the repair treatment of infected and non-infected wounds. For diabetic foot patients with lower limb vascular disease, reconstructing the lower limb blood supply is beneficial for disease control, and lower limb vascular reconstruction and lower limb microcirculation reconstruction can be performed. Among them, in the microvascular reconstruction surgery of diabetic foot, the team adopted extracorporeal circulation perfusion therapy. This method perfuses the ischemic limb and perfuses under high pressure, which can expand the narrowed part of the diseased blood vessel, increase the blood flow through the cross-section of the blood vessel per unit time, increase the tissue blood supply, and promote the reconstruction of the peripheral vascular network during the perfusion process. This technique can reconstruct the lower limb microcirculation in diabetic foot, promote wound healing, effectively delay the progression of diabetic peripheral vascular disease, and reduce the disability rate of diabetic foot (Figs. B.1, B.2, and B.3).

The extracorporeal circulation perfusion technology we mentioned is the application of extracorporeal circulation technology in heart-lung

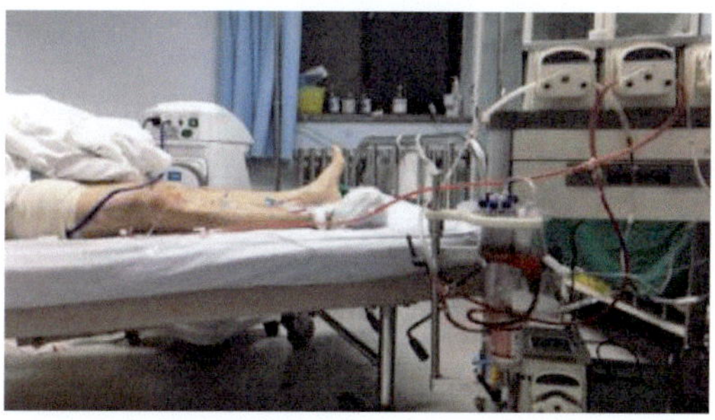

Fig. B.1 Application of extracorporeal circulation perfusion technology in ischemic lesions of the lower extremities in diabetic foot

L. Gao · J. Wang
Department of Orthopedics, Beijing Shijitan Hospital, Capital Medical University, Beijing, China
e-mail: gaolei3337@bjsjth.cn; wangjn@bjsjth.cn

J. Wang, L. Gao (eds.), *Refractory Wounds*, Experts' Perspectives on Medical Advances,
https://doi.org/10.1007/978-981-96-2067-8

transplantation or extracorporeal membrane oxygenation (ECMO) technology in severe heart and lung failure to the human limbs. This device can perform blood oxygenation and removal of toxic substances in the blood. Regarding this treatment method, the earliest in China was proposed by the project mentor Professor Wang Jiangning in 2004, who proposed the concept of extracorporeal circulation perfusion of severed limbs and began to conduct related animal experimental research. In 2008, this technology was used to remove toxins in limbs caused by earthquake-induced crush syndrome. In 2011, the extracorporeal circulation perfusion system was used to perfuse and preserve severed limbs (limb amputation caused by trauma), and this method was used to carry out clinical research on limb replantation and limb preservation cases. From 2014, related research on local limb perfusion of Chinese medicine Mai luo ning was started. From 2015, the extracorporeal circulation perfusion technology was used to treat peripheral arterial disease, especially for patients with diabetic foot and peripheral arterial disease. By improving the blood flow shear force in fluid dynamics, the mechanical stimulation induces the formation of collateral circulation, and the rich capillary network is rebuilt, thereby effectively improving the distal microcirculation of the limb (Fig. B.4).

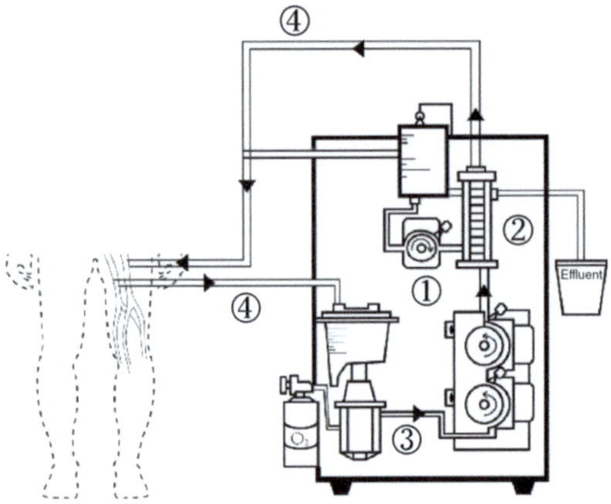

Fig. B.2 Principle of extracorporeal circulation perfusion technology. ① Extracorporeal circulation power pump (roller pump), ② blood filtration device [废液 (Effluent)], ③ artificial heart-lung machine membrane oxygenator (infant type), and ④ extracorporeal circulation blood route (arterial end, venous end)

In addition, the research team has done a lot of work using latissimus dorsi flaps, radial artery flaps, abdominal flaps, cross-leg flaps, lateral femoral rotation flaps, posterior tibial muscle flaps, and peroneal nerve nourishing skin flap transplantation to repair joint exposure and bone exposure patients (Fig. B.5). These are all applications of vascularized flaps for repair, utilizing the principle of capillary reconstruction, and then

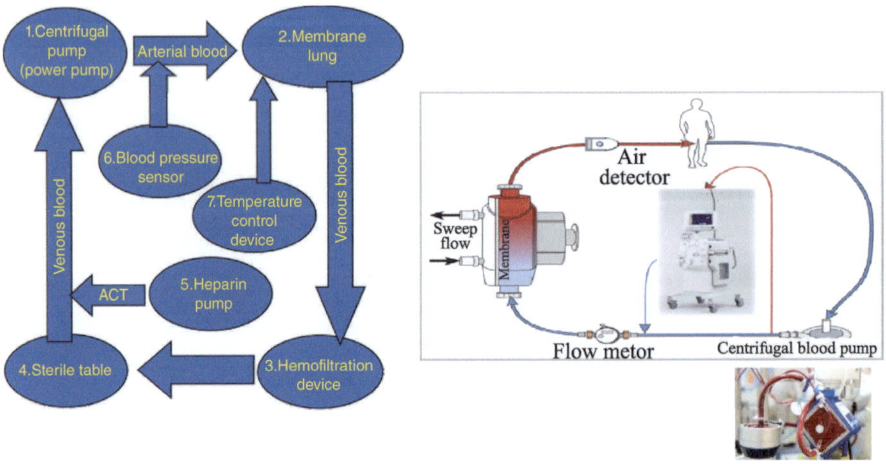

Fig. B.3 Principle of extracorporeal circulation perfusion system. (1) 离心泵(动力泵) [Centrifugal pump (power pump)]; (2) 膜肺 (Membrane lung); (3) 血滤装置 (Hemofiltration device); (4) 无菌台 (Sterile table); (5) 肝素泵 (Heparin pump); (6) 血流压力传感器 (Blood pressure sensor); (7) 温控装置 (Temperature control device); 动脉血 (Arterial blood); 静脉血 (Venous blood)

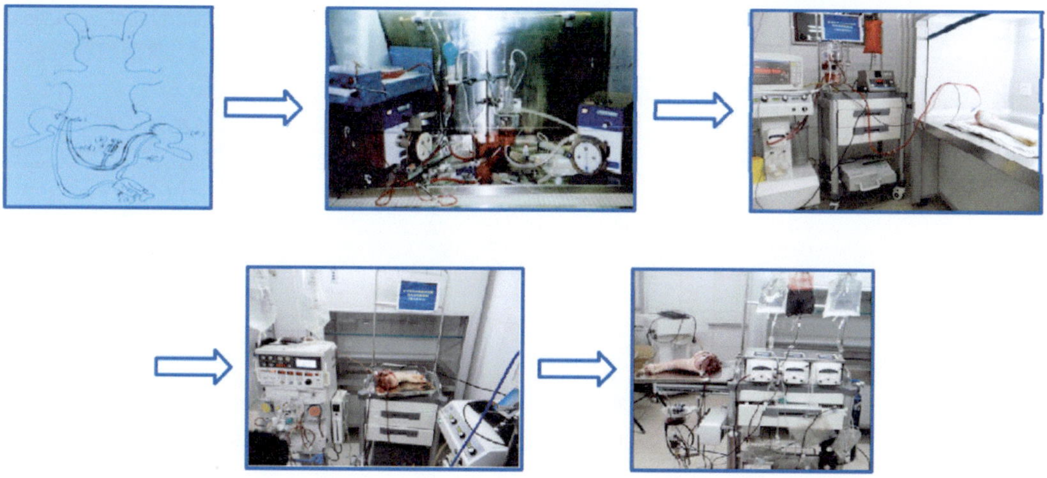

Fig. B.4 Experimental study of extracorporeal perfusion of amputated limbs from 2004 to 2015

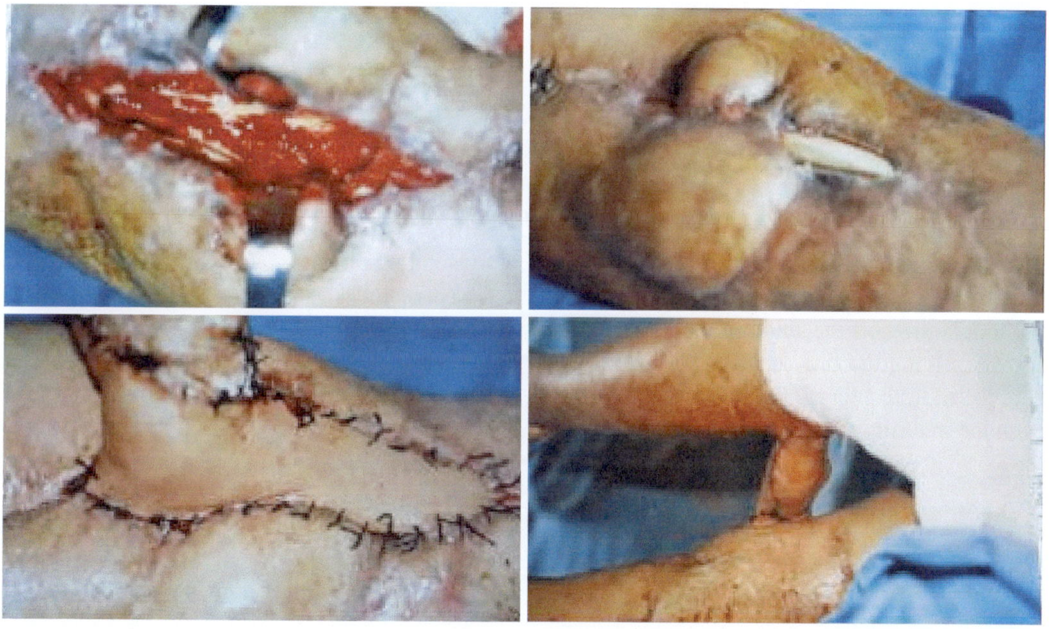

Fig. B.5 Flap transplantation to repair patients with exposed joints and bones

cutting off the pedicle after 21 days to ensure the survival of the flap. However, for patients with diabetic foot, the above flaps are difficult to survive due to vascular problems. Therefore, we have expanded the use of extracorporeal perfusion technology for the first time, applying it to flap grafting (Fig. B.6).

Due to severe vascular disease in the late stage of diabetic foot, it is impossible to find vascularized flaps that can be transferred, and free flaps cannot find selectable vessels at the distal end of the foot. Vascularized flaps cannot be implemented, such as exposed joints and bones that cannot be repaired by skin grafting. They can only be repaired by transferring flaps or free flaps. Some patients face the risk of amputation, but due to limb blood circulation disorders, the survival rate of flaps is low or some are even unable to survive. Therefore, we want to separate the vascularized flaps from the distal end and connect them with the large arteries and distal veins with good physiological

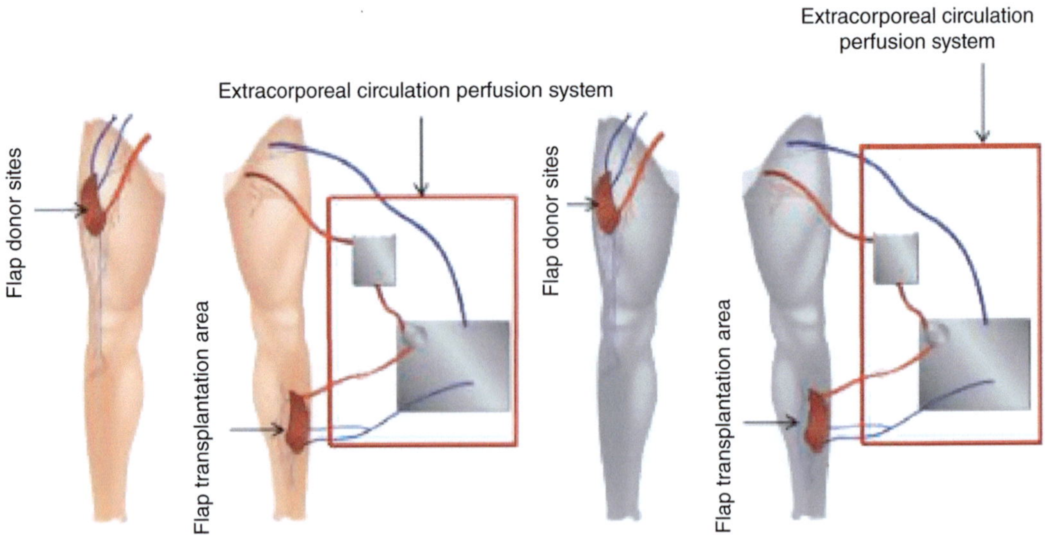

Fig. B.6 Extracorporeal perfusion system for flap grafting. 皮瓣供给区 (Flap donor sites); 皮瓣移植区 (Flap transplantation area); 体外循环灌注系统 (Extracorporeal circulation perfusion system); 皮瓣供给区 (Flap donor sites); 皮瓣移植区 (Flap transplantation area); 体外循环灌注系统 (Extracorporeal circulation perfusion system)

conditions in the lower limbs through the pressure of the arteriovenous pump, to ensure the blood supply of the flaps and ensure the survival rate of the flaps. After the flap survives, it is grafted onto the wound of the diabetic foot without cutting off the autologous blood supply, further solving the low survival rate of the flap caused by limb blood circulation disorders, or even the inability to survive, thereby improving the survival rate of the flap.

Diagnosis of Diabetic Foot

Diabetic foot is a type of complication of diabetes, a local manifestation of the overall condition: including abnormal distal limb sensory, varying degrees of peripheral vascular disease-related foot infection, ulcers, and (or) deep tissue damage. The diagnosis of infection should be made after removing calluses and necrotic tissue, based on the range and depth of the wound and the overall condition to evaluate the severity of the infection. (International Working Group on the Diabetic Foot Prevention and Treatment Guidelines and the Chinese Diabetic Foot Prevention and Treatment Guidelines [2019 version]).

Assessment After Admission for Diabetic Foot

1. Overall Condition Assessment: The assessment includes age, expected lifespan, underlying diseases, occupation, economic conditions, etc., as well as monitoring of blood glucose, blood pressure, blood lipids, nutritional status, etc., to determine whether there are comorbidities such as cardiovascular disease, retinopathy/kidney disease, smoking, etc.
2. Routine Check-up upon Admission: After admission, the patient can be evaluated through hematological assessment, which can detect inflammation indicators, protein levels, heart, liver, kidney function, blood glucose levels, etc. Imaging examinations can provide a comprehensive understanding of the soft tissue and bone conditions of the affected foot. The evaluation of lower limb blood vessels is beneficial for understanding the treatment and prognosis of the wound. The evaluation of heart function is beneficial for a comprehensive understanding of the patient's surgical anesthesia risk. The use of an 18-lead dynamic electrocardiogram can provide a comprehensive understanding of the electrical activity of

various parts of the heart, and has a unique effect on the comprehensive evaluation of myocardial blood supply in multiple parts, reflecting a huge advantage.

3. Hematological Examination: Routine blood test; ABO blood type; full ward biochemistry; hepatitis B four items + hepatitis B surface antigen; routine antibody three items; thromboelastogram; coagulation four items + D-dimer + AT-III; CRP; PCT; BNP; myocardial injury markers; glycated hemoglobin; dry chemistry blood glucose monitoring.
4. Imaging Examination: Digital chest X-ray; foot anteroposterior, lateral X-ray; foot CT scan + three-dimensional reconstruction; foot MRI.
5. Heart Function Assessment: 18-lead dynamic electrocardiogram; echocardiogram.
6. Vascular Assessment: Lower limb vascular ultrasound (artery); lower limb vascular ultrasound (vein); lower limb vascular computed tomographic angiography (CTA); ABI; transcutaneous oxygen pressure; vascular Doppler blood flow detection.
7. Wound Assessment:
   (a) Wound area and depth: The wound area is measured using the eKare inSight system (E KARE company, USA), which includes an intelligent measurement and analysis system. After circling the wound range on the system display screen, it can analyze the wound model and automatically calculate the area, depth, and volume of the wound (Fig. B.7).
   (b) Measurement of foot skin temperature: The foot skin temperature is measured with a non-contact Flir One Pro (FLIR Company, USA) infrared imager. The detection method is for the patient to lie flat, the infrared imaging probe is aimed at the skin between the first and second toes, and kept in a vertical direction, the skin temperature is taken 5 times at the same point, and the average value is calculated (Fig. B.8).
   (c) Transcutaneous oxygen tension measurement: The PeriFlux5000 (PERIMED Company, Sweden) system is used for non-invasive transcutaneous oxygen tension (TcPO2) monitoring (Fig. B.9).

Based on: Clinical Practice Guidelines for the Diagnosis and Treatment of Diabetic Foot Infections by the Infectious Diseases Society of America 2012; 2019 International Working Group on the Diabetic Foot Prevention and Treatment Guidelines; China Diabetic Foot Prevention Guidelines (2019 Edition); China Diabetic Foot Diagnosis and Treatment Guidelines.

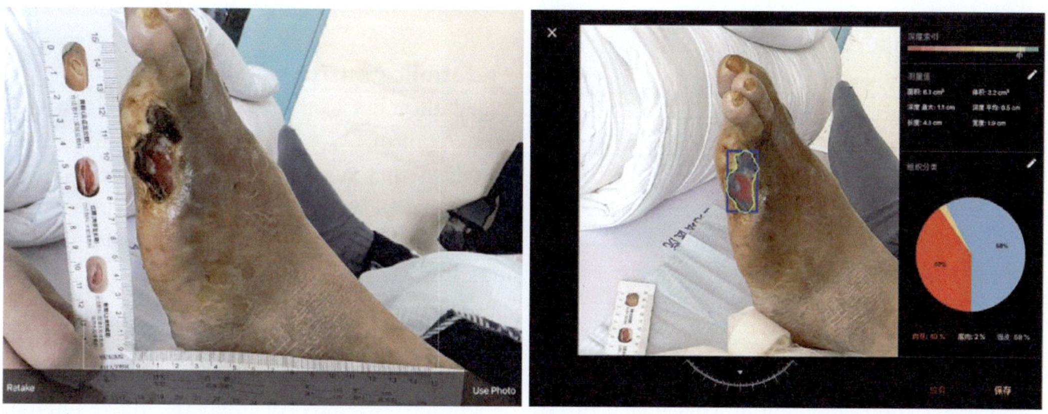

Fig. B.7 Measurement of wound area and depth

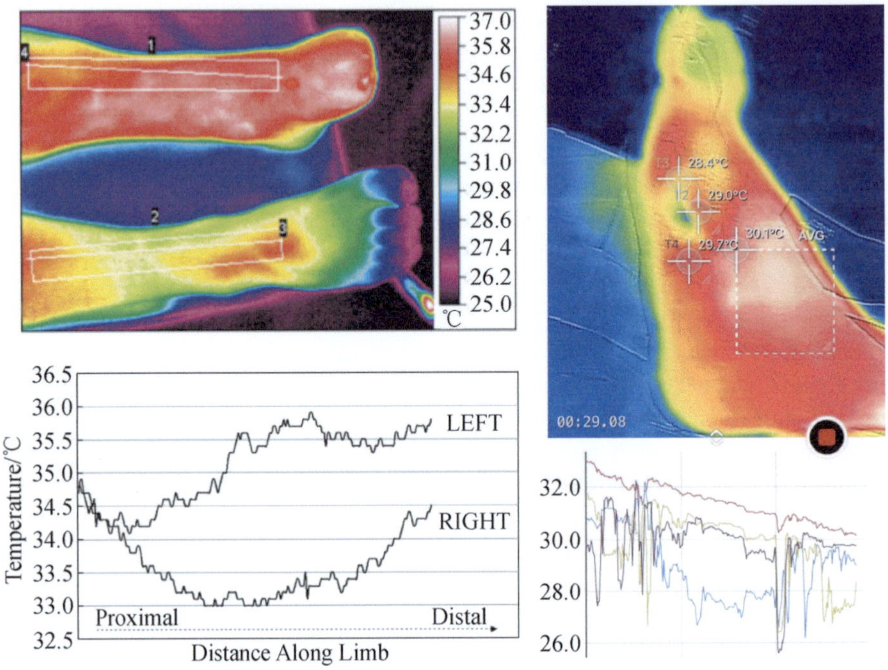

Fig. B.8 Infrared thermal imaging of foot skin temperature

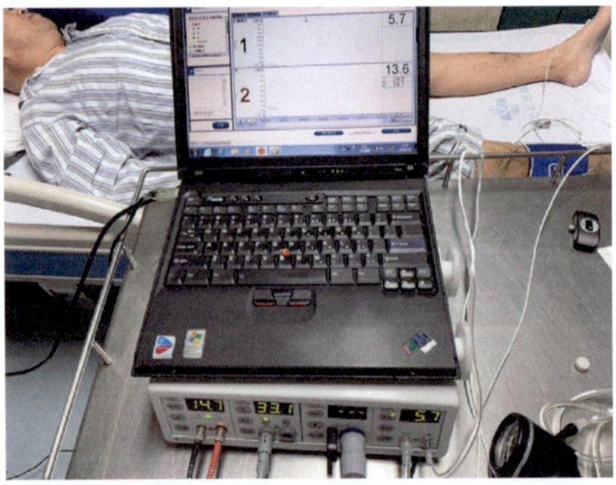

Fig. B.9 Transcutaneous oxygen tension measurement of the foot

Measures for the Treatment of Diabetic Foot Wounds

The key to managing diabetic foot disease is to avoid lower limb amputation. This goal can be achieved through the following three strategies: identifying high-risk foot disease, treating acute changes in foot disease, and preventing further deterioration. A systematic diabetic foot management program must include each of these measures and also cover patient and family education, only then is it possible to successfully avoid amputation. Generally, the choice of treatment plan for diabetic foot disease includes basic treatment (metabolic control, nutritional support, symptomatic treatment, etc.) and local treatment (cleaning, improving blood supply, anti-infection, decompression, dressing selection, etc.).

Metabolic Control

Metabolic control is based on good blood glucose control. Considering the condition of patients with foot ulcers, insulin treatment should be chosen in most cases. This involves needle-free injectors and dynamic blood glucose monitors.

Drug Treatment and Selection

1. Internal Medicine Drug Treatment: For chronic wounds of diabetic foot, internal medicine treatment plays an indispensable role, especially in the application of systemic anti-infection drugs for patients and the use of nutritional nerve circulation improvement

drugs, providing a guarantee for wound healing. For patients with diabetic foot, the control of blood lipids, anticoagulant drugs, nutritional nerve drugs, and microcirculation improvement drugs play an irreplaceable role in the development of surgical treatment and postoperative patient management.

2. Use of Antimicrobial Drugs: Choose drugs based on possible pathogens and susceptibility; initially use parenteral treatment for severe infections, switch to oral drugs when the condition stabilizes (if applicable); use oral drugs to treat mild and most moderate infections; treatment time: soft tissue generally 1~2 weeks; bone infection ≤6 weeks (osteomyelitis excision 5~7 days). For patients who have not recently received antimicrobial treatment, only target aerobic Gram-positive cocci (GPCs; *Staphylococcus aureus*, β-hemolytic streptococcus); or if antimicrobial drugs have been used recently, add coverage for aerobic Gram-negative rods (GNRs; possibly including *Pseudomonas*) and obligate anaerobes (especially in cases of limb ischemia); do not use antimicrobial drugs to treat clinically uninfected wounds.
3. Drugs to Improve Peripheral Neuropathy in Diabetic Root: Alpha-lipoic acid, suitable for abnormal sensations caused by diabetic peripheral neuropathy, taken orally, once a day, 0.6 g/time (2 pills), half an hour before breakfast. For more severe symptoms, it is recommended to start with injection treatment. Since diabetic peripheral neuropathy is a chronic disease, it generally needs to be taken for a long time. Pharmacological explanation: Alpha-lipoic acid is a B vitamin, and it is part of the pyruvate dehydrogenase system and α-ketoglutarate, the coenzyme of the dehydrogenase system. In vitro tests show that alpha-lipoic acid can reduce lipid oxidation in nerve tissue, inhibit protein glycosylation, and inhibit aldose reductase. In the body, alpha-lipoic acid has antioxidant effects and participates in the recycling of antioxidants such as glutathione and coenzyme Q10. Alpha-lipoic acid can chelate certain metal ions (such as copper, manganese, and zinc).
4. Improving Microcirculation Drugs: Alprostadil, used for the treatment of chronic arterial occlusion diseases (thromboangiitis obliterans, occlusive arteriosclerosis, etc.) causing limb ulcers and microvascular circulation disorders causing limb rest pain. Adults 1 time/day, 5~10 μg/time (0.5~1 dose) alprostadil 1~2 mL + saline (or 5% glucose solution) 10 mL, intravenous injection, or directly into a small pot for slow intravenous drip. Pharmacological explanation: Exogenous alprostadil (PGE1), has the effect of inhibiting platelet aggregation, thromboxane A2 production, arterial atherosclerotic plaque formation and immune complex, and can dilate peripheral and coronary vessels; it is a vasodilator and platelet aggregation inhibitor. Alprostadil increases cyclic adenosine monophosphate (cAMP) levels in platelets and vascular smooth muscle cells by activating intracellular adenylate cyclase, resulting in inert platelets and vasodilation. This product is a lipid emulsion, which can reduce the pulmonary inactivation of alprostadil, effectively deliver alprostadil to the lesion site, and control the release of the drug, targeting the damaged vascular site, which is beneficial to the vasodilation and platelet aggregation inhibition effects of this product.

Application of Extracorporeal Circulation Perfusion of Free Flaps in the Treatment of Diabetic Foot Wounds

1. Extracorporeal Circulation Pressurized Perfusion Therapy: The application of an extracorporeal system simulating the physiological environment in the body to perfuse ischemic limbs, and perfusion under high pressure, can expand the narrowed part of the diseased blood vessels, increase the blood flow through the cross-section of the blood vessels per unit time, increase tissue blood supply, and promote peripheral vascular network reconstruction during perfusion. This technology can rebuild the lower limb microcirculation in diabetic foot, promote wound healing, effectively delay the progression of

diabetic peripheral vascular disease, and reduce the disability rate of diabetic foot.

2. Indications and Contraindications: ① Indications: Diabetic patients; lower limbs show ischemic manifestations (numbness of limbs, rest pain, distal end of limbs feel cold), ulcers at the end of the foot (ulceration, infection); after the patient is admitted, imaging data (lower limb arterial CTA) shows different water level segmental stenosis rate is between 50% and 75%; ankle-brachial index (ABI) 0.5 < ABI <0.7. ② Contraindications: Patients with poor overall symptoms, multiple underlying diseases, cachexia, or in a state of severe multi-organ failure; acute phase of foot infection; allergy to iodine; Charcot foot ulcer (neuropathy); after admission, lower limb arterial CTA assessment shows lower limb vascular stenosis rate >75%.
3. Extracorporeal Circulation Perfusion of Free Flap: The day before the patient's flap transplantation repair surgery, extracorporeal circulation perfusion femoral artery and vein catheterization is performed. The patient is in the supine position, the groin area is routinely disinfected and draped, and the strongest pulsating part of the affected side's femoral artery is chosen as the puncture point, 1.5 cm above it. The Seldinger method is used for puncture, and 1% lidocaine is used for local anesthesia at the puncture point. After the anesthesia takes effect, the femoral artery of the affected side is punctured anterogradely. After successful puncture, a 6F arterial microsheath is placed, and 3000 units of low molecular weight heparin sodium are given intravenously for systemic heparinization. A Fogarty 13/40 mm balloon catheter is inserted into the same side femoral vein to serve as the blood return route for circulation perfusion (venous end). The extracorporeal circulation perfusion system's arterial and venous routes are connected to the femoral artery and vein puncture catheters.
4. Taking the Anterolateral Femoral Flap as an Example: On the day of flap transplantation repair surgery, the anterolateral femoral flap is connected to the extracorporeal perfusion machine, the wound defect is repaired, and the extracorporeal circulation machine is removed 21 days later. The skin perforation point marked by preoperative color Doppler blood flow detector is taken as the center, and the flap is designed according to the "point, line, surface" principle of free flap. The pattern is made according to the size and shape of the wound, and the flap is enlarged by 1~2 cm compared to the pattern. The lateral femoral cutaneous nerve is dissected and separated, and the musculocutaneous perforator of the lateral circumflex femoral artery is dissected and separated by the "convergence method." The femoral nerve branches are separated and properly protected. After confirming the reliable blood supply of the flap, the vascular pedicle is cut. After the flap is detached, it is moved to the recipient area and temporarily fixed with a few stitches at the wound edge. Under the surgical microscope, the arterial tube of the extracorporeal circulation machine is anastomosed with the descending branch of the lateral circumflex femoral artery, and 1~2 accompanying veins are anastomosed with the venous tube of the extracorporeal circulation machine. The lateral femoral cutaneous nerve is sutured with the saphenous nerve or the peroneal nerve, the fascia lata is sutured and fixed with the remaining plantar fascia or calcaneal periosteum. After confirming the reliable blood supply of the flap, the wound is closed, and a drainage tube is placed under the flap. After hemostasis of the flap donor area wound, the intermuscular space is closed, and a medium-thickness skin graft is taken from the opposite thigh for repair.
5. Extracorporeal Circulation Pressurized Perfusion System:. This system is mainly based on the Japanese JUN55X device, including the following main parts: ① Extracorporeal circulation power pump (Roller pump) (Japanese JUN 55X), which forms a local circuit for the blood of the affected limb, providing sufficient circulation power, and at the same time, by adjusting the speed, it increases the blood pressure of the entire circulation. ② Artificial heart-lung

machine membrane oxygenator (Infant type) (China Xi Jian Medical), which plays a role in blood oxygenation during the circulation perfusion process, providing oxygen and energy for limb muscle tissue. ③ Blood filtration device, a continuous blood filter (Japanese Nipro UT-500S), which filters out creatinine, urea nitrogen, and other metabolic wastes in the blood of extracorporeal circulation, while adjusting the acid-base balance of circulating blood, and adjusting electrolyte disorders, etc. ④ Disposable extracorporeal circulation blood circuit (Japanese Lai Fu En CH-CHF), which ensures the blood of extracorporeal circulation does not coagulate, and the red blood cells do not undergo mechanical impact, thus ensuring normal blood perfusion. ⑤ Heparin pump, which continuously pumps sodium heparin into the circulation to prevent blood coagulation.

Anticoagulation Issues During Treatment

1. Regular Heparin: It is currently the most commonly used anticoagulant in blood purification. Regular heparin is a heterogeneous compound of polysulfate polysaccharides, with a molecular weight of 530KD, all of its functions are mediated by their binding with anticoagulant thrombin in circulation. Therefore, the anticoagulant effect of heparin is affected by antithrombin III (AT-III). The concentration of AT-III in critically ill patients is usually decreased, which affects the activity of heparin. The decrease in AT III is usually due to excessive consumption of activated coagulation system and decreased synthesis due to liver function decline. Other factors affecting heparin include the patient's weight and coagulation function status. The action of heparin can be neutralized by fish sperm protein.

The application of heparin anticoagulation in continuous blood perfusion (continuous blood purification) is mostly: ① First, inject heparin into saline to treat the pipeline and filter. ② After the treatment starts, heparin is injected into the blood circuit at regular intervals. Add 12500 U of heparin to 3000 mL of saline to pre-flush the pipeline and filter. After the treatment starts, the first dose of heparin 1250~2500 U is injected from the blood circuit, and then 250~500 U of heparin is injected every hour, and the dosage of heparin is adjusted according to the monitoring results. During the treatment, it is necessary to: ① Monitor the activated partial thromboplastin time (APTT), to keep it at 1~1.5 times the normal value. ② Observe the various pressure indicators of the pipeline and filter, through the monitoring system of the machine, to detect early signs of blockage in the pipeline and filter. ③ Monitor the filtration efficiency of the filter, by using urea nitrogen as an indicator. Regularly compare the concentrations in the blood and filtrate. If the filtration rate decreases, it means that the efficiency of the filter has decreased, indicating insufficient anticoagulation.

When using heparin for anticoagulation, the principle of individualization should be observed. Careful observation is needed to find the appropriate dose for the patient as early as possible, and the dosage of heparin should be adjusted according to the monitoring results and treatment needs.

2. Low Molecular Weight Heparin: Ordinary heparin can be cleaved into shorter polysaccharides—low molecular weight heparin in several ways. Low molecular weight heparin has significantly different pharmacological characteristics. Its molecular weight is 4~6.5 KD, and its inhibitory effect on factor Xa is 2~4 times that of inhibiting thrombin. Compared with ordinary heparin, low molecular weight heparin can better predict the dose-effect relationship, has a longer half-life, and has less impact on platelet function. Protamine does not affect it. Low molecular weight heparin is also commonly used for anticoagulation in continuous blood purification. Some hospitals start with 3000 U injected into the blood circuit, then inject 1000~2000 U every 4 h, and adjust according to the monitoring results and treatment needs.
3. Local Heparin Anticoagulation: This anticoagulation method uses protamine to neutralize the anticoagulant activity of heparin, thereby

eliminating the systemic effect of heparin and reducing the complications caused by heparin. The specific practice is to inject heparin into the blood circuit before the filter to prevent coagulation in the extracorporeal blood circuit, and inject protamine into the blood circuit after the filter to eliminate the effect of heparin. Regarding the ratio of heparin to protamine, it is generally believed that 1000 U of heparin to 10 mg of protamine is ideal, considering the half-life of heparin. The larger the dose of heparin, the longer the half-life, and therefore the dosage of heparin and protamine should be adjusted according to the monitoring results.

4. Local Citrate Anticoagulation: Citrate is injected into the blood circuit before the filter. It binds to the ionized calcium in the blood, acting as an anticoagulant, and then calcium chloride is injected into the blood circuit after the filter to replenish the ionized calcium in the blood. This is local citrate anticoagulation. Local citrate anticoagulation is mainly used for patients with a high tendency to bleed. For patients with a high tendency to bleed, sometimes heparin-free blood purification can be used, but the requirements for blood flow are higher. Local citrate anticoagulation does not require high blood flow and may cause metabolic alkalosis, which should be noted.

Flap Perfusion and Arterialized Venous Flap

The venous flap is a flap whose main blood supply enters and exits through the venous system. Compared with traditional arterial flaps, venous flaps have their own advantages, including: easy design, no need for deep dissection, no sacrifice of the main blood vessels of the flap supply area, the position of the flap supply area is not restricted, and the complications of the flap supply area are less.

Based on the direction of blood vessels entering and leaving the flap and the direction of blood flow in these vessels, three types of venous flaps have been proposed. Type I: single pedicle venous flap; Type II: double pedicle venous flap; and Type III: arterialized venous flap, which is perfused after the proximal artery and the proximal vein of the flap are anastomosed, and flows out from the distal vein. The technique of extracorporeal circulation perfusion is used to nurture free flaps. After the collateral circulation is established, the flap is cut off, and the flap finally survives. There is a risk of failure, and the selected flap is an arterial flap, such as the selected anterolateral thigh flap, which has a large dissection range and damages the main blood vessels of the flap supply area. Therefore, in order to simplify the operation procedure and be more conducive to flap survival, later research chose venous flaps, imitating the principle of Type III venous flaps. The arterial end of the extracorporeal perfusion system is connected to the vein of the flap, and the autologous venous blood is drawn out for oxygenation, and then perfused by the vein of the venous flap. The theoretical basis for arterialized venous perfusion is: after arterialized venous, the main route of early tissue blood flow is that arterial blood flows into small veins, and then flows back to small veins with reflux function through inter-venous communication branches; after venous diversion, micro-veins can replace capillaries. It is currently believed that arterialized venous can effectively dilate venous vessels through blood pressure, close or make venous valves ineffective, and cause blood to flow through the ischemic area for circulation, and then open micro-venous shunts, effectively providing blood supply for peripheral tissues. As the vascularization of ischemic tissue is completed, the blood flow gradually becomes physiological blood flow circulation, thereby effectively ensuring tissue survival.

Bibliography

1. Lechleitner M, Abrahamian H, Francesconi C, et al. Diabetic neuropathy and diabetic foot syndrome (Update 2019). Wien Klin Wochenschr. 2019;131(Suppl 1):141–50.
2. Yazdanpanah L, Shahbazian H, Nazari I, et al. incidence and risk factors of diabetic foot ulcer: a population-based diabetic foot cohort (ADFC Study) - two-year follow-up study. Int J Endocrinol. 2018;2018:7631659.
3. Wang A, Xu Z, Mu Y, et al. Clinical characteristics and medical costs in patients with diabetic amputation and nondiabetic patients with nonacute amputation in central urban hospitals in China. Int J Low Extrem Wounds. 2014;13(1):17–21.
4. Jiang Y, Ran X, Jia L, et al. Epidemiology of type 2 diabetic foot problems and predictive factors for amputation in China. Int J Low Extrem Wounds. 2015;14(1):19–27.
5. Xu Z, Ran X. Diabetic foot care in China: challenges and strategy. Lancet Diabetes Endocrinol. 2016;4(4):297–8.
6. Chinese Medical Association Diabetes Branch. China type 2 diabetes prevention and treatment guidelines (2017 edition). Chin J Pract Intern Med. 2018;38(4):292–344.
7. Jiangning W, Lei G. New progress in the treatment of chronic wounds of diabetic foot. Chin J Repair Reconstr Surg. 2018;32(7):832–7.
8. Alexandrescu VA, Brochier S, Limgba A, et al. Healing of diabetic neuroischemic foot wounds with vs without wound-targeted revascularization: reliminary observations from an 8-year prospective dual-center registry. J Endovasc Ther. 2020;27(1):20–30.
9. Khin NY, Dijkstra ML, Huckson M, et al. Hypertensive extracorporeal limb perfusion for critical limb ischemia. J Vasc Surg. 2013;58(5):1244–53.
10. Lei W, Xin N, Yefeng Y, et al. Application of Vascular Ning in the treatment of crush injury and crush syndrome in pigs under extracorporeal perfusion system. Chin J Tissue Eng Res. 2019;23(11):1723–9.
11. Lei Y, Lei G, Lei W, et al. Pressurized perfusion under extracorporeal circulation system improves lower limb blood flow in model pigs. Chin J Tissue Eng Res. 2018;22(4):553–7.
12. Wang F. Interpretation of China's diabetic foot prevention and treatment guidelines (2019 edition). J Hebei Med Univ. 2019;40(11):1241–5, 1250.
13. Lei G, Jiangning W, Yefeng Y. Interpretation of the 2019 "International Working Group on Diabetic Foot Prevention and Treatment guidelines". Chin J Repair Reconstr Surg. 2020;34(1):16–20.
14. Firnhaber JM, Powell CS. Lower extremity peripheral artery disease: diagnosis and treatment. Am Fam Physician. 2019;99(6):362–9.
15. Mendes-Pinto D, Rodrigues-Machado MDG, Navarro TP, et al. Association between Critical Limb Ischemia, the Society for Vascular Surgery Wound, Ischemia and Foot Infection (WIfI) classification system and arterial stiffness. Ann Vasc Surg. 2020;63:250–8.
16. Cherviakov IV, Kha KN, Gavrilenko AV, et al. Differentiated approach to treatment of decompensated lower limb ischemia with the use of the WIFI classification system. Angiol Sosud Khir. 2019;25(1):9–16.
17. Lane RJ, Phillips M, McMillan D, et al. Hypertensive extracorporeal limb perfusion (HELP): a new technique for managing critical lower limb ischemia. J Vasc Surg. 2008;48(5):1156–65.
18. Kueckelhaus M, Fischer S, Sisk G, et al. A mobile extracorporeal extremity salvage system for replantation and transplantation. Ann Plast Surg. 2016;76(3):355–60.
19. Taeger CD, Lamby P, Dolderer J, et al. Extracorporeal perfusion for salvage of major amputates. Ann Surg. 2019;270(1):e5–6.
20. Schmidt CA, Rancic Z, Lachat ML, et al. Hypothermic, initially oxygen-free, controlled limb reperfusion for acute limb ischemia. Ann Vasc Surg. 2015;29(3):560–72.
21. Namgoong S, Yang JP, Yoo KH, et al. Comparison of perfusion values after percutaneous transluminal angioplasty according to the severity of ischemia in the diabetic foot. Int Wound J. 2019;16(1):176–82.
22. Cildag MB, Koseoglu OFK. The effect of Charcot neuroarthropathy on limb preservation in diabetic patients with foot wound and critical limb ischemia after balloon angioplasty. J Diabetes Res. 2017;2017:5670984.

J. Wang, L. Gao (eds.), *Refractory Wounds*, Experts' Perspectives on Medical Advances,
https://doi.org/10.1007/978-981-96-2067-8

23. Bills JD, Berriman SJ, Noble DL, et al. Pilot study to evaluate a novel three-dimensional wound measurement device. Int Wound J. 2016;13(6):1372–7.
24. Staffa E, Bernard V, Kubicek L, et al. Using noncontact infrared thermography for long-term monitoring of foot temperatures in a patient with diabetes mellitus. Ostomy Wound Manage. 2016;62(4):54–61.
25. Staffa E, Bernard V, Kubicek L, et al. Infrared thermography as an option for evaluating the treatment effect of percutaneous transluminal angioplasty in patients with peripheral arterial disease. Vascular. 2017;25(1):42–9.
26. Zubair M, Al Amri M, Ahmad J. A retrospective study of ABI and TBI during the healing of ulcers among diabetic patients. Diabetes Metab Syndr. 2019;13(1):78–83.
27. Kalani M, Brismar K, Fagrell B, et al. Transcutaneous oxygen tension and toe blood pressure as predictors for outcome of diabetic foot ulcers. Diabetes Care. 1999;22(1):147–51.
28. Reiber GE, Raugi GJ. Preventing foot ulcers and amputations in diabetes. Lancet. 2005;366(9498):1676–7.
29. Akbari CM, Logerfo FW. Diabetes and peripheral vascular disease. J Vasc Surg. 1999;30(2):373–84.
30. Brownrigg JR, Hinchliffe RJ, Apelqvist J, et al. Performance of prognostic markers in the prediction of wound healing or amputation among patients with foot ulcers in diabetes: a systematic review. Diabetes Metab Res Rev. 2016;32(Suppl 1):128–35.
31. Lowry D, Saeed M, Narendran P, et al. The difference between the healing and the nonhealing diabetic foot ulcer: a review of the role of the microcirculation. J Diabetes Sci Technol. 2017;11(5):914–23.
32. Tao W, Xuan Z, Jiacai M, et al. Study on the effect of wound healing after lower limb vascular recanalization in patients with diabetic foot and peripheral vascular disease using WIFi grading. Chin J Pract Surg. 2016;36(12):1293–7.
33. Wenchao Y, Xuan Z, Jiacai M, et al. Using WIFi grading to analyze the risk factors related to minor amputation of diabetic foot. Chin J Vasc Surg (Electron Ed). 2017;9(1):37–9.
34. Zhang P, Lu J, Jing Y, et al. Global epidemiology of diabetic foot ulceration: a systematic review and meta-analysis (dagger). Ann Med. 2017;49(2):106–16.
35. Morbach S, Furchert H, Groblinghoff U, et al. Long-term prognosis of diabetic foot patients and their limbs: amputation and death over the course of a decade. Diabetes Care. 2012;35(10):2021–7.
36. Junrungsee S, Kosachunhanun N, Wongthanee A, et al. History of foot ulcers increases mortality among patients with diabetes in Northern Thailand. Diabet Med. 2011;28(5):608–11.
37. Hinchliffe RJ, Brownrigg JR, Andros G, et al. Effectiveness of revascularization of the ulcerated foot in patients with diabetes and peripheral artery disease: a systematic review. Diabetes Metab Res Rev. 2016;32(Suppl 1):136–44.
38. Jeffcoate WJ, Bus SA, Game FL, et al. Reporting standards of studies and papers on the prevention and management of foot ulcers in diabetes: required details and markers of good quality. Lancet Diabetes Endocrinol. 2016;4(9):781–8.
39. Ricco JB, Thanh Phong L, Schneider F, et al. The diabetic foot: a review. J Cardiovasc Surg. 2013;54(6):755–62.
40. Adam DJ, Beard JD, Cleveland T, et al. Bypass versus angioplasty in severe ischaemia of the leg (BASIL): multicentre, randomised controlled trial. Lancet. 2005;366(9501):1925–34.

MIX
Papier aus verantwortungsvollen Quellen
Paper from responsible sources
FSC® C105338

If you have any concerns about our products,
you can contact us on
ProductSafety@springernature.com

In case Publisher is established outside the EU,
the EU authorized representative is:
Springer Nature Customer Service Center GmbH
Europaplatz 3, 69115 Heidelberg, Germany

Printed by Libri Plureos GmbH
in Hamburg, Germany